D1543698

WITHDRAWN

Global Challenge of AIDS
— Ten Years of HIV/AIDS Research

Global Challenge of AIDS
—Ten Years of HIV/AIDS Research

Proceedings of the Tenth International Conference on AIDS/International Conference on STD
Yokohama, August 7-12, 1994

Edited by

Yuichi Shiokawa   Professor Emeritus,   *Juntendo University, Tokyo, Japan*
Takashi Kitamura   Director Emeritus,   *National Institute of Health, Tokyo, Japan*

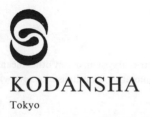

KODANSHA
Tokyo

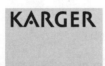

Basel · Freiburg · Paris · London · New York · New Delhi · Bangkok · Singapore · Tokyo · Sydney

THE LIBRARY
UNIVERSITY OF GUELPH

Copublished by
KODANSHA LTD., Tokyo

and

S. KARGER AG, Basel

Exclusive sales rights in Japan, Taiwan, Hong Kong, Republic of Korea and People's Republic of China
KODANSHA LTD
12–21, Otowa 2-chome, Bunkyo-ku, Tokyo 112, Japan

for the rest of the world
S. KARGER AG
Allschwilerstrasse 10, P. O. Box, CH-4009 Basel, Switzerland

Library of Congress Cataloging-in-Publication Data

ISBN 4-06-207359-5 (Kodansha)

ISBN 3-8055-6222-5 (Karger)

Copyright© 1995 by Kodansha Ltd., Tokyo (Japan)
All rights reserved
No part of this book may be reproduced in any form, by photostat, microfilm, retrieval system, or any other means, without the written permission of Kodansha Ltd. (except in the case of brief quotation for criticism or review)

Printed in Japan

THE LIBRARY
UNIVERSITY OF GUELPH

Committee Members

International Steering Committee

T.M.P. Bagasao, *Philippines*
A. Benslimane, *Morocco*
T.J. Coates, *USA*
D.A. Cooper, *Australia*
J.W. Curran, *USA*
J. Dwyer, *Australia*
A.S. Fauci, *USA*
L. Fransen, *EC*
D. de Gagné, *Canada*
E. Guerrero, *Dominican Republic*

K-O. Habermehl, *Germany*
C. Ikegami, *Japan*
N. Kaleeba, *Uganda*
L.O. Kallings, *Sweden*
T. Kitamura, *Japan*
Y.H. Kouri, *USA*
Y. Kumamoto, *Japan*
J.M. Mann, *USA*
M.H. Merson, *WHO*
I. Montagnier, *France*
Y-F. Ngeow, *Malaysia*

E.N. Ngugi, *Kenya*
J. Paavonen, *Finland*
G. Peterson, *WHO*
P. Phanuphak, *Thailand*
R. Philpot, *Australia*
P. Piot, *WHO*
L.G.M. Rodrigues, *Brazil*
A. Ronald, *Canada*
Y. Shiokawa, *Japan*
J. Slootbeed, *Netherlands*
S. Yamagata, *Japan*

Organizing Committee

Y. Shiokawa (Chair.)
Y. Hinuma
G. Hiraiwa
K. Inaba
T. Kitamura

S. Matsumoto
W. Mori
T. Murase
T. Nagano

K. Nagasu
S. Nakahara
A. Oya
T. Ozawa

K. Takagi
H. Takahide
S. Tani
K. Toyoshima

Steering Committee

Y. Shiokawa (Chair.)
Y. Kumamoto (Vice Chair.)
M. Fujimaki
K. Higuchi
Y. Hinuma
H. Hirose
C. Ikegami
K. Kamiya

J. Kawamoto
K. Kiikuni
T. Kitamura
T. Kurimura
M. Minamitani
T. Miyamoto
M. Naruse

M. Nishimura
K. Nishioka
Y. Saito
N. Sakamoto
K. Shimada
S. Shiraogawa
K. Soda

B. Takeda
K. Toyoshima
K. Yamada
S. Yamagata
S. Yamazaki
M. Yauchi
Y. Yoshimoto

List of Contributors

Numbers in parentheses refer to the pages on which a contributors paper begins.

Altman, Dennis (245) *Asia/Pacific Council of AIDS Service Organizations, Politics Department, La Trobe University, Bundoora, Victoria 3083, Australia*

Banda, Mazuwa A. (211) *Churches Medical Association of Zambia, P.O. Box 34511, Lusaka, Zambia*

Bertozzi, Stefano M. (251) *Health Economist, Planning & Policy Coordination, WHO, Global Programme on AIDS, CH-1211 Geneva 27, Switzerland*

Blanche, S. (15) *Hôpital Necker, 149, rue de Sèvres, 75743 Paris Cedex 15, France*

Bolognesi, Dani P. (147) *Duke University Medical Center, LaSalle St. Ext., SORF Building, Room 204, P.O. Box 2926, Durham, NC 27710, USA*

Cao, Yunzhen (65) *The Aaron Diamond AIDS Research Center, New York University School of Medicine, 455 First Ave., New York, NY 10016, USA*

Cornelissen, Marion (123) *Human Retrovirus Laboratory, University of Amsterdam, Academic Medical Center, Meibergdreef 15, 1105AZ Amsterdam, The Netherlands*

Fauci, Anthony S. (49) *National Institute of Allergy and Infectious Diseases, Building 31, Room 7A04, 31 Center Dr. MSC 2520, Bethesda, MD 20892-2520, USA*

Filgueiras, Ana (205) *Brazilian Center for the Defense of the Rights of Children and Adolescents, Rua Barao da Torre, 81-402 CEP: 22411-000-Ipanema, Rio de Janeiro, Brazil*

Gallo, Robert C. (263) *Laboratory of Tumor Cell Biology, National Cancer Institute, National Institutes of Health, Building 37, Room 6A09, Bethesda, MD 20892, USA*

Gatell, José M. (225) *Infectious Disease Unit, Hospital Clinic, Villarroel, 170, 08036 Barcelona, Spain*

Gayle, Helene D. (309) *Centers for Disease Control and Prevention (CDC), NCPS, Bldg. 11, Room 2104, Atlanta, GA30333, USA*

Gissmann, Lutz (113) *Department of Obstertrics and Gynecology, Loyola University Chicago, Cancer Center, 2160 South First Avenue, Maywood, IL 60153, USA*

Goudsmit, Jaap   (123) *Human Retrovirus Laboratory, University of Amsterdam, Academic Medical Center, Meibergdreef 15, 1105AZ Amsterdam, The Netherlands*

Gu, Zhengxian   (179) *Lady Davis Institute for Medical Research, Jewish General Hospital, 3755 Chemin de la Côte-Ste-Catherine, Montréal, Quebec H3T 1E2, Canada*

Haase, Ashley T.   (103) *Department of Microbiology, University of Minnesota, 420 Delaware Street S.E. Minneapolis, MN 55455, USA*

Hatanaka, Masakazu   (77, 290) *Institute for Virus Research, Kyoto University, Sakyo-ku, Kyoto 606-01 and Institute for Medical Science, 5-1 Mishima 2-chome, Settsu, Osaka 566, Japan*

Hernandez, Juan Jacobo   (298) *Colectivo Sol, Cerrada Miguel Hidalgo, #11 Col. Pueblo Quieto, Tlalpan, Maxico, D.F. CO 14040, Mexico*

Himmich, Hakima   (237) *Medical School of Casablanca, Faculty of Medecine, 19, Rue Tarik Bnou Ziad, Casablanca, Morocco*

Ho, David D.   (65) *The Aaron Diamond AIDS Research Center, New York University School of Medicine, 455 First Ave., New York, NY 10016, USA*

Kallings, Lars Olof   (312) *National Institute of Public Health, Box 27848, S-115 93 Stockholm, Sweden*

Kuiken, Carla   (123) *Human Retrovirus Laboratory, University of Amsterdam, Academic Medical Center, Meibergdreef 15, 1105AZ Amsterdam, The Netherlands*

Levy, Jay A.   (275) *Cancer Research Institute, School of Medicine, University of California, San Francisco, San Francisco, CA 94143-0128, USA*

Lukashov, Vladimir   (123) *Human Retrovirus Laboratory, University of Amsterdam, Academic Medical Center, Meibergdreef 15, 1105AZ Amsterdam, The Netherlands*

Mann, Jonathan, M.   (291) *François-Xavier Bagnoud Center for Health and Human Rights, Epidemiology and Iinternational Health, Harvard School of Public Health, 8 Story Street, Cambridge, MA 02138, USA*

Marty-Lavauzelle, Arnaud   (233) *AIDS Fédération Nationale, 247, rue de Bellevile, 75019 Paris, France*

Mellors, Shaun Erland   (307) *Global Network of People (GNP), P.O. Box 27262, Rhine Road 8050, S.A., 209 Broadway Center, Hertzog Blvd., Foreshore, Cape Town, South Africa*

Merson, M.H.   (3) *WHO, Global Programme on AIDS, CH-1211 Geneva 27, Switzerland*

Montagnier, L.   (287) *Institute Pasteur, Unité d'Oncologie Virale, 28 rue du Dr. Roux, 75724 Paris Cédex 15, France*

Montaner, J.S.G.   (179) *St. Paul's Hospital, University of British Columbia, Vancouver, B.C., Canada*

Msiska, Roland   (320) *National AIDS/STD/TB and Leprosy Programme, Lomie House, 6th Floor, Cairo Road, Norshand, P.O. Box 32346, 1010 Lusaka, Zambia*

Nagai, Kazushige   (179) *Lady Davis Institute for Medical Research, Jewish General Hospital, 3755 Chemin de la Côte-Ste-Catherine, Montréal, Quebec H3T 1E2, Canada*

Narayanan, Palaniappan   (201) *Pink Triangle, P.O. Box 11859, 50760 Kuala Lumpur, Malaysia*

Ngeow, Yun-Fong   (21) *Dept. of Medical Microbiology, Faculty of Medicine, University of Malaya, 59100 Kuala Lumpur, Malaysia*

O'Malley, Jeffrey   (316) *International HIV/AIDS Alliance, Barratt House, 341, Oxford Street, London W1R 3BH, UK*

Patkar, Priti   (193) *Prerana Municipal School, 7th Lane, Sukhlaji Street, Kamathipura, Bombay 400 008, India*

Paul, William E.   (57) *National Institutes of Health, Office of AIDS Research, Building 31, Room 4C02, 31 Center Drive, MSC 2340, Bethesda, MD 20892, USA*

Piot, Peter   (35) *Division of Research and Intervention Development, Joint United Nations Programme on AIDS, WHO, CH-1211 Geneva 27, Switzerland*

Qin, Limo   (65) *The Aaron Diamond AIDS Research Center, New York University School of Medicine, 455 First Ave., New York, NY 10016, USA*

Saez, Helga V.   (219) *HIV Center for Clinical and Behavioral Studies, New York State Psychiatric Institute, 722 West 168 Street, New York, NY 10032, USA*

Safrit, Jeffrey   (65) *The Aron Diamond AIDS Research Center, New York University School of Medicine, 455 First Ave., New York, NY 10016, USA*

Salomon, Horacio   (179) *Lady Davis Instituté Jewish General Hospital, 3755 Chemin de la Côte-Ste-Catherine, Montréal, Quebec H3T 1E2, Canada*

Smith, Marilyn   (179) *Lady Davis Instituté for Medical Research, Jewish General Hospital, 3755 Chemin de la Côte-Ste-Catherine, Montréal, Quebec H3T 1E2, Canada*

Spira, Avrum   (179) *Lady Davis Instituté Jewish General Hospital, 3755 Chemin de la Côte-Ste-Catherine, Montréal, Quebec H3T 1E2, Canada*

Stein, Zena A.   (219) *HIV Center for Clinical and Behavioral Studies, New York State Psychiatric Institute, 722 West 168 Street, New York, NY 10032, USA*

Stockfleth, Eggert   (113) *Department of Obstertrics and Gynecology, Loyola University Chicago, Cancer Center, 2160 South First Avenue, Maywood, IL 60153, USA*

Suwunjundee, Junsuda   (303) *Wednesday Friends' Club, Program on AIDS, c/o Thai Red Cross Society Program on AIDS, 1871 Rama IV Road, Bangkok 10330, Thailand*

Tan, Michael L.   (27) *Health Action Information Network (HAIN), 9 Cabanatuan Rd., Philam Homes, Quezon City 1104, Philippines*

Vella, Stefano   (159) *Retrovirus Department, Laboratory of Virology, Instituto Superiore di Sanità, Viale Regina Elena 299, 00161 Rome, Italy*

Volberding, Paul A.   (145) *University of California San Francisco, 995 Potrero Ave., Bldg. 80, Ward 84, San Francisco, CA 94110, USA*

Wainberg, Mark A.   (179) *Lady Davis Instituté for Medical Research, Jewish General Hospital, 3755 Chemin de la Côte-Ste-Catherine, Montréal, Quebec H3T 1E2, Canada*

Wong-Staal, Flossie   (169) *University of California, San Diego, Clinical Science, 9500 Gilman Drive, 0665, La Jolla, CA 92093-0665, USA*

Zhang, Linqi   (65) *The Aron Diamond AIDS Research Center, New York University School of Medicine, 455 First Ave., New York, NY 10016, USA*

Preface by Y. Shiokawa

The Tenth International Conference on AIDS International Conference on STD took place 7–12 August, 1994, in the Pacifico Yokohama complex in the city of Yokohama, Japan.

Although there were initial worries that the conference would be poorly attended because of the great distances between Japan and Western countries, coupled with Japan's high prices and strong currency, we were very fortunate to weicome 12,623 participants from 143 countries to what proved to be a large, productive international conference.

Although AIDS continues to spread worldwide at a rapid pace, we have yet to develop a drug cure or preventive vaccine for the discase despite intensive and ongoing research efforts. Consequently, AIDS now presents humanity with one of its most formidable challenges. Furthermore,those intectcd with HIV or living with AIDS (PWAs) arc bcing subjected to discrimination and prejudice in many countries. Clearly, AIDS has become more than a medical issue; it has evolved into a multifaceted social issue related to politics, economics, ethies, education, and other domains.

Internationally, we invited the World Health Organization (WHO) and the International AIDS Society (IAS) to participate as sponsors, and the Global Network of People Living with AIDS/HIV (GNPL) and the International Council of AIDS Service Organizations (ICASO) to take part as cosponsors.

To enlist support from organizations in the field of sexually transmitted diseases (STD), we requested that the International Society for STD Research (ISSTDR), and the International Union Against the Venereal Diseases and Treponematoses (IUVDT) become involved as cooperating research organizations.

The conference proved to be unique in the extent of participation of people with AIDS/HIV and the cooperation of NGOs from around the world, despite the great distances involved, Within the Organizing Committee, the Cominunity Liaison Committee was established to support NGO activities and persons living with AIDS/HIV while encouraging the representation of all related individuals and organizations.

The conference comprised 30 presentations in plenary sessions, 32 presentations in round-table sessions, 583 oral presentations of abstracts, 2,716 poster presentations, and associated exhibitions and events. To commemorate the conference's first decade, Tenth Anniversary Special Sessions were also held in which participants reviewed the progress anchieved in AIDS research and prevention during the preceding decade and discussed directions for the decade to come.

This was the first International Conference on AIDS to be held in Asia. WHO predicts that the highest rate of increase in AIDS this decade will occur in Asia. The conference therefore took up, 'AIDS in Asia' as the main topic. Asian participants were invited to make an appropriate number of presentations on this issue. I believe that the participation of Asian countries led to increased global awareness of the seriousness of AIDS in Asia and inspired all participants to unite in the Asian effort against AIDS.

Although the Tenth International Conference on AIDS/International Conference on STD achieved its goals of presenting the results of recent research and providing an opportunity for the exchange of opinions, its end does not mean that our responsibilities have ended. We must avoid any sense of self-satisfaction as a result of the productive presentations and discussions held at this conference, or it will have been nothing more than a 'Midsummer Night's Dream' in Yokohama, I would like to emphasize that we must ensure that this conference marks a starting point by initiating a new global light against AIDS that affins the conference theme of 'International Cooperation in the Fight against AIDS: Together for the Future.'

Acknowledgments

The conference was made possible through the substantial support and contributions of the sponsors and cosponsors, particularly WHO and the Ministry of Health and Welfare and other Japanese ministries.

We are grateful to leading scientists and clinicians, government officials, and others for the willing acceptance of our invitations, despite their busy schedules, and for contributing generously to this conference with excellent presentations. Finally, we wish to express deep appreciation for the dedication of all the others involved in the conference whose names for limitation of space I am not able to mention here.

Yuichi Shiokawa, M.D.
Chair, Organizing Committee
The Tenth International Conference on AIDS/International
Conference on STD, Yokohama, Japan

Preface by T. Kitamura

This volume, *Global Challenge of AIDS: Ten Years of HIV/AIDS Research,* is a collection of papers presented at the plenary and tenth anniversary sessions of the Tenth International Conference on AIDS/International Conference on STD (Xth-ICA), held 7–12 August, 1994, in Yokohama, Japan. The conference was organized and supported by numerous governmental and non-governmental organizations working in AIDS research, prevention, control and support of affected society and individuals, as described by the Organizing Committee chair.

Under the set theme, "The Global Challenge of AIDS—Together for the Future," the programming of the Conference put special emphasis on: 1) HIV infection of women and its impact on future generations, 2) HIV/AIDS pandemic in developing countries, and 3) community-based support of people with HIV/AIDS (PWA). With increasingly larger voices of those working on the non-science side of AIDS control and PWA support, the Program Committee (PC) was put in the rather difficult position of balancing the scientific quality of the ICA and its social nature, the public relations opportunity for AIDS control and PWA support activities, and serious concerns were, indeed, expressed by a number of scientists who insisted on the tradition of ICA as a meeting place for broad aspects of HIV/AIDS research.

The Organizing Committee established the Community Liaison Committee to work in liaison activities, including communication and coordination with such support organizations, and the Program Committee entrusted this liaison committee to provide programming advice in four scientific tracks, i.e., A. basic science, B. clinical science and care, C. epidemiology and prevention, and D. impact, social response and education. The track chairs (Drs. Takashi Kurimura (A), Dr. Kaoru Shimada (B), Kenji Soda (C), and Hirotada Hirose (D) were assisted by internationally renowned cochairs (Drs. Flossie Wong-Staal, David Ho, Jean-Baptiste Brunet, Werasit Sittitrai respectively) as well as more than 80 principal HIV/AIDS researchers in- and outside Japan as Program Committee members.

The major scientific features of the Tenth ICA program can be summarized as follows: 1) epidemiology of the serious, unexpected, rapid dissemination of HIV/AIDS in developing countries, especially in Asia; 2) long-term non-progressors who have been HIV-infected for a long period without practical progression of HIV disease, a thorough study of which is giving significant insights into the protective immunity; 3) a new approach to genetic therapy by hairpin ribozyme; 4) HIV protease inhibitors as new therapeutic agents under clinical trial; 5) new approach to a protective HIV vaccine with special reference to eliciting cytotoxic T lymphocyte response; 6) synergistic effects of combined therapy with available HIV therapeutics.

In parallel with 97 sessions of nearly 1,000 oral abstract presentations of representative research reports from more than 3,500 accepted abstracts, the Program Committee invited the 30 speakers for plenary sessions to provide a state-of-the-art summary of progress in the topics of the above four tracks and 11 speakers for three sessions of Tenth Anniversary Special Sessions to review the progress in the last decade.

The editors rearranged the 26 papers presented at the plenary session: according to scientific topic.   As for the four invited speakers from whom the editors did not receive completed papers by the end of March 1995, abstracts from the conference program or excerpts given to the conference chairs have been included as alternatives.   The editors express sincere gratitude for the cooperation of the authors, devoted editorial work by Ms. Shigeko Yoshida, Kodansha Scientific, and Dr. Yoshiki Sakurai, National AIDS Medical Information Center, for his hard work in program coordination during ICA and the editorial work thereafter.

As the program chair, the editor wishes to express his personal congratulations for the successful completion of Tenth ICA and scientific progress reported in both plenary and abstract sessions.   The Tenth ICA should be regarded as the first ICA which dealt with HIV/AIDS in women on a scientific basis.   The editors hope the present volume will serve as a scientific overview of HIV/AIDS research conducted over the ten years the ICA has been in existence.

Takashi Kitamura
Chair, Program Committee
The Tenth International Conference on AIDS/International
Conference on STD, Yokohama, Japan

Contents

Care and Preventive Activities

Counseling/Social/Psychology/Support

Tenth Anniversary Special Sessions

Epidemiology

Global Status of the HIV/AIDS Epidemic and the Response

M. H. Merson

WHO, Global Programme on AIDS, CH-1211 Geneva 27, Switzerland

Since we met last in Berlin, I have had the privilege of visiting some 20 nations — countries as diverse as China, Zambia, Honduras and Sweden — to see the pandemic first-hand. Two facts are undeniable. Despite the heroic efforts of countless individuals, community groups and organizations, more people were infected with HIV in the past year than ever before. And despite the best efforts of health workers and researchers, more people than ever died an untimely death because of AIDS. Never has the pandemic been so visible, never has its impact on individuals and society been greater.

In my talk, I will first update you on the pandemic's current magnitude and trends for both HIV and AIDS. I will then discuss the global response and outline the challenges I see ahead. What must we do better — and, just as important, what must we stop doing — if we are to reduce the scope and impact of the pandemic?

But before starting let me say a special word about Asia. Holding the International AIDS Conference here in Yokohama could not be more timely. HIV and AIDS are challenging this continent as never before. Enormous population movements, the inferior status of women and a reluctance to acknowledge the huge threat posed by AIDS make many Asian countries very vulnerable. But for all its vulnerability, Asia is in a position of unique strength to curb the epidemic, given clear vision and strong political will. I will say more about this later.

Current Magnitude, Trends and Impact

In the past 12 months, we estimate that another 3 million men, women and children have been infected with HIV. The cumulative total stood at around 14 million a year ago. It now exceeds 17 million. Please remember that our estimates are conservative. The percentage distribution of cumulative infections by region has not changed very much except in Asia, where it increased from 12% to 16% with a corresponding decrease in North America and Europe. A little over 60% of all infections to date have occurred in Sub-Saharan Africa (fig. 1).

Let me turn to the regional infection trends among adults and adolescents (fig. 2). In South and South-East Asia, HIV infections are now estimated at over 2.5 million — a million more than just a year ago. The HIV epidemic here is growing at an alarming rate.

3

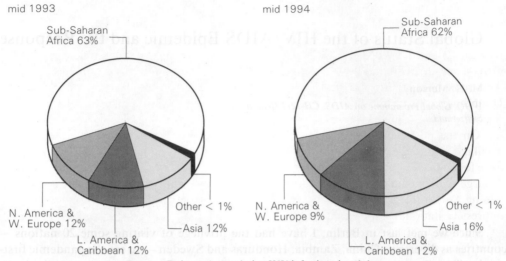

Fig. 1. Estimated cumulative HIV infections in adults.

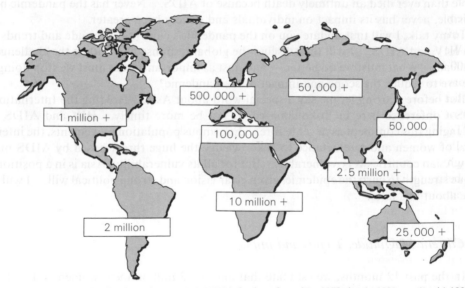

Fig. 2. Estimated distribution of total adult HIV infections from late 1970s/early 1980s until mid-1994.

For example, estimated infections in Thailand have risen tenfold since early 1990. In India they have tripled since 1992.

Many studies have shown how rapidly infections have increased in injecting drug users and sex workers during the past five years—for example, in Cambodia, India, Thailand and Viet Nam. But as we all know, HIV never remains confined to any "risk" group but eventually diffuses into the wider population.   This is already visible in Thailand, where we see a steady rise in HIV prevalence among young men recruited into the military and pregnant women attending antenatal clinics.   In the country as a whole, the rates have reached 4% and 1.5% respectively.   But in Chiang Rai, in northern Thailnd, 20% of young men — one in five — and 8% of young women — one in twelve — are infected (fig. 3). And remember, there was little in the way of HIV infection in Thailand until 1987. Doubtless it is just a matter of time before we see a similar diffusion in other countries of the region.

On the positive side, we are seeing definite signs of change in sexual behavior in Thailand.   As an example of this, reported cases of sexually transmitted disease (STD) have fallen by 77% between 1986 and 1993 (fig. 4).   Most of this decline can be attributed to large scale media campaigns promoting condom use and intensive educational efforts among vulnerable population groups.   Thailand is one of the few countries putting impressive national resources into AIDS prevention and it is getting impressive results.

Turning to East Asia and the Pacific, we see that the estimated number of infections have reached 50,000—this is a doubling in the past year.   Here in Japan HIV rates are still relatively low but climbing steadily in both men and women.

One recent phenomenon has been a steep rise in the rate of reported STDs in China (fig. 5).   This tells us how vulnerable this country is to HIV spread, especially given the massive population movements under way as a result of economic expansion.   If the HIV epidemic takes hold in this giant of a country, it could have an enormous impact not only on China but on Asia as a whole.

We estimate that the countries of Eastern Europe and Central Asia have so far had over 50,000 infections.   But this figure may be misleading.   These countries have many of the factors associated with rapid HIV spread — economic crisis, rising unemployment, armed conflicts and major population movements.   Once we get HIV data on people practising high-risk behavior, we will have a better idea of how big the problem really is.

To date, there have been an estimated 100,000 infections in North Africa and the Middle East — another region where the AIDS threat once seemed remote and cases were thought to come from abroad.   Rising HIV levels are being seen in individuals with high-risk behavior.   For example, in Djibouti prevalence reached 14% two years ago among men attending STD clinics and is now nearly 4% in women seeking antenatal care.

In Latin America and the Caribbean, there have been an estimated 2 million infections so far.   On the positive side, we are seeing evidence of sexual behavior change in the form of declining STD rates, for example in Costa Rica.   But certain Caribbean countries continue to have some of the highest AIDS rates in the world.   And in Brazil, which may hold the key to the ultimate extent of the epidemic in this region, increasing HIV prevalence is being seen in STD clinics in more and more parts of the country.

Moving north, we estimate that North America has had over a million infections to date.   Along with the infections in Western Europe, Australia and New Zealand, this means that cumulative infections now total more than 1.5 million in these industrialized countries.   The decline in the rate of new infections in homosexual and bisexual men is for the most part holding, though there is concern about increasing risk behavior among younger men.   One route that is still growing in importance is heterosexual transmission, especially in urban areas with high rates of STDs and drug injecting.

When it comes to drug injectors, the cities that have averted an epidemic are those

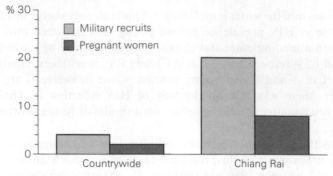

Fig. 3. HIV prevalence among military recruits and antenatal clinic attenders, Thailand, 1993.

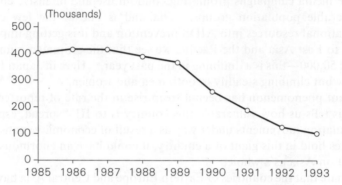

Fig. 4. Incidence of reported STD, Thailand, 1985–1993.

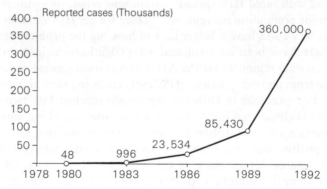

Fig. 5. Number of reported cases of sexually transmitted diseases, 1980–1992, China.

where drug injectors have had legal access to sterile injection equipment, and benefited from AIDS information and a climate of trust established through community outreach programmes. Unfortunately, there have been far too few cities that have committed themselves to such harm reduction programmes.

In Sub-Saharan Africa the estimated total now exceeds 10 million infections. So far, this is the only part of the world where there are more women infected than men—11 to 12 women for every 10 men.

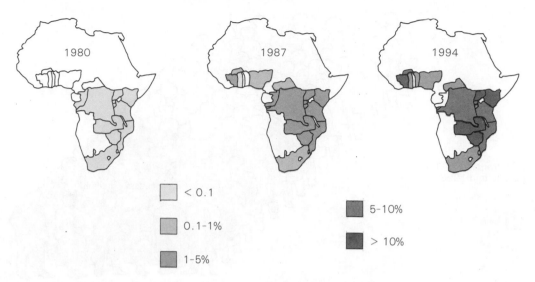

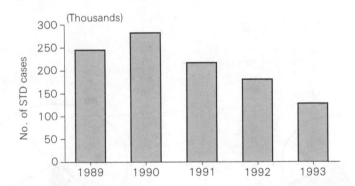

Fig. 6.   Estimated nationwide adult HIV prevalence in selected Sub-Saharan African countries, 1980–1994.

Fig. 7.   Incidence of STD reported from primary health clinics, Harare, Zimbabwe, 1989–1993.

Looking back historically it appears that in 1980 HIV prevalence was less than 0.1% in just a few areas.   By 1987, prevalence in the central and eastern parts of the continent had risen to 1% or even 5%.   As of today, not only does prevalence exceed 10% in the countries affected early on, but the virus is becoming firmly established in the west and south (fig. 6). In fact, these are the areas which account for much of the past year's jump from 8 to 10 million infections.

Despite this increase, as is the case in Thailand and Costa Rica, there are growing signs that control efforts in sub-Saharan Africa are having an impact.   More and more condoms are being sold and distributed, and there is increasing anecdotal evidence that bars and discos that serve as sex trade centers are losing clientele.   STD rates reported from primary health clinics in one city — Harare, Zimbabwe — decreased 63% between 1990 and 1993 (fig. 7).   Taken together, all this points to encouraging changes in sexual behavior.

I turn now to the epidemic of illness — the AIDS epidemic.   As of mid 1994, 190

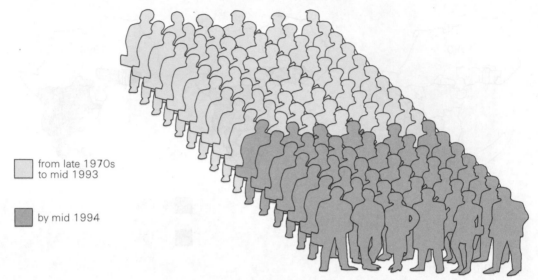

from late 1970s
to mid 1993

by mid 1994

Fig. 8. Estimated cumulative AIDS cases in adults.

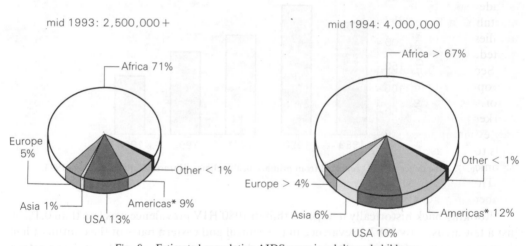

mid 1993: 2,500,000 +

Africa 71%

Europe
5%

Other < 1%

Asia 1%

Americas* 9%

USA 13%

mid 1994: 4,000,000

Africa > 67%

Other < 1%

Europe > 4%

Asia 6%

Americas* 12%

USA 10%

Fig. 9. Estimated cumulative AIDS cases in adults and children.

countries worldwide have reported close to 1 million AIDS cases to WHO. But reporting is always incomplete, and we estimate that as of today, around 4 million adults and children have developed AIDS since the start of the pandemic. This is an increase of a staggering 60% in the past year alone (fig. 8). By the year 2000, the cumulative case total is projected to more than double, reaching nearly 10 million.

AIDS cases have increased everywhere in the past year. But proportionately the increase has been greatest in places where the HIV epidemic is newest, such as Latin America and Asia. Asia now accounts for 6% of the cumulative global total, representing

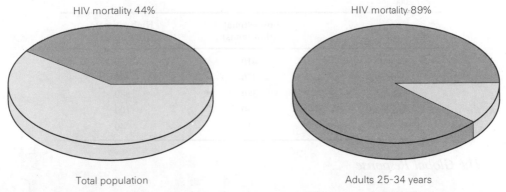

Fig. 10. Mortality attributable to HIV infection, Masaka district, Uganda, 1989–1990.

an eightfold increase in AIDS cases in just one year (fig. 9). The increased burden on hospitals is considerable in such cities as Chiang Mai, Bombay and Yangon.

The AIDS epidemic is having impacts of other kinds, too. First, it is making an appalling contribution to mortality, especially in areas where the epidemic is more than a decade old. In the Masaka district of Uganda, AIDS accounts for close to half of all mortality in the total population. In young adults under 35 — those who are raising families, working the fields, running the schools and hospitals — 9 out of 10 deaths are HIV-related. Or to put it another way, only one death in ten is not HIV-related (fig. 10).

Secondly, because of the age group affected, AIDS is having an economic impact out of proportion to the numbers of people dying. This has serious implications for the private sector. AIDS causes illness, disability and death among employees and their families. Worker productivity declines, firms have higher medical costs and survivor payments and they eventually lose staff with valuable training or skills. This disrupts production and leads to increased training and labor costs. At the same time, as more of the population becomes ill and personal income drops, consumer markets shrink (table 1).

Thirdly, the pandemic has an intensely personal impact on children, increasing numbers of whom will lose one or both parents to AIDS (table 2). Their torment begins with the long illness of their parents. On their death, the children lose not only love and support but, all too often, their home and property, friends, school — everything that has made up their small world.

Table 1. Private sector impact of AIDS

- Decline in worker productivity
- Higher medical costs and survivor payments
- Loss of staff
- Increased training and labor costs
- Shrinking consumer markets

Table 2. Cumulative number of motherless AIDS orphans under age 15 by the year 2000

Country	Low estimate (thousands)	High estimate (thousands)
Uganda	410	880
Zambia	320	490
Kenya	380	580
Thailand	30	100
Dominican Republic	12	40

The Global Response

I started this presentation by talking about the heroic efforts of individuals, community groups and organizations.   Many are present in this hall.   Your achievements are an inspiration to us.

But let us not delude ourselves.   HIV marches on.   No wonder our world is filled with sceptics — if we know so much about preventing AIDS, why is the epidemic continuing to expand?   What should be the priorities of our global response?

I believe there are three major challenges facing us.

First, we must deal better — much better — with the three societal forces that are driving the spread of HIV and blocking effective prvention and care—denial, discrimination and disempowerment.

Denial is what keeps society's leaders from taking the pandemic seriously and investing the resources needed.   Denial even takes the form of outright misinformation; misinformation that today can get from one side of the globe to the other in seconds; misinformation like the persisting myth that HIV is not the cause of AIDS.   I hate to imagine how many people get infected each day because myths like this are put forward as facts.

Discrimination is the basis of misguided efforts to identify and sideline infected individuals in the belief that this can somehow control spread of the virus.   I am thinking, for example, of mandatory screening for HIV — a violation of human rights and an action which is at best futile and more often harmful to true prevention.   Besides, wherever you look, it is usually the less powerful who wind up getting tested — patients more than doctors, women more than men, sex workers more than their clients.   And let me ask a question.   How long will countries go on using HIV tests to screen out visitors and migrants?   How long will it take them to understand that AIDS is not a disease of foreigners, that HIV does not travel on passports?

Then, there is disempowerment.   Disempowered people are vulnerable people. Think of the millions of Rwandan refugees whose desperate faces have recently crossed our television screens.   Or the millions of powerless street children increasing in our cities.   Or the untold numbers of women who fear infection from their partner — but do not have the power to insist on condom use, or the economic ability to leave the relationship.   For people to avoid infection there must be a supportive, enabling environmnt that provides them with knowledge on how to protect themselves and with the motivation and power to do so.

It is clear that until we overcome these social factors—denial, discrimination and disempowerment — we will never bring the epidemic under full control. Political leaders must find the courage to provide leadership despite the sensitivities and taboos around AIDS, discriminatory laws and practices must be abolished and those who are powerless must be given the means to protect themselves.

Our second major challenge is to prioritize and expand our research. Let me mention a few of our priorities. I start with the urgency of finding better drug regimens for keeping HIV-infected people alive and healthy, and learning more about the immune response of long-term survivors and the HIV strains they carry.

With regard to prevention, we have learned in the past year that zidovudine can reduce the risk of mother-to-infant transmission. This looks like the first real technological breakthrough in HIV prevention since the pandemic started. The challenge now is to come up with effective antiretroviral regimens that are affordable, feasible and sustainable in developing countries. Primary prevention would be even better, of course — keeping women uninfected in the first place. We have made some progress in developing vaginal microbicides since Berlin, but we need to move faster.

A vaccine, of course, would be an invaluable complement to our behavioral approaches in bringing this pandemic under control. But to accelerate vaccine development, we must find innovative ways to increase public and private sector collaboration, and the vaccine we seek must be a vaccine for everyone. Decisions on vaccines to be tested must be made by the countries of the north and south together, always remembering that there can be no unethical or scientifically unacceptable short cuts.

Our final challenge is to do now, everywhere, what we already know how to do. In the first instance, this means providing the best possible care for people with HIV infection. What is needed is a continuum of care from the home to the community to the hospital. Unfortunately, in many countries, it would take a great investment in health care— especially at the periphery — to achieve this continuum, since care for people with HIV can only be as comprehensive as the health system itself.

The health care crisis over AIDS has exposed the colossal gaps in health systems worldwide, the lack of equity in access to health professionals and to vitally needed drugs. The solutions are not easy, especially for developing countries facing many health problems. At a minimum they must reorient national spending so that health care gets its due. And donor agencies supporting AIDS control efforts in these countries must provide more resources for care, for if care activities are not supported, prevention programmes will not be credible.

In this regard, we have recently undertaken a retrospective analysis of the epidemic in four countries in East and Central Africa — Uganda, Tanzania, Rwanda and Zambia — which has provided us with insights into how to apply our preventive efforts more effectively.

We believe that during the first 3 – 4 years of the epidemic in these countries there was an "explosion" of new infections. The burst was so intense that almost half of all people who acquired HIV during the first 12 years of the epidemic did so in this initial explosive phase. In other words, those individuals across the population practising high-risk sexual behavior quickly became infected. Then, perhaps 5 or so years later, after this burst was over, prevalence stabilized. We moved from an explosive period to a more endemic situation (fig. 11).

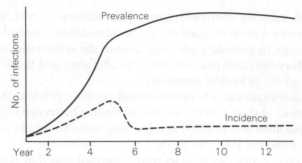

Fig. 11. Hypothesized patterns of HIV incidence and prevalence, mature East African epidemics.

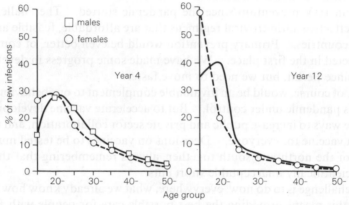

Fig. 12. Change in hypothesized distribution of HIV infections by age and sex, mature East African epidemics.

But this does not mean the problem is over. For as those infected in the initial phase fall ill and die of AIDS, their places are taken by newly infected individuals, thus keeping the number of people alive with HIV — or the HIV prevalence — at the same level. The point is that in such countries stable prevalence can mask continuing high incidence.

What is actually happening becomes even clearer when we look at the age distribution of new HIV infections. During the early explosive phase, say year 4 of the epidemic, newly infected individuals ranged in age from the mid-teens to the forties. Newly infected females tended to be slightly younger than newly infected males, reflecting the fact that women often have sex with older men. By the 12th year of the epidemic, the situation looks radically different. Now new infections cluster more among youth who are just becoming sexually active. Youngsters under 25 account for up to three-quarters of all new infections. And up to 60% of all infections in females occur by age 20 (fig. 12).

We are currently examining the applicability of this analysis to other parts of the world. If it turns out to be applicable — and we have no reason to think it will not—in countries where the epidemic is well-established, one thing is clear. Boys and girls must be given the information, skills and support they need for AIDS prevention before they become sexually active. This is the only way to help keep them uninfected and ensure they do not become the engine that drives the epidemic.

In places where the epidemic is just moving into the early explosive phase — like much of Asia — the overriding need is to act now, without delay, to prevent or blunt the rise in infections.   I appeal to all Asian leaders to face reality and make AIDS prevention a national priority.   Do whatever you need to do to overcome denial, and fight discrimination.   Provide your most vulnerable citizens the information and means — including condoms — to protect themselves.   And do not believe, as many others have believed, that it will not happen to you.

And, please, let us not use cost as an excuse.   We calculate that implementing basic prevention programs in Asia would cost between three quarters and one and a half billion US dollars a year.   This represents less than 0.03% of Asia's economic output.   Or to put it another way, it is the equivalent of what Japan's workers produce in less than one hour. An investment of this kind would avoid an estimated 5 million infections by the year 2000 alone.   And the preventive effect would be even stronger as Asia moves into the twenty-first century.

The economic benefit that could result from prevention on such a scale is difficult to estimate, but it is clearly massive in comparison with the investment needed.   Consider that, by the year 2000, a Thai estimate puts the loss to Thailand's economy alone at nearly $11 billion, and that analysts McGraw Hill estimate that AIDS will cost Asian economies between $38 and $52 billion.

Dear colleagues, ladies and gentlemen, I hope the challenges are clear.   Over 6000 people are becoming infected with HIV every day, more and more of them in Asia.   How big does this number have to get before we take the pandemic seriously and invest the necessary resources?   How much do people with HIV have to suffer before the world acknowledges that AIDS is a viral disease, not a moral judgment?   How long must women wait for equal status with men?   How long are we going to tolerate a world in which only the lucky few get humane medical care?   How many youngsters have to die out of ignorance before we stop pretending that young people do not have sex?

The answers—the global response — are up to us: researchers, government officials, clinicians, journalists, citizens of all nations, men and women living with and without AIDS.   As we move forward, let us seek out and link up with all possible allies — people fighting for development, for equality, for human rights, for fairness, in whatever sphere of life.   If we act together, we can persuade the powers that be that action cannot wait — in Africa, in the Americas, in Europe and not least in Asia, where time is fast running out.

May our meeting this week prove to be, to paraphrase Nehru, India's great Prime Minister, a land-mark which divides the past from the future.

Mother to Child HIV Infection

S. Blanche

Hôpital Necker—Enfants Malades, Paris, France

The mother to child HIV transmission rate has been extensively studied over recent years in prospective cohorts of infants born to seropositive mothers. The reported rates of transmission are lower in industrialized countries than in the developing countries. It is difficult to compare the results of the different cohorts because of the various methods used to calculate the transmission rate. The main reason for the difference between the industrialized and developing countries is probably breast feeding. However, this mode of transmission must not be over-estimated, as the transmission rate in certain African and Haitian surveys, in which all women breast feed, is similar to or even slightly lower than that in certain industrialized countries where breast feeding is uncommon.

Apart from breast feeding, the precise mechanisms of viral transmission remain a matter of speculation, although they are probably multiple. HIV can probably cross the placenta, but the role of the placenta is probably only passive; despite the results of in vitro culture experiments, it seems unlikely that HIV replicates significantly in placental structures in vivo; the most probable vector is maternal blood, which frequently passes to the fetus during labor. Passage of free virions through the intact placenta is still hypothetical. Ascending infection across the amniotic membrane is feasible, by contact with contaminated cervical secretions and finally contamination during passage through the birth canal is suggested by the fact that first-born twins have a significantly higher risk of infection.

Regardless of the mechanisms involved, several lines of evidence point to late transmission in most cases, towards the end of pregnancy. Brossard showed last year that infection before 20 weeks of gestation was exceptional in a very large series of 100 fetuses, a finding which contradicted some older studies. In addition, morbidity and immuno-deficiency are very rare at birth. But the main argument for late transmission is the fact that the virus can not be isolated at birth by culture or PCR in 60 to 70% of casees, whereas all infected children are positive by these methods after a few weeks or months of life.

Our latest contribution to this important question of timing is a Markov analysis of early diagnostic markers in about 100 infected infants enrolled in the French prospective cohort and longitudinaly analyzed in a single virological laboratory. This mathematical model, produced the following hypothesis: 65% of these children would be infected during birth, compared to only 35% in the preceding weeks: this clearly confirms indirect arguments that transmission usually occurs at delivery.

Despite uncertainties as to the mode and precise timing of mother to child transmission, we now know that several parameters can influence the risk for a given infant.   Some of these factors are still preliminary or controversial, such as the mother's age, various maternal co-infections, the conditions of delivery, the presence or absence of certain anti-HIV antibodies, and more recently the mother's nutritional status.   By contrast, the link between the risk of transmission on the one hand and the mother's viral load and immune deficiency on the other hand is now well etablished.   Many markers, ranging from the simplest to the most complex — and costly — such as quantitative DNA PCR can be used to determine the level of viral replication, and each is individually associated with the risk of transmission as shown in this subgroup of women extensively studied for various parameters.   In multivariate analyses, complex markers correlate far better than p24 antigenemia and other simple tests but the CD4 cell count also remains significantly related to the transmission rate in this type of multivariate analysis, despite the statistical power of quantitative DNA PCR.   Actually, the transmission rate correlates very well with the CD4 cell count: women with counts of less than two hundred have a 45% risk of transmitting the virus, compared to 16% in women with counts over 500.

It is interesting to cross these data with those on the timing of transmission: if we take the Markov data mentioned earlier, it appears that the risk of early transmission is significantly linked to the mother's viral load: p24 antigenemia for example is more frequent in mothers whose children are infected in utero than in those whose children are infected at birth.

The most important development over the past year in the field of mother to child HIV transmission and, in AIDS as a whole, is the results of the American-French study ACTG 076-ANRS 024.   The aim was to cut the risk of maternofetal transmission by treatment with zidovudine during pregnancy.   To simplify, the women were given either zidovudine or a placebo during the pregnancy and delivery, and all the neonates were treated for 6 weeks.   The results are clear: the transmission rate was below 10% in the treatment group compared to more than 20% in the placebo group, regardless of the calculation method or the definition of infection.   This is a very exciting result which opens up the hope of preventing mother to child transmission of HIV just as effectively as hepatitis B. Obviously a great deal of work remains to be done.   One problem is to ensure that treatment is safe in the long term for the infant, and another is to determine whether these results can be extended to other women, especially those who have already take zidovudine or have CD4 cell counts lower than 200.   It also remains to be shown that the same degree of efficacy can be obtained in every-day conditions of clinical practice and not just in a strictly conducted trial.

Above all, we must make sure that such treatment is made available to women in poorer countries and those hardest hit by the pandemic.

Clearly, we will have also to find ways of cutting the transmission rate still further. One possibility may be to discourage breast feeding, but this risk must not be overestimated. In contrary, we perfectly know the potential risk of artificial feeding in developing countries.   Another alternative is to use treatments more effective than zidovudine alone. The third possibility is active and/or passive immunotherapy, as long as the antibodies induced have neutralizing potential.   Finally the last approach concerns the delivery with disinfection of the birth canal and, in industrialized countries, Caesarean section.

The possible protection afforded by Caesarean section has long been a matter of debate.

Contradictory results have been published, and a recent meta-analysis of most cohort studies carried out in the industrialized countries has been recently pulled.   The largest two studies were the Collaborative European survey and the French survey: The first showed a positive effect, *i.e.* a significant reduction in the risk of transmission, while the second showed no effect.   The other surveys showed positive on neutral effect, but have quite large confidence intervals.   The meta-analysis concluded that Caesarean section had a slight beneficial effect, falling at the threshold of statistical significance.   But it is difficult to conclude (In short, we simply do not know if Caesarean section is beneficial or not), for three main reasons.   First, the rate of Caesarean section varies widely from one country to the next; second, clinical and laboratory parameters in women who are delivered in this way differ from those of women who give birth naturally.   Third, the indications and techniques are extremely variable.   A large international prospective study may soon be started to obtain a clear answer to this question.

With regard to the course of HIV infection in infants and children, 1994 will see the application of a far more logical classification system.   It is based on both clinical and laboratory parameters.   Clinical manifestations are divided into four classes, N, A, B, C. C group represents a good clinical description of AIDS since all symptoms of this class are associated with a very high mortality risk.   Clinical axis is crossed with CD4 cell count, which varies widely according to age in childhood.   This system will help to standardize data in different surveys, registers and clinical trials.

The risk of AIDS, which corresponds to class C, apparently differs in children and adults.   An analysis of nearly 250 infected children in the french prospective study showed that the cumulative risk of AIDS increases very rapidly in the first year of life to about 20%, then more slowly at a rate of about 2 or 3% a year.   It is the shape of this curve that revealed the bimodal progression of HIV disease in children.

About 15 to 20% of children rapidly develop a severe immune deficiency, opportunistic infections and, in most cases, encephalopathy.   There is a very high morbidity rate in this group of children, most of whom die before the age of 3 or 4 years.   In contrast, 80 to 85% of children only become immunodeficient after a relatively long period, which is similar to or perhaps even longer than that in adults.   Neurological manifestations are far less frequent and, above all, occur far later.

We now know that the risk of developing the early severe form is linked to the mother's disease stage during pregnancy: on this curve, the risk of AIDS at 1 year is around 50% in children born to mothers at CDC stage IV and only 10% in those whose mothers were asymptomatic.   The risk of early onset is also linked to virological status at birth: it is about 25% when the virus can be isolated by PCR or culture at birth, VS 10% when a such research is negative.   The risk is even higher when p24 antigenemia is detectable at birth: children with positive antigenemia have a four fold higher risk of early AIDS than those who are negative at birth.

Several explanations have been proposed, but the most widely accepted again involves the timing of transmission.   Transmission would appear to occur in uterus when the mother's viral load is high and her CD4 cell count is low.   In this case, free virus would be able to infect the fetus by crossing the placenta and amniotic membrane.   Replication would thus begin during fetal life, and the virus would influence the development of the immune system, particularly the thymus.   HIV probably crosses the fetal blood-brain barrier, leading to rapid development of severe illness with encephalopathy and marked immune deficiency.   In contrast, in the case of women with a low viral load, transmission would mainly occur during delivery.   Intracellular virus would be transmitted by maternofetal blood exchanges during labor, but the infant would be able to mount an immune response similar to that in adults, especially in terms of specific anti-HIV cytotoxicity.   However, this explanation is not entirely satisfactory, as experience shows that some children infected at birth by blood transfusion develop the early severe form of HIV disease with encephalopathy during the first few months of life and others hypothesis are also open to discussion.

Although we are beginning to understand the early phase of HIV infection in children, the long-term outcome is still unknown.   In the French prospective pediatric cohort, 70% of the infected children are alive at 6 years of age.   Most deaths before two or three years of life were due to the early severe form of the disease.   More than one-third of the children who are alive at 66 months have no signs of the infection.   If we extrapolate these prospective data, it appears that a large number of children will reach adolescence and that some will reach adulthood.   There is still a great deal to learn about the course of HIV infection in later childhood and adolescence.   It is likely that opportunistic infections will be the same as in adults, and that the incidence of lymphomas will largely be dependent of encounter and replication of Epstein-Barr Virus.

A very important question is the potential impact of HIV infection on these children's psychomotor and cognitive development, as this will largely determine the quality of their social insertion.   We have recently analyzed the school performance and psychomotor development of all children monitored in our institution who were infected at birth and are now at least six years old.   The results are less negative than we feared: most of the children are able to follow the normal school curriculum and their psychomotor test results are almost in the normal range, with the exception of time/space orientation evaluated through the Bender test.   Contrary to widely held beliefs, the results are not influenced by the children's social environment, such as whether or not their mother was infected through HIV drug use.   In contrast, they are strongly influenced by the CD4 cell count at the time of the tests, suggesting that performance may well deteriorate in parallel to the decline in this parameter.   However, what is true at 6 – 8 years of age may not apply when the same children reach adolescence.

These children infected at birth are faced not only by the prospect of AIDS, but also by the likelihood that they will lose their mothers, also through AIDS.   We have studied this problem in the French prospective cohort, although it must of course be borne in mind that the situation in industrialized countries differs in many ways from that in the developing countries.   The risk of separation related to maternal HIV infection is about 2% to 3% a year, as shown by this curve representing cumulative data since birth.   The risk is influenced by the mother's clinical status during pregnancy, but obviously not by whether or not the child is infected.

In general, children separated from their mothers are cared for by the family, or by public and private care institutions.   In this prospective cohort, 43% of these children are taken in by their family and 57% are placed by care institutions.   The risk of institutional care is not influenced by the way in which the mother was infected, nor her age, nor her clinical status; it is not affected either by whether the child is infected.   In contrast, the risk is higher when the parents are immigrants, probably because of the fragility of these uprooted families.   A very important finding is that the child's age at the time of separation has a major impact on the subsequent care setting.   Put simply, the younger the child, the greater the risk of institutional care.   In fact the role played by the family increases gradually with the child's age at separation; the balance tips in favor of care within the family when the child is 24 months old or more when separation occurs, and in this cohort none of the children separated from their mothers after 4 years of age had to be taken into institutional care.   Cross-generation family solidarity is clearly the best answer to this growing individual and social catastrophe, but both the authorities and care groups must provide specific and effective support for family members who are willing to take up the challenge.

Epidemiology of STD and AIDS in Asia

Yun-Fong Ngeow

University of Malaya, Kuala Lumpur, Malaysia

Asia is a vast continent of diverse cultures, religions, socio-economic and political systems and home to more than half the world's population. It has gone through many turbulent times and its strive towards modernization has been set back by numerous wars, natural disasters and diseases. Now, once again, it is the center of world attention as the battle ground against a little virus that strikes fear in the human heart, the HIV.

HIV and AIDS came to Asia later than in the Western world but in less than a decade, they have reached all countries in the region except for some islands in the South Pacific. Although the actual numbers of AIDS cases reported to the WHO are still comparatively low, estimates of HIV seroprevalence from various surveys are staggering: more than 1.5 million affected in India, 600,000 to 800,000 in Thailand, 150,000 in Myanmar and at least 50,000 each in Indonesia and the Philippines [1]. The most perturbing statistics are those showing sharp increases in incidence in some communities. Seropositivity rates jumped from 2 to 54% among commercial sex workers (CSWs) in Bombay (1984 – 1992) and from 2 to 55% among intravenous drug users (IVDUs) in Manipur, Northeast India (1989 – 1990) [2]. Within a year (1991 – 1992), seropositivity increased 10 fold among blood donors in Cambodia (0.076 – 0.75%) [3] and almost tripled among IVDUs in Northeast Malaysia (11 – 30%) [4].

All modes of HIV transmission have occurred in Asia. The infection is still mainly transfusion-related in Japan, predominantly a male homosexual problem in Australia and New Zealand and largely restricted to IVDUs in Southwest China, Malaysia and Viet Nam [5]. However, it is evident that in most parts of Asia, HIV has become an important STD and increasing heterosexual transmission is moving the epidemic from high risk groups into the general population.

In Thailand, for instance, HIV affects up to 72% CSWs, 6% male STD clinic patients and 20% military recruits. The extent of HIV infiltration into the general population can also be seen in seroprevalence rates of up to 7% among antenatal women and 0.23% among blood donors [6, 7]. In India, transmission is 75% heterosexual and 2 – 3% mother to infant [2]. In the city of Bombay alone, between 1992 and 1993, seropositivity increased from 0.7 to 1.2% among pregnant women and from 0.15 to 5% among blood donors. Elsewhere, heterosexual transmission of HIV has exceeded homosexual transmission in Japan, Singapore, Philippines, Korea, Macao and Brunei [5] and has become more noticeable in Hong Kong [8]. In Papua New Guinea, transmission has always been predominantly heterosexual [9].

Why is HIV rampaging through Asia in such a manner?

The epidemiology of HIV infection shares many similar features with that of other STDs and there is a high level of endemic STDs in Asia which could have facilitated HIV transmission. In India alone, an estimated more than 10 million cases of STD occur every year. Despite gross under-reporting, annual incidences of 200 to 700 per 100,000 are recorded in Malaysia, the Philippines and Thailand. In China, although the per capita infection rate is still low, there has been a rapid increase in annual incidence in recent years (46.6% overall annual increase from 1987 to 1990; 71.41% in the Yangtse Valley cities) [10]. Gonorrhoea is the commonest notifiable STD in the region. Reported detection rates range from 0.5 [11] to 12% [12] among antenatal women and 1 [13] to 38% [14] among male STD clinic patients. Facilities for chlamydial diagnosis are very limited but from clinical presentations, non-specific urethritis appears to be at least as common as gonococcal urethritis in many countries. In a Taiwan study, 16.1% of a group of pregnant women were culture positive for cervical chlamydia while 29% were positive by a more sensitive test, the polymerase chain reaction [15]. Among women with genital discharge, detection rates vary from 2% in Bangladesh [12] to over 40% in New Delhi [16]. Herpes genitalis is found in almost 40% of CSWs in the Malaysian capital [14] and in up to 80% of brothel-based CSWs in N. Thailand [17]. In Singapore, its incidence doubled between 1977 and 1987 [18]. Genital warts have become the commonest STD in New Zealand, forming 19% of new cases seen in STD clinics [13]. Lymphogranuloma venereum, chancroid and granuloma inguinale remain tropical diseases, being found in parts of India, Southeast Asia, Papua New Guinea and in the tropical north of Australia [19, 20]. The prevalence of reactive serological tests for syphilis among antenatal women ranges from 0.4% in New Zealand [13] to 9.1% in Fiji [21].

Although STDs tend to be concentrated in urban centers, rural and tribal people are not spared. In Papua New Guinea, the incidence of gonorrhoea increased from 13.2 per 100,000 in 1971 to 61.6 per 100,000 population in 1988. In the same period, syphilis seroreactivity also increased from 6.1 to 19.4 per 100,000 [9]. In recent surveys, it was found that up to 30% of women attending antenatal clinics had STDs and one third of babies had perinatal infections of which 80% were gonococcal, chlamydial or congenital syphilis. Besides alcoholism and drug abuse, STDs are also major problems for Australia's aboriginals. In the Northern Territory, STD rates are up to 40 times higher than those of other Australian states and more syphilis, gonorrhoea and chlamydial infections are seen among aboriginals than non-aboriginals [22]. Both HIV and AIDS are established in the aboriginal community. Among hill tribes in Southeast Asia, HIV and other STDS are brought back to remote villages by young women who contract the diseases in city brothels where they work and are sent back to their homes when they are known to be HIV positive.

Antimicrobial resistance is a major therapeutic problem. Low level resistance to multiple antibiotics has long been an earmark of Southeast Asian gonorrhoea. Superimposed on this, high level resistance to penicillin and tetracycline spread rapidly in the last 2 decades. Currently, the prevalence of high level plasmid-mediated penicillin resistance (PPNG) has established at 40 – 60% in Taiwan, Viet Nam, Thailand, Malaysia, Singapore, Brunei, Philippines and the Solomon Islands and high level chromosomally-mediated penicillin resistance (CMRNG) is most prevalent in China (62%), Hong Kong

(44%) and Korea (38%). Gonococci with plasmid-mediated resistance to tetracycline (TRNG) which were first reported in the USA in 1985, are now seen in 20 – 40% of isolates from Singapore, Malaysia and the Philippines and are also found in Australia, New Caledonia, Fiji, China, Korea and Vietnam [23 – 25]. Resistance to second line antibiotics like spectinomycin and kanamycin is causing treatment failures with standard doses [26] and decreasing susceptibility to fluoroquinolones which have only been recently introduced for therapy, has been reported from Japan, Hong Kong, Thailand, Australia and Papua New Guinea [23, 27, 28].

Delayed and inappropriate treatment leads to serious sequelae which are all seen in Asia where infertility rates range from 1.3% in Korea to 6.7% in Indonesia [29]. The percentage of infertile women with evidence of infective tubal damage is 12% in Singapore, 26% in India and 35% in Indonesia. In various Indian studies, chlamydia are associated with 36% of female infertility [16] and 35 to 50% of pelvic inflammatory diseases [30]. Ectopic pregnancy still presents as a surgical emergency and congenital syphilis occurs where antenatal screening is not available to all pregnant women [31].

The most frequently cited source of infection for male STD patients is the CSW. Prostitution flourishes in Asia where there are millions of impoverished women and a social attitude that turns a blind eye to male promiscuity. While some countries have reached developed nation status and others are enjoying booming economies, in the midst of the Asian opulence, there is plenty of abject poverty. For the destitute, prostitution is a means of avoiding starvation and this is capitalized by pimps and organized crime [32].

CSWs find ready clientele among all strata of society. The rich who get infected can afford private medical care at home or abroad and are usually not relected in official STD or HIV statistics. In newly industrialized countries, rapid economic growth has attracted migration to urban areas from villages and brought in large populations of male labor from poorer neighboring countries to work in the building industry, plantations, forestry or mining camps. Away from their families and lonely, these single migrant workers turn to CSWs. War in Southeast Asia brought in soldiers who needed Rest & Recreation and helped to build up large entertainment industries in favorite resorts.

International travel and sex tourism have also been great boons to prostitution. Sex tourism was popularized in the 1970s and 1980s when it was not uncommon for sex tours to be organized for workers as a reward for high production. Sex tourists may take home HIV and other STDs but often also bring these diseases to the casual partners they leave behind. In Australia, outside Sydney and Melbourne, most PPNG infections are imported from Southeast Asia [33]. Among Japanese men who are HIV positive, 58.1% were infected overseas [34]. The first case of AIDS in Indonesia was a Dutch tourist who died in Bali and the most recent HIV infection in Sabah, East Malaysia was identified in an Italian. In Nepal, male tour guides have been exposed to female HIV positive tourists.

Asia's 150 million malnourished children are easy prey to pedophils and men looking for virgins to avoid HIV. In Sri Lanka, UNICEF estimated that about 15,000 boys, many less than 14 years old, may be engaged in homosexual prostitution. Street children in the Philippines and Bombay are similarly selling their bodies to fill their bellies. In Thailand and Cambodia, tribal girls as young as 10 to 11 years old are being sold into brothels by family members or kidnappers.

CSWs go where their clients beckon and in so doing, help to change local STD statistics. In the 19th century, poverty-stricken Japanese farmers used to send their daughters to fill the flesh pots in Asia.   Today, thousands of Asian women are pouring into Japan to work in the sex-related entertainment industry.   Among foreign hospitality girls in Japan, the HIV seroprevalence is 2 to 6% [35].   In Singapore, Malaysians make up 92.7% of CSWs and account for STD incidences of 45 to 60 per 100 [36].   There are more than 20,000 Nepali girls working in Bombay brothels, up to 30% of whom may be HIV positive.   When these girls return to Kathmandu they take back with them STDs and HIV as do the Laotian girls who return to Laos with diseases contracted in Thailand.   Along the highways of India, Indonesia and Thailand, CSWs service long distance truck drivers who become potential vehicles of spread for STDs and HIV to all parts of the country [37, 38].

Sexual transmission is also linked to substance abuse which has been responsible for high rates of HIV infection particularly in the Northeast of India, Myanmar, Thailand, South China and Malaysia.   These areas are in the neighborhood of the famous "Golden Triangle" of Southeast Asia where opium is cultivated and often used for medicinal and recreational purposes by various hill tribes.   Heroin has been locally produced and refined since the early 1960s but it was only in the 1980s that injecting drug use increasingly replaced opium smoking as a form of addiction.   It is the sharing of needles and syringes which causes rapid spread of HIV infection among IVDUs but addicts also have regular or casual sexual partners whom they can infect and who can, in turn, pass on the infection to others, often through prostitution.   In South Asia, heroin injectors are mostly young men from the slums.   In some other countries like Australia, homeless youths who turn to drugs and prostitution can come from all social classes.

Certain developments in Asia do not augur well for the control of HIV and STD. Asian youths, like their counterparts in the west, are getting sexually experienced at an earlier age.   Surveys among secondary school children in various Asian countries showed that 10 to 85% of boys and girls in urban and rural centres are sexually active.   Casual sex is becoming more common as a source of infection among young adults and adolescents, as reflected by significant STD rates among the 13 to 24 year olds [39, 40].   Yet, sex education, particularly on safe sex, is almost non-existent in schools.   Increasing numbers of young women are turning to prostitution not out of real economic necessity but to earn extra pocket money.   In many places, the ratio of male: female infected is approaching 1 : 1.   In Myanmar and parts of China, young women are actually getting infected at higher rates than young men [10].   More infected women means more infected children and more AIDS orphans.   Tuberculosis is endemic in Asia and its incidence is expected to increase because of the interaction between TB and HIV.   This link is already seen in India, Viet Nam, the Philippines where TB occurs in more than 60% of AIDS patients and in Chiang Mai where HIV coinfection with TB has increased from 5.4% in 1989 to 20.6% in 1992 with an average increase of 3% every 6 months [41].   Multidrug resistant TB is also present and causing therapeutic problems.   In 1990, a total of 30,000 TB deaths in Asia were attributed to HIV [42].   There is one consolation, however, in that blood-related transmission of HIV is on the decline, as more countries step up their screening of blood and blood products. This is particularly important in India, where, in the country's many private blood banks, the sterility of blood collection equipment is suspect and a large proportion of the blood collected is from paid donors, many of whom are HIV positive [43].

It is evident that STDs and HIV in Asia are strongly associated with poverty, ignorance, sexual exploitation of women and drug addiction.   Control strategies must focus on immediate actions to disrupt transmission via behavioral change while working towards longer term objectives such as eradication of socio-economic, cultural and political factors which promote prostitution and drug dependency. Unfortunately, many Asians are uncomfortable talking about sex, unwilling to prioritize HIV and STD for major public health spending and vigorously oppose anything which may appear to encourage promiscuity and drug abuse, like condom distribution and needle exchange. Attitudes, laws and regulations still discriminate against HIV-positive individuals, forcing many to keep their infection status secret, thus preventing them from participating in harm reduction programmes.

I have painted a rather grim picture of STDs and HIV in Asia but I would like to end my presentation on an optimistic note. Asia was not exactly totally unprepared for the onslaught of HIV. We have benefitted from the scientific knowledge and social experience of the Western world and we do have some success stories. Aggressive strategies carried out in some communities have increased condom use among CSWs and their clients and have encouraged the adoption of harm reduction practices among IVDUs [44, 45]. In Australia, for instance, as a result of effective preventive measures, HIV incidence which was comparable with that in the USA 10 years ago, has steadily dropped to a fairly stable level which is lower than that for most European countries. Declining incidences of gonorrhoea and chlamydial infections have been documented in Japan, Australia, New Zealand, Thailand, Hong Kong and Malaysia and syphilis is said to be fast disappearing in South Korea [8, 13, 46 – 49]. These trends may not be sustained but they have given hope that HIV is not invincible. It is now up to the governments and the people of Asia to pool our resources together to rescue future generations from the tragedy of STD and AIDS.

References

1   DataFile, Panos WorldAIDS 1994; 34:8.
2   Hira S: Venereology 1993; 6:83.
3   WHO Weekly Epidemiol Record 1993; 68:(50)371.
4   Singh S, Crofts N: AIDS Care 1993; 5:273.
5   WHO Western Pacific Region AIDS Surveillance Report 1993; 1:5.
6   Viravaidya M: 1st SE Asia HIV Management Workshop, Bangkok, 1992.
7   Min Public Health, Thailand 1990.
8   Fung HW, Ng WS: Venereology 1993; 6:63.
9   WHO Weekly Epidemiol Record 1991; 66:(49)361.
10   Chung Kuo I Hsueh ko Hsueh Yuan Hsueh Pao 1993; 15:6.
11   Goh TH, Ngeow YF, Teoh SK: Sex Transm Dis 1981; 8:67.
12   Wasserheit JN: Int J Gynaecol Obstet, suppl. 3 1989; 145.
13   Lyttle H: Venereology 1993; 6:112.
14   Ramachandran S, Ngeow YF: Genitourin Med 1990; 66:334.
15   Pao CC, Kao SM, Wang HC, Lee CC: Am J Obstet Gynaecol 1991; 164:1295.
16   Mittal A, Kapur S, Gupta S: Indian J Med Res 1993; 98:119.
17   Mastro TD, Limpakarnjanarat K, Nopkesorn T, Korattana S, Satten GA: presented at 8th IUVDT Regional Conference, 1993, Thailand.
18   Ang CB, Chan R, Goh CL: Venereology, 1993; 6:95.
19   Wiesner P, Brown S, Kraus S, Perine P: In: International perspective on neglected sexually transmitted diseases: impact on venereology, infertility and maternal and infant health, Hemisphere Pub., 1983, p219.
20   Garg BR, Baruah MC, Oudeacoumar P, Kumar V: Indian J Sex Transm Dis, 1989; 10:62.
21   Rowe PJ: In: Challenges in Reproductive Health Research, Biennial Report (1992 – 1993), WHO, 1994, p83.
22   Bowden FJ, Sheppard C, Currie B: Venereology, 1994; 7:50.
23   Tapsall JW: Annual Report of the WHO/WPRO Gonococcal Antibiotic Susceptibility Programme, 1992.
24   Clendennen TE 3rd, Hames CS, Kees ES, Price FC, Rueppel WJ, Andrada AB, Espinosa GE, Kabrerra G,

Wignall FS: Antimicrob Agents Chemother, 1992; 36:277.
25 Chu ML, Ho LJ, Lin HC, Wu YC: Clin Infect Dis 1992; 14:450.
26 Fu YL: Chinese J Obstet Gynaecol, 1990; 25:262.
27 Tanaka M, Kumazawa J, Kobayashi I: Genitourin Med 1994; 70:90.
28 Kam KM, Lo KK, Lai CF, Lee YS, Chan CB, Antimicrob Agents Chemother 1993; 37:2007.
29 Meheus A, In: Reproductive Health Education and Technology: issues and future directions, p73.   Johns Hopkins Program for International Education in Gynaecology and Obstetrics, Baltimore 1988.
30 Lal H, Rathee S, Sharma D, Chaudhary S, Indian J Med Res 1992; 95:77.
31 Wang YJ, Chen CH, Wang TM, Chi CS, Acta Paediatr Sin 1993; 34:191.
32 Ford N, Koetsawang S, Soc Sci Med 1991; 33:405.
33 Tapsall J, Venereology 1991; 4:99.
34 Ozaki S, The Asia-Pacific Venereologist 1992; 1(2):6.
35 Soda K, The Asia-Pacific Venereologist 1992; 1(2):10.
36 Wong ML, Tan TC, Ho ML, Lim JY, Wan S, Chan R, Int J STD AIDS 1992; 3:332.
37 Singh YN, Malaviya AN, Int J STD AIDS 1994; 5:137.
38 Ruddick A, In: AIDS Executive Summary, Indonesian Epidemiology Network 1993.
39 Urmil AC, Dutta PK, Sharma KK, Ganguly SS, India J Public Health 1989; 33:176.
40 Hart G, Int J STD AIDS 1993; 4:204; ibid 1993; 34:191.
41 Upham G, TB & HIV, SidAlerte International Jan-Mar 1994; (suppl No. 2), p10.
42 MMWR 1993; 42(49).
43 Bhattacharya R, Dalwadi V, Parekh V: VIII International Conference on AIDS/III STD World Congress, Amsterdam, 1992, abstract PoD5165.
44 Tanne JH: BMJ 1991; 302, 1557.
45 Hedge K, Miller M, O'Connor D, Buzolic A, Venereology 1991; 4:112.
46 Donovan B: Med J Aust 1992; 2:156.
47 Mugrditchian D, Benjarattanaporn P: World Bank, AIDS in Asia Newsletter 1994; 3:6.
48 Kawana T: The Asia-Pacific Venereologist 1992; 1(2):3.
49 Lee JB, Byeon SW, Chung KY, Lee MG, Whang KK, Genitourinary Med 1992; 68:60.

Recent HIV/AIDS Trends among Men Who Have Sex with Men

Michael L. Tan

Health Action Information Network (HAIN)
Quezon City 1104, Philippines

Epidemiological Trends

The first reports of AIDS cases in the early 1980s involved mainly homosexual men in North America, Western Europe, Australia, and New Zealand. This led to an early association of HIV and AIDS with homosexuality.

Globally, it is estimated that about 15 percent of cumulative adult HIV infections occurred through homosexual transmission. By regions, the range of estimates is very wide, from less than 1 percent in Sub-Saharan Africa to 56 percent in the Americas to more than 80 percent for Eastern Europe and the Oceania [1].

Table 1. Estimates of percentage of adult HIV infections occurring through homosexual transmission [1]

North America	56
Western Europe	47
Oceania	87
Latin America	54
Sub-Saharan Africa	<1
Caribbean	10
Eastern Europe	80
South East Mediterranean	20
North East Asia	20
South East Asia	8

These figures need to be taken for what they are: rough estimates. We will return to these statistics later in the paper.

In Europe and the United States, the percentage of AIDS cases involving homosexual and bisexual transmission, in relation to the total, has gradually declined over the years. In Europe Community (EC) nations, for example, homosexual and bisexual transmission accounted for two thirds of cumulative AIDS cases in 1984. By 1993, the figure was about a third [2].

27

Table 2. Percentage of adult/adolescent AIDS cases reported as male homosexual/bisexual transmission, European Community (with adjustments for reporting delays) [2]

1984	66.6
1985	62.7
1986	57.3
1987	51.2
1988	44.6
1989	41.6
1990	39.2
1991	37.1
1992	35.4
1993	32.2

In the late 1980s, researchers noted that several U.S. cities with high rates of HIV infection among gay men — San Francisco, New York, Los Angeles — had registered significant declines in the annual AIDS incidence [3].   These declines were attributed to a decline in HIV infection itself and a slowing in the progression to AIDS among HIV-infected persons.   The decline in HIV infection has, in turn, been attributed in part to an increase in risk reduction activities [4, 5].

Much of the optimism over explanations for the decline in infection was, unfortunately, based on studies using self-reported behavior [4, 6 – 9].   The epidemiological data has not always been as encouraging.   For example, a study [10] of more than 3,000 gay men in four large US cities, found that declines in seroconversion only occurred during the first 3 years of a 5-year study period.

There are well-grounded fears of a rebound in the epidemic among gay men in developed countries.   The decade of the 90s in fact ushered in references to the biomedically-framed concept of "relapse" and the need to consider maintenance of risk reduction behaviors [7, 11 – 14].   Fears of a rebound have centered on younger gay men, and among gay men from ethnic minorities.

In areas outside North America and Western Europe, the epidemiological picture remains unclear.   In several Latin American countries, early reports involved mainly homosexual and bisexual transmission but such cases have reportedly declined as cases of heterosexual transmission increase.   In the Central American isthmus countries for example, homosexual and bisexual transmission accounted for 61 percent of AIDS cases in 1987 but declined to 25 percent by 1990 [1].

Great caution is needed in interpreting these figures.   It seems that early reports in many developing countries often identified returning homosexual or bisexual residents who had acquired their infection while living in developed countries.   As the epidemic became more "indigenous", the numbers of homosexuals and bisexuals seem to decline while the numbers of "unknowns" increase.   In the World Health Organization's Western Pacific Region, only 4.3 percent of cumulative AIDS cases as of the end of 1993 were classified as "unknown/other".   In contrast, almost 30 percent of cumulative HIV cases fall under this "unknown/other" category, many of them men.   This "unknown" category among HIV cases can be sizeable — 51.7 percent in Cambodia; 38.5 percent in Australia, 27.4 percent in the Philippines, and 23.1 percent in China [15].   Contrast these figures with a figure of 5 percent classified as "other/undetermined" for cumulative reported HIV cases in the European Community as of the end of 1993 [2].

There are many possible explanations for these unclassified cases but one must keep in mind the possibility that some of these cases may in fact involve transmission through men having sex with men.   Many men who have sex with men do not self-identify as "gay", "homosexual" or "bisexual" and would probably prefer to cite sex with a female sex worker, or even injecting drug use as their risk factor rather than admitting to having had sex with other men.

The epidemiological picture, no doubt, is affected by many cultural factors.   In Africa, for example, the official figures would suggest that only South Africa has a problem of homosexual and bisexual transmission of HIV and that even there, such transmission would occur only among whites.   (In South Africa, about 18 percent of 2,296 reported AIDS cases involved homosexual and bisexual men: 368 homosexuals (344 white) and 49 bisexual (36 white) [16].

Clearly, more attention needs to be given to "men who have sex with men", rather than self-identified "gay" or "bisexual" men.   In India, for example, eunuches or hijras constitute a population at risk because they have to do sex work.   One study among 100 hijras aged 20 to 35 found five to be positive for HIV infection, compared to an estimated 0.3% incidence of HIV infection among homosexual men in India [17].

Social and Behavioral Aspects

The unclear epidemiological picture of HIV among men who have sex with men reflects deeper problems, including a wide gap in our knowledge about the situation of this population, especially those in developing countries.

The term "men who have sex with men", despite its shortcomings, is more useful for HIV prevention strategies.   At the same time, the size of this population is almost impossible to estimate.   Recent sexuality surveys in the U.S., the United Kingdom, and France [18 – 20] give low figures for persons who have had homosexual experiences but the researchers themselves agree that under-reporting is to be expected.

Many segments of the population of men who have sex with men remain invisible, and cannot be reached even by preliminary need or situation assessment studies.   Cohort studies, so essential both for epidemiological and sociobehavioral research, are even more difficult to do and has in fact been limited to a few urban centers in developed countries, quite often focusing on the dominant ethnic group.

It should not be surprising then to find that recent surveys indicate continuing knowledge gaps among men who have sex with men, even in developed countries.   For example, a recent survey of Australia men who have sex with men showed that a quarter of their respondents still did not consider unprotected anal or vaginal intercourse without ejaculation to be unsafe.   Moreover, 12 percent of the sample had unprotected anal intercourse with casual male partners [21].

There is a need to understand the context of homosexuality and bisexuality in different societies but there is a dearth of published literature on societies outside of North America, western Europe and Australia.   A collection of research studies on bisexuality in developed and developing countries [22], sponsored by the World Health Organization, provided a useful start but there has been little support to continue such studies.

The available studies show that sharp differences are to be found across cultures, even in the definitions of what a "homosexual" is, and what a "gay identity" might mean.   Many societies do not even have indigenous terms for "heterosexual", "homosexual" or "bisexual", reflecting the fact that these terms were coined only in the last century in Europe. It is interesting that even in the British sexuality survey, the terms "homosexual" and "heterosexual" were not used because of various reasons including homosexuality's "stigmatizing identity" as well as a lack of understanding of the term "homosexual" itself [20].

The position taken in the British study has, however, its dangers.   The researchers write: "The use of a term denoting a sexual identity is irrelevant in the context of HIV and STD, since it is sexual practice and not identity which is relevant to understanding the dynamics of transmission" [20].

Precisely, the lack of studies of sexual identity, of such identities are shaped and shape sexual behavior between men, has been a major deficiency that adversely affects the planning of effective prevention strategies.

The population of men who have sex with men consists of many subcultures and sexual identities.   These subsultures cannot be simplistically defined as those who are "out" and those who are not or as "covert" and "overt" as is still done by some psychologists and sociologists.   The subcultures are much more complex.   For example, age can be a sharp boundary marker for the subcultures, and their behavior.   In the Philippines, what would otherwise be effective intervention programs by a gay organization, The Library Foundation, have still been unable to reach older men who have sex with men, who seem to "retire" by marrying or by limiting sexual activities with male sex workers.   The matter of age also draws boundaries in sexual networks.   Older Filipino male homosexuals will tend to maintain "traditional norms" of having sex with "straight men" while younger counterparts prefer other gay or bisexual men.

In Australia, the Project Male-Call study found a trend of younger gay men considering AIDS as a problem of older men, accompanied by perceptions that as long as they had sex with men of their own age, they could reduce their risks for HIV [21].

Among the sociodemographic variables, projects reaching men who have sex with men in Malaysia and the Philippines have found that class is perhaps the most significant determinant for subcultures and differences in knowledge, attitudes, and behavior, as well as the prospects for changes in knowledge levels following interventions [23].

One consequence of "high-risk group" characterizations, including the generic category of "men who have sex with men" is the creation of a mythological monolithic population that obscures the risk factors faced in different situations.   For example, using existing categories, where do we put male sex workers—men who have sex with men, sex workers, or perhaps in other instances, intravenous drug users?   Labels also tend to create blind spots.   One forgets, for example, that studies of the "heterosexual male" population could yield valuable information on sex between men [24, 25].

While cross-cultural differences are important, we also need to look into the striking similarities that are found across cultures.   There is, for example, an increasing internationalization of the concept of "gay", the term itself now integrated into many languages.   No doubt, there will be variance in local interpretations of the term but there is at least a common term around which distinct gender identities are developing for men who have sex with men (as well as women who have sex with women).

In behavioral terms, studies in cultures as diverse as the Philippines [23], Australia [21], the United Kingdom [26] and Canada [27] show that risk-taking and risk-reduction activities among men who have sex with men revolve around the types of sexual partners one has.   In all the studies, researchers have found that consistent condom use in anal sex was far more likely with casual rather than regular partners, a pattern which certainly has parallels with heterosexual couples.

More cross-cultural studies may yield other important similarities.   For example, one could examine how machismo shapes common patterns of sexual behavior — including such behavior between men — in different cultures.   Another important area for research would be societies' perceptions of homosexuality, and how such perceptions impact on risk behavior as well as risk reduction.

HIV as a Chronic Disease and Its Impact on Men Who Have Sex with Men

Ten years into the HIV epidemic, there are still many gaps in our knowledge about biomedical and sociobehavioral aspects of the epidemic among men who have sex with men.

It is clear that the epidemiological picture varies in different countries.   One recent study [28] using stored sera from homosexual and bisexual men who participated in hepatitis B vaccine trials in 1978 to 1980 showed that the cumulative incidence of HIV-1 infection was 7.5 percent in Amsterdam, 26.8 percent in New York City and 42.6 percent in San Francisco.   The researchers attribute the differences to a combination of differences in sexual activity at the time the HIV-1 epidemic began and a later introduction of HIV-1 in Amsterdam.   This multi-site study also suggests that there will be differences in stable prevalences.

Future trajectories of the epidemic will depend on the success of risk-reduction strategies.   There are, however, continuing obstacles that have to be overcome.   Some of the problems relate to continuing gaps in the biomedical information, as is the case for orogenital sex.   Two recent studies [27, 29] analyze problems with the inconsistencies in gay men's health information campaigns when it comes to risks involved in oral sex.   A literature review will show several dozen studies relating to orogenital sex, and to correlations between Kaposi's sarcoma and analinglus; yet, there is no conclusive position on the risks of these sexual activities for HIV and other STDs.   Perhaps reflecting the dilemmas faced, as well as the differences in gay cultures, two "western" magazines came out simultaneously in June 1994 with diametrically opposed views on oral sex: in the U.S., the gay magazine 'Out' [30] features an article on the 'Facts about Oral Risk for HIV', adopting a highly alarmist viewpoint that fell short of accusing the medical establishment of suppressing the facts about the risks in oral sex.   In contrast, the Australian National AIDS Bulletin [29] featured an article which calls for a perspective that recognizes oral sex as not being a significant transmission risk especially in relation to the principal modes of transmission.

In other instances, the gaps lie in an understanding of risk-reduction behavior itself. Theories about risk-reduction behavior have generally clustered around those developed in health psychology, and have not been too useful in addressing important structural issues. An example comes with the individual-centered concept of 'relapse', which fails to consider how the larger social milieu contributes to, or prevents, effective risk-reduction strategies.

The temporal impact of the epidemic also needs to be considered. One research team in Australia [31] has emphasized the need to distinguish between 'negotiated safety' and 'relapse', with 'negotiations' shaped in the context of relationships and sexual partnerships and with a consideration of serostatus. It is interesting that in Malaysia, questions have started to crop up about the possibilities of dropping the use of condoms among same-sex couples who have been monogamous or 'safe' and who have hurdled the 'window period' with HIV antibody testing. Such questions will have to be addressed, and educational messages modified, but with a careful consideration of differences among countries with regard to access to testing and social support systems.

The importance of community-based programs has been raised, based mainly on the experiences of developed countries. These cover a wide range of strategies from outreach programs to peer-education. There is no lack of reference to the need for such social support but it is not always clear how this can be operationalized in different situations.

The impact of these programs are often limited to the superficial without probing into serious questions about access to information; appropriateness of materials, and sustainability of risk-reduction strategies.

Community-based activities among men who have sex with men are evolving. There have been changes in community activism, including a decline in mulitant approaches. The debates within the communities are important, including the long-standing one over professionalism versus voluntarism [32]. One which takes on more significance as gay communities shift into support activities for people living with HIV/AIDS. The forms of advocacy, and militance, also evolve. The International Gay and Lesbian Human Rights Commission, for example, has been effective in the inclusion of people living with HIV in the agenda of human rights campaigns.

In most countries, community participation remains rhetorical, often because the conditions for community organizing are not present. Ironically, AIDS activists and workers may have contributed to this probem by "de-gaying" the epidemic supposedly to remove the stigma attached to AIDS. As a result, men who have sex with men have dropped in the order of priorities for many donor agencies and governments or, in other instances, have never even made it into the order of priorities.

The result is a potentially disastrous situation because there is no support for HIV prevention activities even as the stigma attached to both AIDS and men who have sex with men remains undiminished.

In the long run, it may yet be the efforts to address the consequences of homophobia, such as denial by individuals; communities, or governments, that will spell a difference in effectively slowing down the epidemic.

References

1   Mann JM, Tarantola DJM, Netter TW: AIDS in the World, Harvard University Press, Cambridge, 1992.
2   European Centre for the Epidemiological Monitoring of AIDS, AIDS Surveillance in the European Community and Cost Countries, Quarterly Report No. 25 (31 December 1993).
3   Karon JM, Berkelman RL: J. Acquired Immune Deficiency Syndromes, 1991; 4: 1179.

4   Joseph JG, et al. Am J Public Health, 1990; 80: 1513.
5   Johnson AM, Gill ON: Philos Trans R Soc Long Biol, 1989; 325: 153.
6   Siegel K, et al: Arch Sex Behav, 1988; 17: 481.
7   Ekstrand M, Coates T: Am J Public Health 1990; 80: 973.
8   Joseph JG, et al: Psychol Health, 1987; 1: 73.
9   Hunt AJ, et al: Brit Med J, 1991; 302: 505.
10 Kingsley LA, et al: Am J Epidemiology 1991; 134: 331.
11 Stall R, et al: J. Acquir Immune Defic Syndr 1990; 3: 1181.
12 Van den Hoek JAR, Van Griensven GJK, Coutinho RA, Lancet, 1990; 336: 179.
13 Riley VC, Lancet, 1991; 337: 183.
14 Hart G, et al: Soc Health and Illness 1992; 14: 216.
15 World Health Organization Western Pacific Regional Office (WHO WPRO).   AIDS Surveillance Report, January 1994.
16 Epidemiological Comments 1993; 20: 184.
17 Lakshmi N, et al: Genitourinary Medicine, 1994; 70: 71.
18 Rogers SM, Turner CF: J Sex Res 1991; 28: 491.
19 ACSF Investigators: Nature 1992; 360: 407.
20 Wellings K, et al: Sexual Diversity and Homosexual Behaviour.   In: Johnson Anne M, et al (eds.): Sexual Attitudes and Lifestyles, 183.   Blackwell Scientific Publications, Oxford, 1994.
21 National Centre for HIV Social Research (Macquarie University), Evaluation Report on Project Male-Call, Department of Human Services and Health, Canberra, 1994.
22 Tielman RAP, Carballo M, Hendriks AC, eds. Bisexuality and HIV/AIDS: A Global Perspective, Prometheus Books, Buffalo, New York, 1991.
23 Tan ML: An Evaluation of HIV Prevention Workshops of The Library Foundation, Quezon City, Typescript, 1994.
24 Nopkesorn T, Sungkarom S, Sornlum R: HIV Prevalence and Sexual Behaviors among Thai Men Aged 21 in Northern Thailand.   Research Report No. 3, Program on AIDS.   Thai Red Cross Society, Bangkok, 1991.
25 Sittitrai W, et al: Thai Sexual Behavior and Risk of HIV Infection.   Thai Red Cross Society, Bangkok, 1992.
26 Hunt AJ, et al: AIDS Care 1993; 5: 439.
27 Myers T, et al. The Canadian Survey of Gay and Bisexual Men and HIV Infection: Men's a Survey. Canadian AIDS Society, Ottawa, 1993.
28 Van Griensven GJP, et al: Am J Epid 1993; 137: 909.
29 O'Donnell D: National AIDS Bulletin, June 1994, 20-22.
30 Rotello G: OUT, June 1994, pp148-168.
31 Kippax S, et al: AIDS, 1993; 7: 257.
32 Altman D: Expertise, Legitimacy and the Centrality of Community.   In: Aggleton P, et al: AIDS: Framing the 2nd Decade, 1-8.   Falmer Press, London, 1993.

Prevention and Control of Sexually Transmitted Diseases: Challenges for the 1990s

Peter Piot

Division of Research and Intervention Development,
WHO, Global Programme on AIDS, Geneva, Switzerland

At previous conferences, the debate around STD has focused mainly on the issue, whether STD increase the risk of HIV transmission.

Today—the agenda is one of action on reproductive health, and it seems more appropriate to focus the debate on how can we prevent and control STD? In this presentation, I will concentrate on public health approaches to STD control, with an emphasis on the situation in the developing world.

Incidence of Various STD

In contrast to HIV/AIDS, figures on the incidence and prevalence of the conventional STD are at best incomplete. At WHO, we recently estimated that annually between 150 and 330 million cases of curable STD occur in the world—for instance, there are annually 52 to 122 million cases of gonorrhoea and 10 to 24 million cases of syphilis (table 1).

Table 1. Curable STD in the World (million)

Disease	New cases/year
Gonorrhoea	52 to 122
Chlamydia	29 to 72
Syphilis	10 to 24
Chancroid	5 to 7
Trichomoniasis	57 to 102

Burden of Disease (World Development Report)

Last year, the World Bank tried to assess the impact of various health problems on the burden of disease in the developing world. The types of health problems that ranked highest were a surprise to many among us.

Among young adults below 45 years of age, both HIV infection and the other STD ranked among the top five health problems, particularly for women (fig. 1).

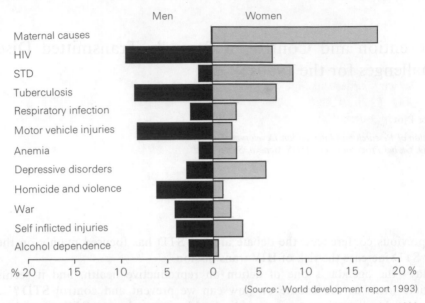

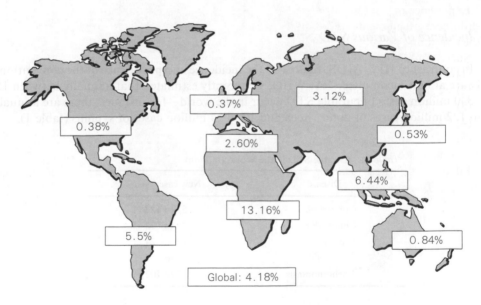

Men   Women

Maternal causes
HIV
STD
Tuberculosis
Respiratory infection
Motor vehicle injuries
Anemia
Depressive disorders
Homicide and violence
War
Self inflicted injuries
Alcohol dependence

% 20   15   10   5   0   5   10   15   20 %

(Source: World development report 1993)

Fig. 1.   Burden of disease in adults 15–44 years in the developing world by gender, 1990.

0.37%

3.12%

0.38%

0.53%

2.60%

6.44%

13.16%

0.84%

5.5%

Global: 4.18%

Fig. 2.   Global incidence of Gonorrhoea (%) (15–49 years).

Incidence of Gonorrhoea by Continent

The burden of STD in the world is also not shared equally among nations.   For example, the annual incidence rates per 100 population of gonorrhoea by continent.   Sub-

Saharan Africa, Latin America and South and South-East Asia have the highest rates, with more than one in ten adults between 15 and 49 years acquiring this infection per year (fig. 2).

For over 40 years we have had antibiotics to cure the common bacterial and protozoal STDs. So why is there still a problem?

Basically, I believe that it is because STD have rarely been approached as a public health problem, but rather as a problem for small group of blameworthy individuals, or as a purely clinical problem.

This brings me to the second part of my presentation: How can we control STD?

Let us consider a very simplified model of STD prevention and care delivery. An infected individual has to go through many steps before he or she is cured of an STD. Whereas the traditional approach to STD focuses entirely on curing an individual seen at a health facility, this clearly affects only a minority of patients. Some people with an STD will be asymptomatic and hence unaware that they need care. Others may have symptoms, but not seek appropriate care. Others may seek care but not be cured, because the drugs available may not be effective. Bridging each step therefore requires a specific solution, including encouraging people to seek care at the slightest suspicion of an STD, ensuring the availability of effective drugs, making treatment financially accessible, and training staff.

Public Health Package

Experience of other health problems has shown that without a mix of well defined and affordable strategies and interventions, there is little hope of having an impact on the disease at the community level.

Such a public health package for STD control, includes the following 5 priorities:

(1) Promotion of safer sexual behavior, including condom use
(2) Provision of comprehensive case management at primary care level
(3) Specific interventions for high-risk populations
(4) Promotion of appropriate health care seeking behavior
(5) Case finding for syphilis during pregnancy, and prophylaxis of ophthalmia neonatorum

First of all, there are the activities to prevent people from becoming infected. Promotion of safer sexual behavior including condom use is the cornerstone of both AIDS and STD prevention programs. Hopefully we will soon have a female-controlled barrier method, as discussed by Zena Stein (See p. 219).

Care Seeking Behavior, Women

Since these interventions will be discussed extensively by other speakers, I will now move to another, much neglected area: the promotion of health care seeking behavior. Firstly, in many countries, a substantial proportion of patients do not go to a qualified health facility for treatment of their STD. For instance, a recent survey among women with a symptomatic reproductive tract infection in Nigeria, found that the majority of them never made it to a proper public or private health facility (fig. 3).

Care Seeking Behavior, Men

Secondly, there may be considerable delay before seeking care. In a study in Zimbabwe, 30% of men with generally painful genital ulcers waited for over a week before

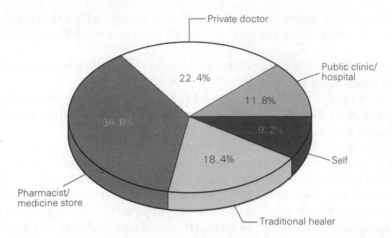

Fig. 3.   Source of treatment for symptomatic women with reproductive tract infection Ado-Ekiti, Nigeria.

seeking treatment, and many continued to have sex.

STD Clinic Visits

Thirdly, the most important factor in health care seeking behavior may well be access to acceptable and affordable services.   The reverse was amply demonstrated by an unfortunate experiment in Kenya.   In late '89, when a user fee was introduced, with no improvement of quality of care, the number of patients at the main STD clinic in Nairobi dropped by over 50%.   There is no doubt that this policy resulted in greatly increased transmission of STD and HIV in the community.   But when effective drugs are made available in health facilities and staff are trained to offer good quality care, the number of STD patients increases significantly—as was shown for instance in a community project in northern Tanzania.

This brings me to the key issue of integrated STD care delivery.   STD care should be offered as an explicit part of a broader reproductive health package.   Making available effective case management at the point of first encounter with the health system will mean integrating STD care in the general health care structure, rather than setting up 'special' vertical clinics.   However, such STD clinics may play an important role as referral, research and training centers.

Quality of STD Case Management

Realistically, we still have a long way to go before we achieve a general acceptable quality of STD case management.   Surveys performed by WHO in three continents demonstrated very low levels of health education, condom promotion, and information for partners during routine STD care.

The potential for improvement in this field is therefore enormous, but this will require a major effort in training and behavior modification of health personnel.

Effective case management is key in the control of STD.   Unfortunately, laboratory support for the diagnosis of STD is rarely availabale at the primary care level, and laboratory tests for most STDs are expensive, and take too long to be of any use when

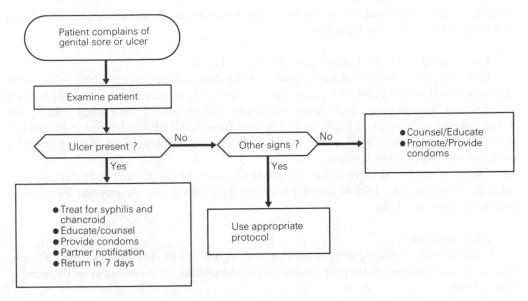

Fig. 4. Flow chart for genital ulcers.

making on-the-spot treatment decisions.

Therefore, many countries now recommend syndromic case management using flow charts.

Genital Ulcer Flow Chart

Figure 4 is an example of such a flow chart for the management of a patient with a genital ulcer. It is currently used in many places. Once the presence of an ulcer is confirmed, a combined treatment for the causes of genital ulcer, usually syphilis and chancroid, is given. Please note also that on this flow chart, case management involves a great deal more than treatment. It involves education/counselling, condom provision, and partner notification.

Cure rates

In general, high cure rates are obtained when such flow charts are correctly used, as shown from a study carried out in health centers in Côte d'Ivoire, where between 87% and 100% of STD patients were cured.

Case Manaagement in Women: Risk Assessment

Flow charts for syndromic case management are difficult to design for genital discharge in women, as this is both a rather insensitive, and non-specific symptom or sign, other than for vaginitis.

The major therapeutic problem here is to distinguish between vaginal and cervical infection. The treatment for these conditions is different, and so are the public health and personal consequences. Recent research suggests that risk assessment for STD based on certain demographic or behavioral characteristics may greatly increase the sensitivity of flow charts. In other words, asking the right questions may tell you more about the risk for gonococcal and chlamydial infection in a woman than a clinical examination, as shown in a study in Zaire by Bea Vuylsteke.

Case Management in Women: Low Predictive Value

However, preliminary results suggest that the diagnostic accuracy of algorithms for reproductive tract infection in women varies widely. It is usually high in symptomatic women, but may have a much lower sensitivity and specificity in women coming for antenatal care as shown in a study by P. Mayaux from AMREF in Mwanza. Because of the low positive predictive value, this may lead to unnecessary treatment of a considerable proportion of uninfected women.

The problem is that there will be no better alternative to syndromic case management until inexpensive and rapid diagnostic tests for gonococcal and chlamydial infection in women become available.

Drug Resistance

Continuously emerging drug resistance and high levels of HIV infection make things even more complicated, as they may diminish the therapeutic effectiveness of recommended algorithms.

Multidrug resistance has now become common in both *N. gonorrhoeae* and *H. ducreyi*, particularly in Asia and Africa, as will be discussed by Dr Ngeou. As a result, older and cheaper antibiotics can no longer be used, and have to be replaced by more effective, but much more expensive drugs such as the quinolones and cephalosporins.

Unfortunately, bacteria are smart, and they are now developing resistance to even the latest generation of drugs for the treatment of STD, as first documented here in Japan by Professor Kumamoto's group, and also in Central Africa, where gonococcal susceptibility to the quinolones is decreasing.

Genital Ulceration by CD4$^+$

HIV infection may affect both the clinical expression and the response to treatment of STD. This is all the more relevant as in many countries today a substantial proportion of STD patients are infected with HIV.

First, HIV-positive persons suffer more often from genital ulcers. For instance, at Project Retro-CI it was found that the prevalence of genital ulcers in a group of female sex workers in Abidjan increased with more profound immunodeficiency (fig. 5). Most of these ulcers are of unknown etiology, and their clinical presentation may be modified—making diagnosis more difficult.

Cure Rate of Chancroid

Several studies from Nairobi suggest that HIV-positive patients with chancroid respond significantly less well to treatment with ceftriaxone, usually a highly effective antibiotic for this disease (fig. 6).

Syphilis Treatment

Finally, there is much debate as to whether we should change recommended treatment for syphilis. There are many anecdotal data, but very few studies on large numbers of patients. In a rare study of syphilis in women in Zaire, the serologic response to standard

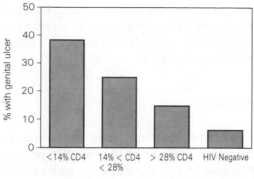

(Source: Ghye P at al: 1994; Projet Retro-C1)

Fig. 5. Prevalence of genital ulcers by HIV status and % CD4⁺ in female sex workers, Abidjan.

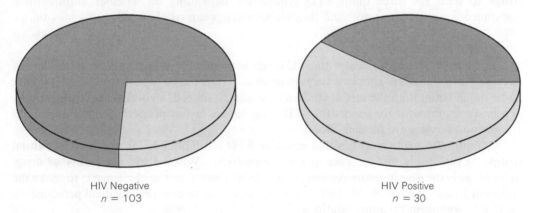

HIV Negative
n = 103

HIV Positive
n = 30

Fig. 6. Outcome of treatment of chancroid with ceftriaxone, Nairobi (Source: Tyndall M. et al, JID 1993; 167 : 469).

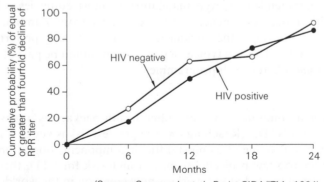

(Source: Goeman J. et al; Projet SIDA/ITM, 1994)

Fig. 7. Serologic response to standard therapy in HIV positive and HIV negative women with syphilis [initial RPR titre equal or greater than 8], Kinshasa.

therapy with benzathine penicillin was similar among HIV-positive and HIV-negative women (fig. 7). This suggests that the response to treatment may not be different in patients with syphilis and concomitant HIV injection. However, we need more data before we can arrive at a firm conclusion.

Costs of WHO Treatment

Let us now turn to the essential but very complex issue of drugs. Without antibiotics, there can be no STD program. It would be like an AIDS program without condoms, but we are facing several dilemmas here. Should people with a communicable disease such as STD pay for their treatment ? Even some hard nosed free market economists say no while invoking Adam Smith. Should we prefer highly effective but rather expensive antibiotics over the cheaper but less effective ones ? There is a 10 to 20 fold difference in the cost of drugs to treat the three main STD syndromes, depending on whether antimicrobial resistance is a problem or not, and thus cheaper drugs can still be used.

Drugs: Drug Peddler
It is hardly possible to deal with STD drugs without addressing the general problem of access to affordable and effective drugs in general. It would be foolish to expect STD care to be much better than the rest of the health system. Indeed, a good general drug supply is a basic requirement for successful STD programme, just as properly functioning blood transfusion services are for safe blood.

A minimum requirement is that effective STD antibiotics be on the list of essential drugs. Even this is not the case in many countries. Where there are plenty of drugs around, as is the case in many American and Asian countries, the challenge is to make the right antibiotics both available and accessible, as well as to convince medical personnel to adhere to treatment recommendations.

Congenital Syphilis
There is one STD intervention that has been around for a long time, but is often poorly implemented: prevention of maternal and congenital syphilis. Testing all pregnant women for syphilis is recommended or even mandatory in most countries. It is an effective intervention, with a high cost-benefit ratio, as shown from Zambia, where not only congenital syphilis but also the incidence of stillbirth and preterm delivery were tremendously reduced. This is a typical activity which should be part of any reproductive health or mother-and-child health programme.

Kinshasa
A final essential component of our public health package is intensified services for people at high risk for STD. Reaching those at greatest risk is key to a successful HIV or STD program, but is also one of its most difficult components operationally.

While there are too few projects for men at high risk for STD, there are many HIV prevention programs targeted at sex workers now going on in the world. However, very few have tried to measure the impact of the intervention in terms of HIV and STD incidence, and very few offer more than education.

In one such clinic-based intervention in Kinshasa, regular use of condoms with clients went up from 11% to 68% after 3 years of intervention. This coincided with a significant decline in HIV incidence from 12/100 woman years during the first 6 months to 4/100 woman years over the last 6 months, 3 years later–as well as to a decline in other STDs.

A similar decline in STDs has been documented in a sex worker project in Sonagachi in Calcutta, India, as discussed by Dr Jana.

SW Intervention

The same study, by Marie Laga, Project SIDA, also provides good evidence that treatment of STDs contributed to the decline in HIV incidence. We can deduce this from figure 8, which not only shows that regular condom users had a lower risk for HIV than irregular condom users, but also that in both categories those women who attended a clinic more frequently had consistently lower rates of HIV infection.

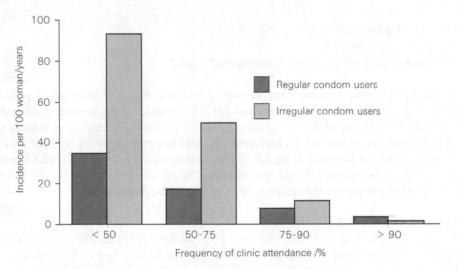

Fig. 8. HIV incidence by frequency of clinic visits and condom use among 531 prostitutes, Kinshasa 1989–91 (Source: Laga M. et al; Lancet 1994; 344:246).

The factor at the clinic that made the difference was STD treatment.

This study shows that a clinic-based intervention consisting of STD care and condom promotion can result in a decline in HIV incidence among highly exposed women. Offering a non-judgmental and accessible service to vulnerable populations such as sex workers can make a considerable contribution to prevention, and is a good investment.

This and some other projects in Africa and Asia provide a strong case for large-scale implementation of combined care and prevention models for HIV prevention for those at greatest risk of HIV and STDs.

Cost of Services – World Development Report

STD control is often called a bottomless pit. I would like to end this discussion with two questions:

Table 2. Estimated costs of selected public health and clinical services in low-income countries (per capita income=$350), 1990

	Per case or participant	Per capita	Per Daily
• Prevention package		4.2	
• Minimum essential package of clinical services			
• Chemotherapy for tuberculosis	500	0.6	3 – 5
• Management of the sick child	9	1.6	30 – 50
• Prenatal and delivery care	90	3.8	30 – 50
• Family planning	12	0.9	20 – 30
• Treatment of STDs	11	0.2	1 – 3
• Limited care	6	0.7	200 – 350

(Source: World Development Report 1993)

One: Can we afford it ?
and two: Can it work ?
The answer to both questions is undoubtedly yes ?

In the 1993 World Development Report, a minimal essential package of preventive activities and clinical services is promoted for all countries.   As you see from table 2, treatment of STDs is one of the five priority areas for clinical services.   The table suggests that STD treatment would on average cost 20 cents per capita, or $1 to 3 per disability adjusted life years—a measure of health.   This compares very favourably with other well accepted and cost-effective clinical interventions listed on this table.   So, STD care is affordable provided we use the rational approaches we have discussed.

Gonorrhoea in Sweden
Finally, there is now good evidence that you can have STD control without stopping having sex.   Western and Northern Europe now have a historic low of STD, as illustrated by the gonorrhoea incidence in Sweden which is at its lowest since 1914.   A supportive social environment, gender equity, sex education at school, and good and accessible health services are the keys to this success story.

STD Rates

Several African countries are also beginning to see declining STD rates.   The best documented case is that of Zimbabwe, which was one of the first countries to fully integrate quality STD care into the general health system.   As of 1992, the number of reported STD cases has been decreasing.

In Asia, a similar trend is being seen in Thailand, where the reported incidence of all STD has been declining for several years now.   In addition, prevalence rates of syphilis and gonorrhoea have been decreasing in prostitutes and in women seen in antenatal clinics.   All this suggests that there is a real decline in STD incidence, most probably due to behavior change and better STD services.

A downside of the picture in Asia is the rapidly rising STD trend in China, which suggests that this country may be very vulnerable to the spread of HIV.

Over the last few years we have learnt a great deal about the prevention and control of STD, I will name just five points:

(1) Large-scale behavior change including condom use is occurring in many populations, and is leading to lower STD incidence rates.

(2) STD care may enhance the acceptability and effectiveness of preventive activities.

(3) Improving services for STD care and making them affordable attracts patients.

(4) Access to effective drugs is critical for a successful STD programme.

(5) Simplified case management based on a syndromic approach is feasible and effective.

To conclude, AIDS has truly revolutionized our approach to STD, although it is disappointing to see how slowly the "STD community" has taken up the lessons of HIV prevention, and how reluctantly the "AIDS community" has recognized that HIV infection is primarily an STD, and that some sound principles of STD control can be applied to HIV prevention.

Pathogenesis

Host Factors in the Immunopathogenesis of HIV Disease

Anthony S. Fauci

National Institute of Allergy and Infectious Diseases,
National Institute of Health, Bethesda, MD., USA.

Introduction

The immunopathogenesis of HIV disease is a multifactorial and multiphasic process [1] with HIV disease being the net result of the interaction between the virus and a variety of host factors including the immune response, cellular activation, cytokine secretion, and immunopathogenicity. All of these factors to a greater or lesser degree, are genetically determined (fig. 1). Our research on these virus-host interactions includes the central role of lymphoid tissue and the endogenous cytokines within these tissues in the pathogenesis of HIV disease, studies on long term non-progressors, and events associated with primary infection. We have been intensively studying lymphoid tissue in HIV disease as a milieu for virus sequestration, cellular activation, cytokine secretion, and ultimately lymphocyte depletion and tissue destruction.

Lymphoid Tissue in HIV Disease

Approximately 2 to 4 weeks after primary infection with HIV, up to 70% of individuals typically experience an acute, self-limited syndrome characterized by fever, rigor, generalized lymphadenopathy, sore throat, retro-orbital pain, arthralgias, myalgias, rash, malaise, weight loss, nausea, diarrhea, and meningitis; the syndrome usually resolves in 1 to 2 weeks [2]. During the acute syndrome there is a burst of viremia that seeds lymphoid tissue with virus and establishes within lymphoid tissue a reservoir for virus burden and replication (see below). The level of $CD4^+$ T cells declines but then rebounds somewhat in most patients [3, 4]. The median time between primary HIV infection and development of AIDS is approximately 11 years [5]. The progression from infection to disease may be affected by genetic differences between individuals [6].

HIV disease can be empirically divided into three stages: early, intermediate, and advanced. The early stage is characterized by lymphoid hyperplasia and highly effective trapping of extracellular virions on the follicular dendritic cells of lymph node germinal centers. At this time virus expression in tissue and viremia are relatively low and partially, but not completely, curtailed by the immune response together with efficient virus trapping. Disruption of the lymphoid tissue occurs as disease progresses and is associated with a

49

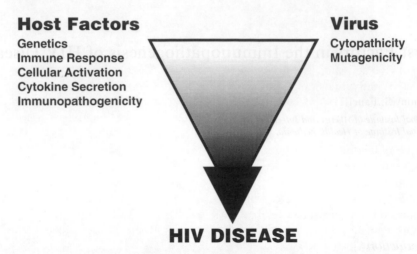

Host Factors

Genetics
Immune Response
Cellular Activation
Cytokine Secretion
Immunopathogenicity

Virus

Cytopathicity
Mutagenicity

HIV DISEASE

Fig. 1. Relationship of virus and host factors in the pathogenesis of HIV disease.

decrease in the competency of virus trapping [2, 7], an increase in the number of lymph node cells expressing virus, and in most patients, an increase in viremia. Finally, in the advanced stage of disease, virtually complete dissolution of lymphoid tissue occurs associated with a relatively complete lack of ability to trap virions. At the same time, virus is produced within the parenchyma of the lymph nodes, which spills over into the peripheral blood producing a high degree of viremia [8].

Cellular Activation in HIV Disease

Activation of the immune system is an important part of an appropriate immune response. Once an antigen is cleared, the immune system normally returns to a state of relative quiescence until the next foreign antigen is introduced [9]. In the early stage of HIV disease, there is intense immune activation as indicated by spontaneous lymphocyte proliferation; monocyte activation; expression of T cell activation antigens on CD4$^+$ and CD8$^+$ T cells; increased cytokine expression, elevated levels of neopterin, β2-microglobulin, acid-labile interferon, interleukin-2 receptors; and autoimmune phenomena [1]. Contrary to a normal immune response, in HIV infection the immune system is chronically activated. Spontaneous hyperactivation of B cells in AIDS patients has been reported [1, 10] as well as persistent activation of multiple components of the immune system. T cells can be activated by exposure to HIV antigen, which leads to a state of chronic persistent immune activation [11]. Spread of infection to adjacent and influxing cells is facilitated by the state of cellular activation and by the presence of large amounts of virus.

Role of Cytokines in HIV Disease

Cytokine secretion accompanies activation. The role of cytokines in HIV disease with respect to the dysregulation of cytokine expression, as well as the regulation of HIV expression by endogenous cytokines [1] is substantial. To examine dysregulation of cytokine expression, we performed reverse transcriptase-polymerase chain reaction (RT–PCR) on in vivo activated and ex vivo studied mononuclear cells from the lymph nodes of HIV-infected individuals and compared the results to those from lymph nodes of individuals without HIV infection who underwent lymph node biopsy for other reasons. Heightened activation and expression of proinflammatory cytokines were observed in HIV-infected individuals at all stages of disease as compared to uninfected individuals. Both constitutive and induced cytokine expression were elevated in HIV-infected individuals [1].

Two populations of $CD4^+$ T cells (TH1 and TH2), first identified in mice and later in humans, mutually exclusively produce certain cytokines [12, 13]. In humans, activation of TH1 and TH2 cells are associated with specific outcomes of infections. TH1 and TH2 cytokines have been shown to correlate with resistance to infection to particular parasitic disease [14], while TH2 cytokines have also been associated with progressive infection in other diseases [15]. Questions about the role of TH1 versus TH2 cytokines in the acceleration of HIV disease [16, 17] from early to advanced stage led us to compare the constitutive expression of various cytokines in lymph nodes of HIV-infected individuals at different stages of disease [18]. IL-2 is generally expressed at low levels, while another TH1 cytokine, interferon-gamma, is highly expressed compared to the lymph nodes of individuals who are uninfected. A low constitutive expression of IL-4 and high expression of IL-10, both TH2-type cytokines, was also observed in all stages of HIV disease. Thus, no obvious major shift in pattern of cytokine secretion from early to late disease was detected. The lack of switch from TH1 to TH2 cytokine patterns was confirmed on longitudinal analysis in three individual patients as they progressed through the different stages of disease.

Despite an intensive degree of cellular activation where approximately 50% of $CD4^+$ T cells and more than 80% of $CD8^+$ T cells are activated, we found an extremely low constitutive expression of IL-2 and IL-4. Furthermore, subset analysis showed that most, if not all, of the interferon-gamma and IL-10 is expressed by $CD4^-$ cells; $CD8^+$ cells; and $CD8^-$, $CD4^-$, non-T cells; rather than by $CD4^+$ cells as might be expected. Substantial modulation of cytokine expression in HIV disease including overexpression of certain cytokines likely reflects a state of heightened cellular activation. Despite this state of activation, IL-2 and IL-4 are poorly expressed. In addition, there is no obvious shift or predominance of TH2 over TH1 cytokine patterns in cells that are taken from infected, activated lymph nodes and studied ex vivo as HIV disease progresses.

We had demonstrated previously that specific cytokines can upregulate HIV expression [19]. In the mid-1980s, our research on bulk mononuclear cell supernatants demonstrated that these supernatants can upregulate HIV expression in chronically infected T cell and monocytoid cell lines. Subsequently, we and others demonstrated that a variety of cytokines can upregulate HIV expression, some in a dichotomous pattern [19].

Several years ago, we reported that HIV expression in both the U1 monocytoid cell line and the ACH-2 T cell line, can be regulated by exogenous cytokines such as TNF-α, GM-CSF, and IL-6 [20, 21]. U1 and ACH-2 are chronically HIV-infected cell lines used as models for studies of immunologic and molecular regulation of HIV expression. Cultures of acutely infected peripheral blood mononuclear cells stimulated with IL-2 alone enabled us to examine in a more physiological manner the autocrine and paracrine loops of

52

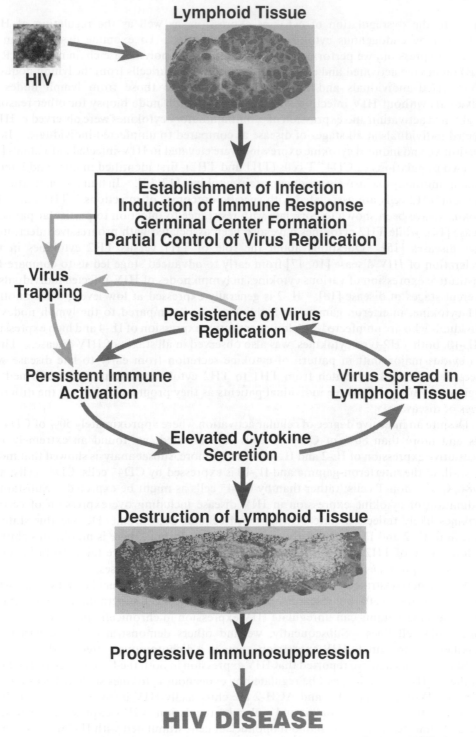

Fig. 2. Virologic and immunologic events associated with the development of advanced HIV disease.

regulation of HIV expression. Antibodies to TNF-α, IL-1β, and interferon-gamma profoundly downregulate the expression of HIV. Similar effects are seen with agents that block IL-1, such as IL-1 receptor antagonist and antibody to type I, but not to type II, IL-1 receptors. Certain cytokines such as IL-10 block HIV replication in acutely infected primary macrophages by inhibiting this autocrine loop of HIV induction by endogenous TNF-α and IL-6. These data indicate that primary infection with HIV sets in motion a series of events characterized by dissemination of virus, seeding of lymphoid tissue, a partially effective immune response, persistent virus replication, trapping of virus in lymphoid organs, chronic immune activation, cytokine secretion, and accelerated virus replication, which leads to further peristence and dissemination of virus and ultimately destruction of lymphoid tissue resulting in advanced HIV disease (fig. 2). This process occurs in most patients despite the emergence of an HIV-specific cell-mediated and humoral immune response during acute infection.

Studies in HIV-Infected Individuals Who are Long-Term Non-Progressors

A number of laboratories are studying HIV-infected individuals termed long term non-progressors, who maintain their immunologic competence foe many years despite the absence of antiretroviral therapy [22]. As with those who experience progressive immunologic deterioration in disease, focusing on host factors in long term non-progressors may shed light on the pathogenesis of HIV disease. We have studied a group of long term non-progressors who have been infected with HIV for approximately 10 years [22].

Because of the correlation between consistent destruction of lymph nodes and progression of HIV disease, we examined the lymph nodes of the long term non-progressors. Despite follicular hyperplasia in some of the individuals, we found that long term non-progressor lymph node architecture is typically well preserved. Other long term non-progressors have very little activation and minimal germinal center formation. The proportion of lymphoid tissue occupied by germinal centers can be determined by morphometric analysis and reflects the state of activation of the lymph node. This proportion was significantly greater in progressors early in their disease as compared to HIV-negative individuals and long term non-progressors. In one case, lymph node biopsics taken 9 years apart demonstrated that despite clear-cut documented HIV infection for several years, the individual's lymphoid tissue was remarkably well preserved. This is in sharp contrast to the state of lymph nodes of individuals with disease progression.

Examination of the deposition of extracellular virions on the follicular dendritic cells, and expression of virus in individual cells demonstrated variable degrees of virus trapping. Comparative analysis by DNA-PCR on mononuclear cells indicated approximately a log lower viral burden in peripheral blood and lymph node of long term non-progressors versus progressors. In addition, RNA-PCR indicated there were much lower levels of virus replication in monoclear cells of long term non-progressors compared to progressors. Comparative analysis of plasma viremia using quantitative competitive (QC) PCR revealed the expected very high levels of plasma viremia in progressors. However, of considerable interest was the presence of generally low, but variable, levels of viremia in most long term non-progressors that are comparable to individuals who are in the early, clinically latent stages of disease [22].

Over time, long term non-progressors consistently maintained their high levels of $CD4^+$ T cells even during transient peaks in viremia.   This suggests that the host's response to the virus plays an important role together with the competency of the virus in the evolution of the state of long term non-progression.   Low level but persistently replicating virus in certain long term non-progressors was associated with a robust immune response to the virus.   Specifically, high levels of neutralizing antibodies were detected in long term non-progressors compared to progressors.   In addition, HIV-specific cytotoxic T lymphocytes could be demonstrated in a limited number of patients we have studied thus far [22].

Virus isolated from most of these patients has been shown to be infectious and replication competent.   While virus isolated from progressors was facilitated by adding PHA to the cultures, the addition of PHA blasts was required for virus isolation in the long term non-progressors.   The need for PHA blasts is likely a reflection of the lower degree of viral burden in the long term non-progressors. $CD8^+$ T cells were able to inhibit replication of virus in non-progressors in a manner similar to the phenomenon demonstrated in certain early progressors as originally described by Levy [23].

Long term non-progressors probably represent a heterogeneous group of patients with variable impact of virus and host factors on the evolution of the state of non-progression. Regardless of the mechanisms, the phenomenon of long term non-progression is associated with a lesser degree of virus trapping; with adequate, but not complete, control of virus replication; modest immune activation; containment of virus spread; and, most importantly, a maintenance of the integrity of the lymphoid tissue, together with a relatively intact immune response.

Host Response in Primary HIV Infection

To examine some of the host factors that may control an individual's T cell-mediated primary immune response to HIV, RNA-PCR was used to study the various T-cell receptor $V\beta$ families in six patients during primary HIV infection [24].   Serial determinations over time demonstrated that $V\beta$ subsets expanded to different degrees in different patients. The magnitude of expansion of certain $V\beta$s was greater than that found in our studies of $V\beta$s in patients at any later stage in the course of the disease [25].   In one case, expansion was transient and the relative proportion of $V\beta19$-expressing cells returned to normal levels within 136 days.   Double-staining cytofluorometry indicated that this $V\beta$ expansion was virtually exclusively within the $CD8^+$ T cell subsets and that a large percentage of these cells were DR^+, or activated; among the $CD8^+/DR^+$ cells, a large percentage were $V\beta19^+$.

We assumed that the $CD8^+$ T cells were expanded either in a polyclonal fashion in response to a superantigen or in a highly restricted manner to a specific antigen.   We obtained nucleotide sequences of recombinant clones of $V\beta19$ derived from this patient at day 20 when $CD8^+V\beta19^+$ cells were dramatically expanded.   Although all the rearrangements were unique with respect to junctional diversity, there was a heavy bias in the usage of the $J\beta2.1$ segment (10 of 11 clones included this segment) suggesting an oligoclonal response.   Of particular interest were the nucleotide sequences of $V\beta19$ from a blood sample of the same patient collected at day 136.   A heavy bias in the usage of $J\beta2.1$ was still present.   More importantly, 9 of 11 recombinant clones now showed identical V–D–J rearrangements, and the rearrengements in these clones were identical to one of the clones present at day 20 indicating the occurrence of a selection process over time in vivo. Supportive evidence for the antigen-specificity of the response was the demonstration that HIV-specific cytotoxic activity was demonstrated within the $V\beta19^+$ $CD8^+$ T cells.

To determine whether there was any correlation between major expansions of $V\beta$ and clinical course of HIV disease, we grouped our initial six patients according to the degree and restriction of $CD8^+$ $V\beta$ expansions. All six patients had an initial downregulation of viremia despite the fact that their later courses were qualitatively quite different. Two patients had major expansions of a single $V\beta$ and fulminant courses of HIV disease; after less than 1 year their $CD4^+$ T cell counts were 200 per µl or less. Two other individuals had moderate expansions of two separate $V\beta$s; these individuals had a more typical course of disease. After 1 1/2 to 2 years their $CD4^+$ T cell counts were approximately 400 µl. The third group of two patients had a much less pronounced and/or more diffuse expansion of $V\beta$s and a clinical course clearly suggestive of slower progression. These patients had CD4 counts of 825 and 1,000 per µl at 2 years and 7 1/2 months, respectively.

We obtained a lymph node biopsy at 30 weeks from an additional patient who manifested major expansion of a restricted $V\beta$ (in this case $V\beta14$), together with a precipitous drop in $CD4^+$ T cell count. The lymph node architecture was disrupted and virus trapping was already compromised in a way similar to that seen in patients after several years of progressive disease. We have now studied more than 12 patients and the phenomena described above are consistent. Although the number of patients studied is small, the results lend themselves to several potential explanations. On the one hand, major expansions of restricted $V\beta$s may reflect an immune response to a virus with low sequence variability and, according to Mullins [26], such viruses have been associated with rapid progression. On the other hand, the restricted expansion may reflect a restricted ability to respond to a mutating virus and this may limit the ability to effectively control virus replication [27]. Finally, major expansions of HIV-specific $CD8^+$ T cells with a predominant $V\beta$ usage may actually lead to clonal exhaustion of CTLs as Zinkernagel [28] described in the lymphocytic choriomeningitis virus (LCMV) model. Whatever the cause, it is clear that events early in the course of infection may provide insight into those types of host factors that contribute to rapid progression, slow progression, or non-progression of disease.

Summary and Conclusions

It is clear that HIV disease is the result of a complex interaction of the virus and the infected host. Host factors differ greatly among individuals and likely play a significant role in the pathogenesis of HIV disease and in the determination of the rate of progression and/or the state of non-progression. Finally, and most importantly, certain of these host factors may actually be amenable to therapeutic intervention.

References

1   Fauci AS: Science 1993; 262: 1011.
2   Tindall B, Cooper DA: 1991; AIDS 5: 1.

3   Gaines H, von Sydow, MA, von Stedingk LV, Biberfeld G, Bottiger B, Hansson LO, Lundbergh P, Sonnerborg AB, Wasserman J, Strannegaard OO: AIDS, 1990; 4: 995.
4   Cooper DA, Tindall B, Wilson EJ, Imrie AA, Penny R: J Infect Dis, 1988; 157: 889.
5   Lemp GF, Payne SF, Rutherford GW, Hessol NA, Winkelstein W Jr, Wiley JA, Moss AR, Chaisson RE, Chen RT, Feigal DW Jr, Thomas PA, Werdegar D: JAMA, 1990: 263: 1497.
6   Goedert JJ: In: AIDS Research Reviews Volume 1, Koff WC, Wong-Staal F, Kennedy RC, eds. Marcel Dekker, New York, 1991; p. 137.
7   Safrit JT, Andrews CA, Zhu T, Ho DD, Koup RA, J Exp Med, 1994; 179: 463.
8   Pantaleo G, Graziosi C, Demarest JF, Butini L, Montroni M, Fox CH, Orenstein JM, Kotler DP, Fauci AS: Nature 1993; 362: 355.
9   Crabtree GR: Science 1989; 243: 355.
10 Lane HC, Masur H, Edgar LC, Whalen G, Rook AH, Fauci AS: N Engl J Med 1983; 309: 453.
11 Pantaleo G, Graziosi C, Demarest JF, Cohen OJ, Vaccarezza M, Gantt K, Muro-Cacho C, Fauci AS, Immuno Reviews 1994; 140: 105.
12 Mosmann TR, Cherwinski H, Bond MW, Giedlin MA, Coffman RL: J Immunol 1986; 136: 2348.
13 Maggi E, Biswas P, Del Prete G, Parronchi P, Macchia D, Simonelli C, Emmi L, De Carli M, Tiri A, Ricci M: J Immunol 1991; 146: 1169.
14 Taylor-Robinson AW, Phillips RS, Severn A, Moncada S, Liew FY: Science, 1993; 260: 1931.
15 Sieling PA, Abrams JS, Yamamura M, Salgame P, Bloom BR, Rea TH, Modlin RL: J Immunol 1993; 150: 5501.
16 Clerici M, Hakim FT, Venzon DJ, Blatt S, Hendrix CW, Wynn TA, Shearer GM: J Clin Invest 1993; 91: 759.
17 Clerici M, Shearer GM: Immunol Today 1993; 14: 107.
18 Graziosi C, Pantaleo G, Gantt KR, Fortin JP, Demarest JF, Cohen OJ, Sekaly RP, Fauci AS, Science 1994; 265: 248.
19 Poli G, Fauci AS, Semin Immunol 1993; 5: 165.
20 Folks TM, Justement J, Kinter A, Dinarello CA, Fauci AS: Science 1987; 238: 800.
21 Folks TM, Clouse KA, Justement J, Rabson A, Duh E, Kehrl JH, Fauci AS: Proc Natl Acad Sci U.S.A 1989; 86: 2365.
22 Pantaleo G, Menzo S, Vaccarezza M, Graziosi C, Cohen OJ, Demarest JF, Montefiori D, Orenstein JM, Fox C, Schrager L, Margolick J, Buchbinder S, Giorgi JV, Fauci AS, N Engl J Med 1995; 332: 209.
23 Mackewicz CE, Ortega HW, Levy JA: J Clin Invest 1991; 87: 1462.
24 Pantaleo G, Demarest JF, Soudeyns H, Graziosi C, Denis F, Adelsberger JW Borrow P, Saag MS, Shaw GM, Sekaly RP, Fauci AS: Nature 1994; 370: 463.
25 Rebai N, Pantaleo G, Demarest J, Ciurli C, Soudeyns H, Adelsberger J, Vaccarezza M, Walker R, Sekaly R, Fauci AS, Proc Natl Acad Sci USA 1994; 91: 1529.
26 Delwart EL, Shpaer EG, Louwagie J, McCutchan FE, Grez M, Rubsamen-Waigmann H, Mullins JI: Science 1993; 262: 1257.
27 Kalams SA, Johnson RP, Trocha AK, Dynan MJ, Ngo HS, D'Aquila RT, Kurnick JT, Walker BD: J Exp Med 1994; 179: 1261.
28 Moskophidis D, Lechner F, Pircher H, Zinkernagel RM, Nature 1993; 362: 758.

A Turning Point in AIDS Research: the Search for New Frontiers

William E. Paul

Office of AIDS Research, National Institutes of Health, Bethesda, MD., USA

Introduction

Last year, many scientists and people living with HIV left the International Conference on AIDS in Berlin with a feeling of deep pessimism. Twelve years into the AIDS epidemic, no cure or vaccine was in sight, and some of our modest hopes for existing therapies were disappointed. At the same time last year, I was in my laboratory at the National Institutes of Health, studying cytokine biology with particular reference to how interleukin-4, a molecule that we had discovered a decade ago, controls the nature of immune responses.

I have been an immunologist all my professional life, but I am new to AIDS research. Six months ago, Harold Varmus, Director of the NIH, asked me to lead the AIDS research effort of the United States as Director of the Office of AIDS Research. I accepted this responsibility for several reasons. As a physician, I felt an obligation to enlist in the battle against AIDS, due to the enormity of human suffering caused by this epidemic. As a scientist, I believe that, while the scientific questions we face in AIDS are exceedingly difficult, they are neither insurmountable nor unanswerable. Finally, I accepted the Directorship of the Office of AIDS Research because I believe we are at a turning point in the history of the disease. It is time for a frank assessment of our previous successes and failures, and time to chart a new course for the future, avoiding the twin perils of an unreflective allegiance to the status quo and an impulsive acceptance of easy answers and solutions.

President Clinton and Secretary Shalala made the battle against AIDS one of their foremost priorities. In its first year, this Administration obtained a 21% increase in funding for AIDS research. Fully 12% of the entire $11 billion NIH budget is now devoted to AIDS research. In fact the NIH budget as a whole is characterized as either AIDS or non-AIDS, a status accorded no other disease. Furthermore, Congress passed new legislation restructuring the way the NIH carries out AIDS research, investing primary responsibility for planning, coordinating and funding all AIDS-related research in the Office of AIDS Research, or, in this era of acronyms, the OAR.

The OAR has a new mandate to evaluate the entire NIH AIDS research program, and to set in place refocused scientific priorities through the development of a comprehensive research plan and budget. As its Director, I take this responsibility extremely seriously. However, I will not surrender to the conceit that I can meet this challenge alone. My first action as OAR Director was to invite distinguished colleagues, both from within the world of AIDS research and from related disciplines, including some, like myself, who had not worked in AIDS before, to join me in crafting a new program for AIDS research.   This morning, I will present to you this new research agenda.   It is our hope that this agenda can provide a foundation for real advances in our common struggle against AIDS.

Clinical Research

I will begin with a discussion of clinical research, if only for the reason that you would have expected me, as a basic scientist, to leave that subject for last.   Clinical research on any life-threatening disease has two equally critical components: the discovery and development of new drugs; and, improving the standard-of-care by optimizing the use of existing agents.   The AIDS research program will maintain a balanced portfolio of both small, laboratory-intensive pathogenesis-based studies and larger, longer studies that measure which treatments are best for prolonging health and life.

Our therapeutic successes against HIV itself have been real, but limited.   The oldest drug in our armamentarium, AZT, may be best at preventing transmission of the virus from mother to infant, where it can reduce that rate by two-thirds.   The data supporting this encouraging result will be presented to you later today.   As we heard last year from the Concorde investigators, and we will hear again this week, the administration of AZT during early HIV disease does not appear to confer a survival benefit.   However, we must remember that AZT does offer such a benefit for patients with full-blown disease, and ddI has been shown to delay progression.   There is as yet little definitive information on the effects of the other nucleoside analogue reverse transcriptase inhibitors on progression or survival.   While combinations of these RT inhibitors had been hoped to provide additive or even synergistic benefit, there is no proof yet of the clinical efficacy of such combination regimens.

Nonetheless, the development of the nucleoside analogues does demonstrate that it is feasible to reduce viral replication, and induce short-term immunologic and clinical benefit. Therefore, the task before us in the coming years is to deepen the magnitude of viral suppression, improve immunological and clinical benefit, and prolong the still tragically limited clinical efficacy of these first-generation antiretroviral agents.   Indeed, as Dr. Stefano Vella discussed on (p. 159), we must pay particular attention to combination therapies with agents directed against distinct molecular targets.

When this epidemic began, we lacked preventive agents against *Pneumocystis carinii* pneumonia, *Mycobacterium avium* complex disease, and opportunistic fungal infections. Now, we can often prevent these conditions, and we have better treatments for them and for cytomegalovirus disease.   Thanks to the dedicated work of clinical researchers, people with HIV infection are living longer now than they did a decade ago.   Indeed, the survival time of people with AIDS has doubled, largely due to our advances in the treatment and prevention of opportunistic infections.   These have been among our greatest successes in AIDS research thus far, and they have provided tangible benefits for people living with the disease.

Pathogenesis-driven clinical trials can teach us a great deal about the virological and immunological aspects of HIV disease in vivo by answering basic scientific questions within the framework of a clinical study.   We will continue to provide strong support for these pioneering efforts.   Similarly, studies of immune-based therapies may provide both new therapeutic approaches to HIV disease as well as clues towards elucidating its pathogenesis.

One of the gaps in our clinical research program is in large phase III randomized studies that are sufficiently powered to reliably answer questions about the clinical benefits of the antiretroviral agents that will be widely used.   Infected individuals and their physicians need to know how best to use the drugs we now offer them.   To examine this, we must call on industry to participate in shouldering the cost of the necessary studies, as the NIH simply does not have the resources to conduct these trials alone and to still meet its other pressing responsibilities.

The NIH AIDS clinical research infrastructure is composed of many networks that grew rapidly and independently of each other in the context of a public health emergency, but in the absence of a broad plan for clinical research.   They now receive a very considerable fraction of the total NIH AIDS research budget.   A more complete, coherent, and cost-effective clinical research effort is necessary and possible.   With better coordination, these various networks must be made to work together to maximize their research productivity.

Drug Discovery

In the area of drug discovery, our efforts to intercede in the viral life cycle have focused primarily on agents directed against the HIV reverse transcriptase and more recently the HIV protease.   Four reverse transcriptase inhibitors are currently approved by the U.S. Food and Drug Administration for the treatment of HIV infection.   Several HIV protease inhibitors are slated to begin phase III efficacy trials in the near future.

We will place special emphasis on and devote resources to the development of therapies based on new molecular targets in order to broaden our arsenal of weapons against the virus.   This will require a more detailed understanding of HIV regulatory proteins, including *nef* and *rev*, and of the less well-studied accessory proteins, as well as the design of biologically relevant screens for inhibitors of these gene products.

AIDS researchers have reached a consensus that our drug discovery efforts cannot be limited to antiretroviral agents alone.   As Anthony Fauci elegantly described to us (see p. 49), the pathogenesis of HIV infection is a multifactorial process that most likely involves both direct viral cytotoxicity, as well as other indirect effects mediated through the immune system itself.   We will intensify our efforts to develop new agents or modalities to intercede in the immunopathogenesis of the disease as well as to find new ways to attack the virus directly.

Currently, several cytokine and anti-cytokine therapies are being tested for their potential value in HIV infection; among them are interleukin-2, interleukin-12 and the tumor necrosis factor-inhibitors, pentoxyfylline and thalidomide.   Clinical investigators are expanding HIV-specific cytotoxic T-lymphocytes for reinfusion into the infected donor of these cells.   Others are examining the usefulness of highly targeted immunomodulatory agents to stem those aspects of immune activation that contribute to the progress of the disease.   There is also great enthusiasm about the potential of gene therapy to limit the capacity of cells to support the growth of the virus.   We are committed to supporting the development of novel approaches based on our latest understanding of the pathogenesis of the disease, and not limiting ourselves strictly to antiviral approaches.

While we have had important successes against opportunistic pathogens, other infections and cancers present us with new challenges: crypto- and microsporidium, Kaposi's sarcoma, non-Hodgkin's lymphoma, progressive multifocal leukoencephalo-pathy...the list goes on.   Furthermore, in this era of increasing antibiotic resistance, many common microbes once thought vanquished are returning with a vengeance.   Multi-drug resistant tuberculosis raises the specter that the monster we thought was slain was merely asleep.   Therefore, our new agenda calls for an intensified effort to discover and develop new anti-infectives and novel antineoplastic agents.

Vaccine Research

Our greatest hope for the eradication of HIV lies in the development of effective preventive vaccines.   Indeed in many parts of the world, vaccines are the only realistic way to deal with the epidemic.   Let me emphasize that vaccine development is an essential element of the OAR research agenda.

As Dr. Bolognesi discussed (see p. 147), an NIH advisory council recently recommended that phase III field trials of two gp120-based candidate vaccines were not yet warranted, due to concern about the ability of these vaccines to stimulate production of antibody capable of neutralizing primary viral isolates and to generate broadly cross-reactive cytotoxic T-cell responses.   This decision has forced us to recognize the urgency of the development of second generation HIV preventive vaccines with enhanced immunogenicity.   We must base this effort on the latest knowledge about the virus and the immune response it evokes.   Large scale testing of vaccines will proceed, when reliable scientific evidence suggests that our new candidates have a reasonable degree of promise. It is essential that we earn the trust of those in at-risk communities worldwide who will be the participants in our vaccine trials.

Until we better understand the nature of protective immunity to HIV and how to measure it, we will not be in a strong position to develop vaccine strategies that will optimize such immunity.   Robbins and Schneerson have argued that virtually every effective vaccine for humans now available is based on the induction of neutralizing antibodies that prevent infection.   Indeed, our understanding of the mechanisms through which neutralizing antibody and effector T cells function indicates that while antibodies can prevent infection, T cells are largely limited to acting after a cell has become infected.   We do know that natural infections with various intracellular bacteria, viruses and parasites are often terminated by T cell responses and that such responses can provide what is essentially a sterilizing immunity.   However, there is still uncertainty as to whether a fully protective preventive vaccine can be based on the principle of post-infection elimination of a pathogen by effector T cells.

We will increase support for studies of the mechanisms of immunological resistance to infection with HIV and related lentiviruses.   Work is now proceeding on several unique cohorts of individuals that may hold important clues in this regard.   In the Nairobi Sex Workers Study, a group of women are being carefully analyzed who, despite repeated apparent exposure to HIV, appear to have resisted injection.   Studies are underway of discordant couples in which the HIV-negative partner has remained uninfected, despite continued high-risk behavior with the HIV-positive partner. These exposed but apparently uninfected individuals may have acquired a form of protective immunity; understanding the nature of this immunity can provide insight into what is required for effective vaccine-based prevention.

Animal models, particularly the SIV-infected macaque, will be important in establishing the nature of protective immunity. What, for instance, is the nature of the immunity to a fully virulent SIV that is induced by vaccination with a *nef*-deleted viral mutant? We are supporting studies of these immune responses and will take an active role in determining if attenuated viruses can be developed that are sufficiently safe to warrant serious consideration as vaccine candidates. As has been discussed, risk/benefit ratios of an attenuated virus vaccine will vary depending upon infection rates and other regional considerations. An attenuated virus vaccine may be entirely appropriate in certain regions, but less appropriate in others.

Post-infection vaccination has been proposed as an immunomodulatory strategy for the treatment of HIV-infected individuals. We may be able to use post-infection immunization or, more likely, other immunomodulatory approaches to usefully redirect the immune response of HIV-infected individuals once we have discovered the kind of response that would be most effective in slowing the progression of disease.

Although considerable controversy surrounds the applicability of the TH1/TH2 paradigm to HIV-infected individuals, the possible benefit of altering the balance of cytokines made in the course of infection will be carefully examined. Heightened production of interferon-gamma and interleukin-2 may have value in slowing progression of immunodeficiency. Suppression of interleukin-4 production may enhance microbicidal action of macrophages.

We must remember that the nature of an immune response that slows progression of an established injection may be very different than one that protects against initial infection with the virus. Long-term non-progressors, those individuals who remain immunologically intact over a decade after seroconversion, may share unique immune responses that are particularly potent against the virus once infection has been established. The analysis of these responses may provide clues for us in the effort to understand the characteristics of an immune response effective in HIV-positive individuals.

Behavioral Research

Currently, behavioral interventions are our only weapon to prevent the spread of the epidemic. Behavioral research is a large and vital part of the NIH AIDS research portfolio. As Director of the Office of AIDS Research, one of my challenges will be to better integrate our biomedical and behavioral research programs. Behavioral components of both vaccine and drug clinical trials will be essential to obtaining reliable results.

Last month, the Institute of Medicine of the U.S. National Academy of Sciences released a report on the state of research in this area. The experts who contributed to the report's recommendations are among the finest in their field, and I will continue to look to them for guidance in re-shaping our efforts in behavioral research. Several key recommendations in the IOM report will be carefully considered as we map the future of behavioral research on AIDS.   Among them is to obtain reliable information of sexual practices and substance abuse in order to more clearly elucidate HIV risk-taking behavior. Investment in behavioral research should provide us with better intervention strategies to prevent HIV transmission.

Other prevention strategies, particularly viricides and female-controlled barriers of HIV and STD infection, are critically needed to give women additional options with which to protect themselves.   NIH has initiated a major program to develop such barriers, and in the coming year will substantially increase the funds devoted to this effort.

Basic Research

The engine that will drive the entire AIDS research enterprise forward is basic research. I believe the current inadequacy of treatments for HIV infection and the absence of a vaccine to protect the uninfected are largely due to the wide gaps in our understanding of the pathogenesis of HIV disease, of the details of the viral life cycle and the function of the viral proteins, and of the interactions of the virus with the immune system.

The list of unanswered, basic questions in AIDS research is a long one: What is the in vivo function of the less well studied protein products of the viral genes, and what are their roles in the regulation of the viral life cycle?   Are there host genetic factors that determine relative susceptibility of individuals to infection; if so, what are they and how do they work? Is cell-associated or free virus more important in establishing infection?   How does the virus cross the mucosal barrier?   What is the first cell that is infected?   What are the cellular co-factors, in addition to CD4, that are critical in determining entry into and infection of a cell?   How does infection result in cell death?   Is there an effective immune response mounted that controls the virus for the long period of time between infection and the development of symptomatic disease?

However, the fact that many would agree on this list of unsolved problems almost certainly means that key questions are still not being asked.   We must rededicate ourselves to basic research to meet these and other challenges.   A vigorous program of creative investigator-initiated work is essential.   Indeed, in our temptation to manage the research effort we must always recall that the pathbreaking work, which has the capacity to tranform our approach to this disease, will come from insights that cannot be planned in any administrative office.   Command science is no more likely to succeed than command economics.

If we do not provide innovative scientists with the resources and opportunities to attack the basic unsolved problems related to AIDS and HIV, we may find that a decade from now, we are no further along in our struggle.   To achieve the revitalization and expansion of basic research on AIDS, I will increase the resources available for support of investigator-initiated work and will use all my powers to persuade a broader pool of basic scientists to join us in this effort.

Only in the context of a healthy, vigorous and broadly-based biomedical research enterprise as a whole can the effort to understand, prevent and treat HIV infection and AIDS have any real hope of success.   Research efforts aimed at solving a problem that is directly or indirectly related to AIDS will, almost inevitably, give rise to insights of great significance in entirely different areas.   Equally, discoveries outside the field of AIDS may have tremendous and immediate impact on research on HIV infection.   We often simply do not know from where our great leaps forward will come.   As a striking example, one of the most important developments in modern cancer biology, the discovery of the p53 tumor suppressor gene, was actually a result of studies by Arnold Levine of the regulation of adenovirus growth.   This forcefully illustrates that pitting one area of science against another, or research on one disease against research on another is short-sighted and supposes that we can predict the trajectory of scientific progress.

The New Partnership

This, then is our agenda:
*A rededication to fundamental science, coupled with a vigorous, highly-efficient therapeutic research program;
*A stronger effort to develop second generation vaccines and to bring them to clinical trial as soon as possible;
*An emphasis upon behavioral science and its integration with biologically-based AIDS research.

OAR now has the authority to shift resources to meet these scientific priorities, and I can assure you we have already begun to do so.

Our efforts cannot fully succeed without partnerships around the world, among researchers and scientists from government, academia, and the private sector, in a true alliance with people living with AIDS and their advocates.   We must build a more effective and collaborative worldwide research effort against this pandemic.

When we leave Yokohama, each of us, from whatever country, whatever scientific discipline, or whichever HIV-affected community, must join in forging a new sense of unity and purpose so that in the second decade of the pandemic we will make important strides toward conquering AIDS.   Just as we have eradicated smallpox and are nearing the elimination of polio, our collective goal must be to accept nothing less than the complete elimination of AIDS from our world.

Virologic and Immunologic Characterization of Long-Term Survivors of Human Immunodeficiency Virus Type 1 Infection

Yunzhen Cao, M.D., Limo Qin, M.D., Linqi Zhang, Ph.D., Jeffrey Safrit, Ph.D., and David D. Ho, M.D.

The Aaron Diamond AIDS Research Center, New York University School of Medicine, New York, NY, USA

The natural history and pathogenic processes of human immunodeficiency virus type 1 (HIV-1) infection are complex and variable, and they depend on a multitude of viral and host factors and thier interactions [1]. Host factors may result in a variable susceptibility to HIV-1 infection and its pathogenic effects, whereas variation in the virus may account for differences in virulence and disease progression. Although symptoms related to the acquired immunodeficiency syndrome (AIDS) or laboratory evidence of immunodeficiency develops in a majority of infected persons within 10 years of seroconversion [2 – 5], a small number (approximately 5 percent) of infected persons, termed long-term survivors or persons with long-term nonprogressive disease, have remained clinically healthy and immunologically normal for more than a decade [6 11]. These long-term survivors have recently become the subject of intensive investigation, because they may yield important information on the determinants of nonprogression that may be useful in designing new interventional strategies to contain the disease.

To obtain a balanced view of the pathogenic proccesses in long-term survivors, we examined host, immunologic, and virologic factors in a cohort of 10 subjects who have remained asymptomatic with normal and stable CD4$^+$ lymphocyte counts despite 12 to 15 years of HIV-1 infection.

Methods

Study Subjects

Ten HIV-1–seropositive subjects from the New York metropolitan area were referred to us because they met our working definition of long-term survivors of HIV-1 infection: they had no symptoms, normal and stable CD4$^+$ lymphocyte counts, no prolonged use of antiretroviral agents, and at least 12 years of infection. The general clinical characteristics of the cohort are summarized in table 1. The subjects ranged in age from 38 to 47 years, and all but one were men. Seven were infected through homosexual contact, two were infected through intravenous drug use, and the one woman was infected heterosexually. Their CD4$^+$ lymphocyte counts have been consistently in the normal range, with no decline over time. The duration of HIV-1 infection was documented by the date of seroconversion in three subjects (Subjects 1, 4, and 9) who participated in a prospective study of the natural

Table 1. Clinical characteristics of long-term survivors[†1]

Subject[†2]	Age(yr)/ Sex	Route of infection	Range of CD4 counts (cells/mm³)	Years of infection	HLA type Class I	Class II
1(+)	38/M	Homosexual sex	600 – 1200	15	A3; B57; Cw3	DR1,7; DQ(ND)
2(○)	38/M	IV drug use	500 – 700	≥12	A24,32; B51,52; Cw1,2	DR15,11,52; DQ6,7
3(△)	46/M	Homosexual sex	560 – 740	≥13	A2,3; B7,14; Cw7,8	DR15,6,52; DQ1(6)
4(□)	40/M	Homosexual sex	500 – 1200	14	A1,2; B51,57; Cw2,6	DR7,11,52,53; DQ7,2
5(◇)	41/M	IV drug use	800 – 1000	≥12	A2,26; B38; Cw3	DR11,13,52; DQ6,7
6(●)	38/M	Homosexual sex	560 – 860	12	A2,19; B44; Cw3,5	DR52; DQ1
7(▲)	42/F	Heterosexual sex	500 – 850	13	A1,2; B8,58; Cw3,7	DR15,3,52; DQ6,2
8(■)	44/M	Homosexual sex	400 – 800	≥15	A2,24; B18,51; Cw1,7	DR52; DQ1,3
9(×)	47/M	Homosexual sex	600 – 1100	14	A11,26; B62; Cw3	DR4,6; DQ(ND)
10(◆)	47/M	Homosexual sex	550 – 850	≥14	A1,25; B18,37; Cw6	DR15,11,52; DQ6,2

†1 IV denotes intravenous, and ND not done.
†2 Each subject is identified by a number and a symbol, which is also used in figures 1, 2, and 4.

history of the disease at the New York Blood Center.   Subject 7 had given birth to an infected child 13 years before the start of our study, and Subject 8 had had unexplained hypergammaglobulinemia and lymphoid hyperplasia on biopsy 15 years before the study began.   The duration of infection in the other subjects was determined on the basis of the year in which they discontinued high-risk behavior, such as intravenous drug use (Subjects 2 and 5) or unprotected homosexual sex (Subjects 3, 6, and 10).   None had received antiretroviral agents for a prolonged period, although some had received short courses of zidovudine (Subjects 2 and 7), didanosine (Subject 2), or recombinant gp160 (Subject 3). No subject was receiving antiretroviral therapy at the time of this study.   As table 1 shows, these long-term serivors had a range of HLA class I and II phenotypes as determined by standard serologic typing (Blood Systems Laboratory, Scottsdale, Ariz.), indicating that they did not share a common HLA type.   In addition, the 10 subjects were not found to have epidemiologic features in common.

Quantitation and Isolation of HIV-1

Infectious HIV-1 in plasma and peripheral blood mononuclear cells (PBMC) was quantitated as described elsewhere [12 – 14].   Particle-associated RNA in plasma was quantitated with a modification of the branched-DNA signal-amplification assay [15, 16], with freshly collected samples.   This ultrasensitive assay has a typical detection limit of approximately 630 copies of RNA per milliliter of plasma [17].   HIV-1 DNA in PBMC was quantitated by the polymerase chain reaction (PCR) as described elsewhere [18]. Briefly, proviral DNA was initially studied with limiting dilutions to a point at which less than 25 percent of the resulting PCR products were positive.   The number of proviral copies was then estimated by the formula—$\ln(F)$, where F is the fraction of negative reactions, assuming that the incidental appearance of positive PCR products follows a Poisson distribution.   Appropriate positive and negative controls were included in all quantitative assays.

When the initial attempt to isolate HIV-1 was unsuccessful, subsequent attempts were made with up to 5 million PBMC that had been subjected to CD8$^+$ lymphocyte depletion with immunomagnetic beads (Dynal, Great Neck, N.Y.).

Susceptibility of PBMC from Long-Term Survivors to HIV-1 Infection in vitro

To assess the susceptibility of cells from long-term survivors to HIV-1 infection in vitro, PBMC (2 million cells) from each of eight study subjects (all except Subjects 1 and 9) and two normal controls were inoculated with 3000 median tissue-culture infective doses (TCID$_{50}$) of the HIV-1 isolate JRCSF [19].   The cultures were then washed extensively on the second day, and the expression of p24 antigen in the supernatant was determined by an immunoassay (Abbott Laboratories, Abbott Park, Ill.) on days 4, 7, and 14 of culture. Similar experiments were carried out in parallel with PBMC that had been largery ($>$98 percent) depleted of CD8$^+$ lymphocytes by the immunomagnetic-bead method.   In these experiments as well as those described immediately below, PBMC from subjects with progressive disease could not be studied in parallel for comparison, because such cells harbor another infections isolate of HIV-1 that would have clouded the interpretation of the results.

HIV-1-Inhibitory Activity Mediated by CD8$^+$ Lymphocytes

A series of experiments were conducted to quantitate the inhibitory activity of CD8$^+$ lymphocytes on HIV-1 replication in CD4$^+$ lymphocytes.   CD4$^+$ and CD8$^+$ lymphocytes were each purified (to 98 percent purity) from PBMC of long-term survivors and normal controls with immunomagnetic beads.   CD4$^+$ lymphocytes were then stimulated for three days by the addition of phytohemagglutinin (2 µg per milliliter), and CD8$^+$ lymphocytes were stimulated for three days with an anti-CD3 monoclonal antibody (12F6), irradiated allogeneic feeder cells, and interleukin-2 (100 units per milliliter).   Two million CD4$^+$ lymphoblasts were then inoculated with 3000 TCID$_{50}$ of the JRCSF isolate alone or together with variable numbers of autologous activated CD8$^+$ lymphocytes (from 1 million down to 320 in fivefold dilutions).   The expression of p24 antigen in the culture supernatant was monitored periodically during the ensuing 14 days.

Neutralizing Activity of Plasma against Primary HIV-1 Isolates

Serial dilutions of plasma samples from nine long-term survivors (all subjects except Subject 1) and four subjects with progressive disease were tested for neutralizing activity against a panel of 13 primary HIV-1 isolates (each containing 100 TCID$_{50}$) obtained after short-term culture of PBMC from long-term survivors or from U.S. patients who had the acute infection syndrome, were asymptomatic, or had AIDS.   The assays were performed according to a published protocol [20, 21], with 2 million activated PBMC from a normal donor used as target cells and the expression of p24 antigen in the supernatant used as a measure of HIV-1 replication.   Extreme care was taken to ensure the complete removal of all added plasma from the cultures before the measurement of p24 antigen, because residual plasma might contain anti-p24 antibodies capable of interfering substantially with the p24 antigen assay, resulting in false evidence of virus neutralization.

Kinetics of Replication and Cytotoxicity of HIV-1 Isolates

HIV-1 was successfully isolated from the PBMC of three subjects (Subjects 8, 9, and 10) by a standard procedure [12, 14] whereas in a fourth (Subject 7) isolation required CD8$^+$

lymphocyte depletion. The kinetics of replication in 2 million PBMC from a normal donor was determined for each viral isolate (3000 TCID$_{50}$) by serial monitoring of p24 antigen expression in the culture supernatant, as described elsewhere. Viral cytotoxicity in purified cultures of CD4$^+$ lymphocytes was assessed by serial counting of viable cells by light microscopy [14].

Results

Levels of HIV-1 in PBMC and Plasma

The levels of HIV-1 in the PBMC and plasma of long-term survivors were determined by several techniques. First, plasma cultures were uniformly negative for infectious virus ($<$1 TCID$_{50}$ per milliliter) in tests of nine subjects involving up to 1 ml of sample (fig. 1). However, particle-associated HIV-1 RNA was detectable in four subjects (Subjects 4, 6, 8, and 10) by an ultrasensitive branched-DNA assay [15 – 17]; the values ranged from 839 to 11,549 copies of RNA per milliliter of plasma. The other five subjects had HIV-1 levels below the limit of detection of the assay ($<$630 RNA copies per milliliter). Overall, the amount of HIV-1 in the plasma of these nine long-term survivors was orders of magnitude lower than that found in subjects with progressive disease. In our experience [12], asymptomatic persons with progressive disease had titers of infectious HIV-1 ranging from 5 to 100 TCID$_{50}$ per milliliter of plasma (mean, 30), whereas patients with AIDS had titers ranging from 5 to 5000 TCID$_{50}$ per milliliter (mean, about 1000). Similarly, subjects with progressive disease in a recent study of ours had plasma counts of viral RNA ranging from 4000 to 90 million copies per milliliter. The mean values were 580,000 copies per milliliter among patients with CD4$^+$ cell counts below 200 per cubic millimeter and 71,000 copies per milliliter among those with counts ranging from 200 to 500 per cubic millimeter [16].

Levels of HIV-1 were also determined in the PBMC of long-term survivors. Infectious HIV-1 was detected and quantified in three subjects (0.2, 50, and 5 TCID$_{50}$ per million cells in Subjects 8, 9, and 10, respectively) by a standard limiting-dilution assay [12 – 14] (fig. 1). In contrast, seven subjects had no detectable infectious virus in 10 million PBMC ($<$0.1 TCID$_{50}$ per million cells). These negative results are particularly striking because in other settings we have isolated HIV-1 from PBMC at a rate approaching 100 percent [12 – 14]. Therefore, additional attemps to recover infectious HIV-1 were made with 2 million to 5 million PBMC depleted of CD8$^+$ lymphocytes, because this maneuver has been shown to improve the efficiency of HIV-1 isolation [22 – 25]. The cultures for Subjects 1 through 6 remained negative, although an HIV-1 isolate was obtained from Subject 7 by this method (data not shown).

The amount of HIV-1 proviral DNA in the PBMC of long-term survivors was determined by an established method of quantitative PCR [18]. As figure 1 shows, all the subjects had detectable viral DNA, but the copy numbers were generally quite low, ranging from 10 to 100 copies per million PBMC, except in Subjects 9 and 10, who had 296 and 1783 copies per million PBMC, respectively. These two subjects also had the highest titers of infectious HIV-1 in PBMC (fig. 1). Once again the amount of HIV-1 in the PBMC of long-term survivors as measured by these two techniques appeared to be substantially lower than the levels that we [12 – 14] and others [18, 26 – 28] have found in patients with progressive disease; such patients had a mean infectious titer of about 1700 TCID$_{50}$ per million PBMC

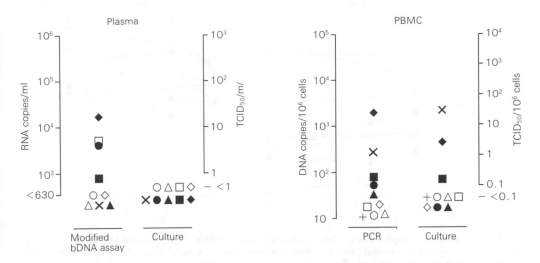

Fig. 1. Levels of HIV-1 in plasma and PBMC of long-term survivors.   Each symbol represents a study subject, identified in *table 1.*   TCID$_{50}$ denotes median tissue-culture infective dose, and bDNA branched DNA. The detection limit of the bDNA signal-amplification assay was 630 copies of RNA per milliliter of plasma.

and a mean count of about 5000 copies of proviral DNA per milliliter.

It therefore appears that in the long-term survivors we studied, HIV-1 replication is well controlled in vivo.   What accounts for this finding?   The experiments described below pursue three possible explanations: that these patients' CD4$^+$ lymphocytes are less susceptible to HIV-1 infection; that they have stronger HIV-1—specific immune responses; and that they harbor strains of HIV-1 that are defective or attenuated.

Susceptibility of PBMC from Long-Term Survivors to HIV-1 Infection in vitro

PBMC from eight long-term survivors (all except Subjects 1 and 9) and two normal controls were examined for their in vitro susceptibility to infectious by JRCSF [19], an exogenous strain of HIV-1, since no infectious virus was found in cells from any of the subjects except Subjects 8 and 10.   As figure 2 shows, the virus replicated efficiently to high levels (>10,000 pg of p24 antigen per milliliter) in the PBMC of two normal donors, whereas its replication in the PBMC of long-term survivors was substantially less.   In fact, only one culture (of cells from Subject 4) reached a level of p24 antigen expression ≥1000 pg per milliliter.   At first glance, these results suggest that cells from long-term survivors were more refractory to HIV-1 infection in vitro.   However, when the cultures were depleted of CD8$^+$ lymphocytes, the remaining CD4-enriched PBMC from each long-term survivor supported HIV-1 replication at levels in excess of 1000 pg of p24 antigen per milliliter, and in five subjects the level exceeded 10,000 pg per milliliter (fig. 2).   On average, CD8$^+$ lymphocyte depletion produced a 22-fold increase in peak HIV-1 replication in PBMC from the eight long-term survivors, as compared with a 3-fold increase in the two normal controls.   Although CD4-enriched PBMC from several long-term survivors (for example, Subjects 6 and 8) were less efficient in replicating the JRCSF isolate (fig. 2), these cells did support the efficient growth of other primary HIV-1 isolates (data not shown).   On the

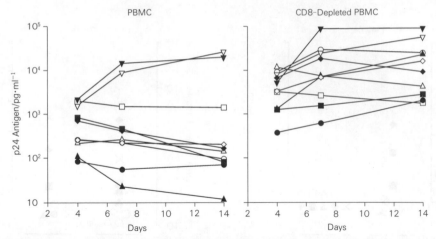

Fig. 2. Kinetics of replication of HIV-1 isolate JRCSF in PBMC and CD8-depleted PBMC from eight long-term survivors and two normal controls. Each symbol represents a study subject identified in *table 1.* Two normal donors are also shown (▽ and ▼).

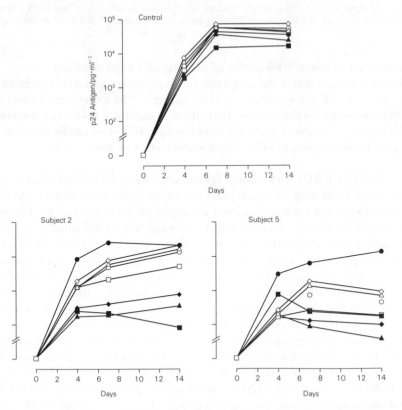

Fig. 3. Kinetics of replication of HIV-1 isolate JRCSF in unfractionated PBMC (■) from a normal control and subjects 2 and 5, as well as in CD8-depleted, CD4-enriched PBMC without CD8+ lymphocytes (●) and with 1 million (▲), 200,000 (◆), 40,000 (□), 8,000 (○), 1,600 (△), and 320 (◇) autologous CD8+ lymphocytes added back to the cell culture.

basis of the findings shown in figure 2, we conclude that the CD4$^+$ lymphocytes from long-term survivors had no gross intrinsic resistance to HIV-1 infection in vitro.   Instead, there is strong evidence to suggest that CD8$^+$ lymphocytes from these survivors had substantial HIV-1–inhibitory activity.

Detection and Quantitation of HIV-1 — Suppressive Activity of CD8$^+$ Lymphocytes

To show conclusively that CD8$^+$ lymphocytes from long-term survivors indeed mediate potent suppression of HIV-1 replication in vitro, a series of experiments were performed in which CD8$^+$ lymphocytes were added back to the sample.   The results of three such experiments are shown in figure 3.   In CD4-enriched PBMC from a normal donor, the JRCSF strain of HIV-1 replicated efficiently to high levels, and the addition of 320 to 1 million autologous CD8$^+$ lymphocytes resulted in only slight reductions in viral replication. In contrast, for Subjects 2 and 5, the addition of autologous CD8$^+$ lymphocytes led to marked reductions (by about two orders of magnitude) in HIV-1 replication.   In quantitative experiments of this type, we were able to determine the minimal number of autologous CD8$^+$ lymphocytes required to inhibit peak HIV-1 replication by 90 percent for eight long-term survivors, as follows: Subject 2, 40,000 CD8$^+$ lymphocytes; Subject 3, 200,000; Subject 4, 200,000; Subject 5, less than 300; Subject 6, 1 million; Subject 7, less than 40,000; Subject 8, 200,000; and Subject 10, 200,000.   These findings show that long-term survivors had a quantitatively greater HIV-1 — suppressive response to CD8$^+$ lymphocytes than did subjects with progressive disease, in whom 1 million autologous CD8$^+$ lymphocytes were generally required to induce substantial inhibition of viral replication [22 – 24].

Neutralizing Activity of Plasma against HIV-1

Having detected evidence of a strong cellular immune response, we next turned our attention to the neutralizing activity of plasma samples from nine long-term survivors against a diverse panel of primary HIV-1 isolates.   The results are shown in table 2. Although primary HIV-1 isolates are known to be relatively resistant to neutralization by antibody and soluble CD4 [21, 29], plasma samples from our long-term survivors had broad neutralizing activity in general, especially when compared with the lack of neutralizing activity of plasma samples from subjects with progressive disease.   These findings suggest that the long-term survivors had vigorous functional antibody responses directed against HIV-1.

Characterization of the Biologic Properties of HIV-1 Isolates in vitro

As has been mentioned, infectious HIV-1 could not be isolated from six subjects despite multiple attempts using optimal protocols.   Nevertheless, HIV-1 was recovered from PBMC of three subjects (Subjects 8, 9, and 10) by a standard method and from a fourth (Subject 7) by a CD8-depleted coculture.   The kinetics of replication in these four isolates was assessed in normal activated PBMC, as shown in figure 4(a).   The isolates from Subjects 9 and 10 replicated to levels similar to that of a wild-type isolate (JRCSF); in contrast, the isolates from Subjects 7 and 8 both replicated to maximal levels of p24 antigen expression that were below 1000 pg per milliliter, a finding consistent with substantial attenuation of growth.   None of the four isolates were capable of infecting a number of T-cell lines, including MT-2 cells, and thus none were considered to have a syncytium-

Table 2. Effectiveness of plasma from long-term survivors and controls with progressive disease in inhibiting infection by primary HIV-1 isolates

Source of plasma (Subject)[†]	Primary HIV-1 isolate												
	From long-term survivors			From patients with acute infections				From asymptomatic patients		From patients with AIDS			
	From Subject 7	From Subject 9	Subject 10	VS	RA	JP	A	WM	N-70	JRCSF	JRFL	LS	AC
	reciprocal of plasma dilution that produced ≥90% inhibition of HIV-1 infection												
Long-term survivors													
2	16	16	—	16	64	—	64	16		32	64	32	32
3	8	16	64	8	64	64	16	32		—	32	256	>256
4	64	—	—	64	64	16	32	128		16	8	16	32
5	256	16	8	16	64	256	64	64		256	64	64	>256
6	256	16	—	64	32	64	16	16		64	—	256	32
7	128	—	8	8	8	32	128	32		64	128	64	32
8	16	8	—	16	256	8	16	128		64	—	64	8
9	—	—	—	—	32	256	8	256		—	16	—	—
10	32	8	—	—	—	>64	—	16		—	—	—	32
Controls with progressive disease													
A								8					
B											32		
C										8		8	
D												8	8

† Subject 1 was not included because of insufficient plasma samples. The control subjects included two asymptomatic carriers with low CD4$^+$ cell counts (Subjects A and B), a patient with AIDS-related complex (Subject C), and a patient with AIDS (Subject D).

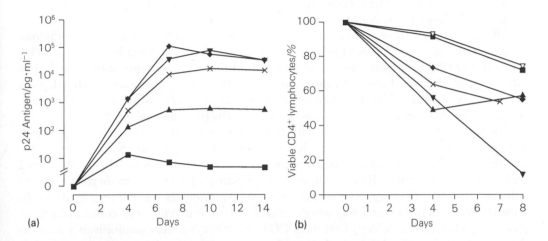

Fig. 4. Kinetics of replication (*a*) and cytotoxic effect on CD4+ lymphocytes (*b*) of HIV-1 isolates from long-term survivors and of the JRCSF isolate (▼).   Each symbol represents a study subject, identified in *table 1.* In (*b*), ▽ denotes a control culture without virus.

inducing phenotype.   The cytotoxicity of these isolates against normal purified CD4+ lymphocytes was also examined in vitro.   As figure 4(*b*) shows, the isolate from Subject 8 had no cytotoxic effect at all, whereas those from Subjects 7, 9, and 10 were somewhat cytotoxic, though less so than JRCSF, which is generally not considered to be one of the more cytotoxic variants among well-characterized HIV-1 isolates.   On the basis of these findings, we believe that viral attenuation was evident in Subjects 7 and 8.

Discussion

In the asymptomatic long-term survivors we have described, HIV-1 replication appeared to be well controlled, with the viral load in plasma and PBMC orders of magnitude lower than those typically found in subjects with progressive disease (fig. 1). Recently, low levels of HIV-1 in lymphoid tissues of other long-term survivors have also been reported [30].   These findings are consistent with those of a large number of published reports suggesting that disease progression is driven by an increasing viral burden [12, 14, 16, 18, 26 – 28, 31 – 33].

In eight of our long-term survivors (all except Subjects 9 and 10) there were distinctive virologic features.   Repeated attempts to isolate infectious HIV-1 from six of the eight subjects were unsuccessful (fig. 1); in the other two (Subjects 7 and 8), viral attenuation was evident (fig. 4).   These findings, coupled with the extremely low viral loads observed, suggest that these subjects may not merely represent one extreme end of the normal distribution of patients with HIV-1 infection.   These eight subjects were phenotypically similar to the long-term survivor reported by Greenough et al. [11].   In contrast, Subjects 9 and 10, who had higher viral burdens and wild-type-like viruses, were more similar to the subjects with long-term nonprogressive disease studied by Pantaleo et al. [30], who found higher viral burdens (mean plasma RNA copy number, 70,000 per milliliter) and obtained higher rates of virus isolation than those reported here.   It is not clear that such subjects, although they meet the current clinical definition of long-term survivors [6], will not have progressive disease in the coming years.

We also studied three potential mechanisms that would account for the low viral load in long-term survivors: host-cell resistance, strong immunity, and weakened virus. Our study of the CD4$^+$ lymphocytes in our subjects did find efficient replication of HIV-1 in vitro and the absence of gross intrinsic resistance to the virus. However, varying degrees of efficiency in viral replication were observed among the CD4$^+$ lymphocytes from these subjects, as we [34] and others [35] have seen with cells from normal donors.

In a manner consistent with an earlier report showing that persons with long-term nonprogressive disease have higher levels of HIV-1—specific antibodies and CD8$^+$ lymphocytes [36], we found evidence of vigorous immune responses to HIV-1. Figures 2 and 3 show a substantial HIV-1—suppressive response by CD8$^+$ lymphocytes in all the subjects studied. This suppressive effect of CD8$^+$ lymphocytes was not restricted to cells with HLA compatibility and was more efficient if there was cell-to-cell contact (data not shown). Therefore, it is likely that these CD8$^+$ lymphocytes were qualitatively similar to those with the virus-inhibitory characteristics described by Walker et al. [22 – 24]. Although the nature of these inhibitory cells remains elusive, it is known that clones of cytotoxic T lymphocytes, when activated in vitro, can mediate similar inhibition [37]. Cytotoxic T lymphocytes that recognize specific HIV-1 envelope, core, and polymerase products have been detected in samples of PBMC from Subjects 1 through 7 and 10 (unpublished data).

These long-term survivors also had potent and broad neutralizing-antibody responses against a diverse panel of primary HIV-1 isolates (table 2). This was in distinct contrast to findings in subjects with progressive disease [29] (and table 2). The presence of a high level of neutralizing-antibody activity and a vigorous CD8$^+$ lymphocyte response indicates that the immune system of the long-term survivors must have been continually exposed to viral antigens.

We obtained mixed results with respect to HIV-1 attenuation in long-term survivors. Subjects 9 and 10 had higher viral loads and harbored HIV-1 isolates that replicated as efficiently as wild-type viruses. In contrast, isolates from Subjects 7 and 8 showed markedly reduced rates of replication in vitro. We speculate that the degree of viral attenuation may have been even higher in the subjects from whom we could not isolate the virus. The viral genome of these long-term survivors is currently being characterized in order to elucidate the possible genetic basis of such attenuation. To date, no evidence of a gross *nef* defect has been found in our 10 subjects [38], although one such case has been identified by others [39]. Recently, defects in the NFκB and Spl sites within the viral long-terminal repeats have been found in two of our subjects (unpublished data).

Two previous reports strongly support the notion that viral characteristics have a critical role in long-term nonprogressive infection. First, Learmont et al. [10] described six recipients of blood transfussions from one HIV-1—infected donor who have remained well and immunologically stable despite a decade of infection. The blood donor has also remained healthy. This cluster of long-term survivors suggests the possibility that an attenuated virus was transmitted. Second, experiments carried out by Kestler et al. [40] showed that monkeys experimentally inoculated with simian immunodeficiency virus with deletions in the *nef* gene had no signs of disease and maintained low viral burdens along with normal CD4$^+$ T-cell counts. This study showed conclusively that viral attenuation can result in long-term nonprogressive infection.

In summary, the long-term survivors we studied had low levels of HIV-1 in the presence of strong virus-specific immune responses combined with some degree of viral attenuation, thereby tipping the balance in favor of the infected host.   The level of virus and the degree of immunity observed in these subjects could serve as important guideposts for our therapeutic and prophylactic efforts against AIDS.   Ideally, therapies should aim to reduce the burden of HIV-1 to the levels seen in long-term survivors or below, and vaccines should attempt to induce the type of immunity found in these subjects.   Most important, perhaps, long-term survivors of HIV-1 infection provide a ray of hope indicating that it is possible to live with the virus for prolonged periods without harm.

Acknowledgment

We are indebted to the study subjects for their participation, to R. Koup and J. Moore for helpful suggestions, and to W. Chen for the preparation of the figures.   Supported by grants (AI24030, AI25541, AI32427, and AI27665) from the National Institutes of Health (NIH) and an NIH contract on Correlates of Immune Protection, the Centers for AIDS Research of New York University, and the Aaron Diamond Foundation.
(N Engl J Med 1995; 332: 201 – 8)

References

1   Pantaleo G, Graziosi C, Fauci AS: The immunopathogenesis of human immunodeficiency virus infection. N Engl J Med 1993; 328: 327 – 35.
2   Lifson AR, Rutherford GW, Jaffe HW: The natural history of human immunodeficiency virus infection.   J Infect Dis 1988; 158: 1360 – 7.
3   Muñoz A, Wang M-C, Bass S, et al: Acquired immunodeficiency syndrome (AIDS)-free time after human immunodeficiency virus type 1 (HIV-1) seroconversion in homosexual men.   Am J Epidemiol 1989; 130: 530 – 9.
4   Jason J, Lui K-J, Ragni MV, Hessol NA, Darrow WW: Risk of developing AIDS in HIV-infected cohorts of hemophiliac and homosexual men.   JAMA 1989; 261: 725 – 7.
5   Rutherford GW, Lifson AR, Hessol NA, et al: Course of HIV-1 infection in a cohort of homosexual and bisexual men: an 11 year follow up study.   BMJ 1990; 301: 1183 – 8.
6   Schrager LK, Young JM, Fowler MG, Mathieson BJ, Vermund SH: Long-term survivors of HIV-1 infection: definitions and research challenges.   AIDS 1994; 8: Suppl 1: S95 – S108.
7   Buchbinder SP, Katz MH, Hessol NA, O'Malley PM, Holmberg SD: Long-term HIV-1 infection without immunologic progression.   AIDS 1994; 8: 1123 – 8.
8   Keet IPM, Krol A, Klein MR, et al: Characteristics of long-term asymptomatic infection with human immunodeficiency virus type 1 in men with normal and low $CD4^+$ cell counts.   J Infect Dis 1994; 169: 1236 – 43.
9   Sheppard HW, Lang W, Ascher MS, Vittinghoff E, Winklestein W: The characterization of non-progressors: long-term HIV-1 infection with stable $CD4^+$ T-cell levels.   AIDS 1993; 7: 1159 – 66.
10   Learmont J, Tindall B, Evans L, et al: Long-term symptomless HIV-1 infection in recipients of blood products from a single donor.   Lancet 1992; 340: 863 – 7.
11   Greenough TC, Somasundaran M, Brettler DB, et al: Normal immune function and inability to isolate virus in culture in an individual with long-term human immunodeficiency virus type 1 infection.   AIDS Res Hum Retroviruses 1994; 10: 395 – 403.
12   Ho DD, Moudgil T, Alam M: Quantitation of human immunodeficiency virus type 1 in the blood of infected persons: N Engl J Med 1989; 321: 1621 – 5.
13   Daar ES, Moudgil T, Meyer RD, Ho DD: Transient high levels of viremia in patients with primary human immunodeficiency virus type 1 infection.   N Engl J Med 1991; 324: 961 – 4.
14   Connor RI, Mohri H, Cao Y, Ho DD: Increased viral burden and cytopathicity correlate temporally with $CD4^+$ T-lymphocyte decline and clinical progression in human immunodeficiency virus type 1-infected individuals.   J Virol 1993; 67: 1772 – 7.

15   Pachl C, Todd JA, Kern DG, et al: Rapid and precise quantification of HIV-1 RNA in plasma using a branched DNA (bDNA) signal amplification assay.   J Acquir Immune Defic Syndr (in press).

16   Cao Y, Ho DD, Todd J, et al: Clinical evaluation of branched DNA (bDNA) signal amplification for quantifying HIV-1 in human plasma.   AIDS Res Hum Retroviruses 1995; 11: 353 – 61.

17   Fultz T, Todd J, Hamren S, et al: Quantitation of plasma HIV-1 RNA using an ultra-sensitive branched DNA (bDNA) assay.   Presented at the 2nd National Conference on Human Retroviruses and Related Infections, Washignton, D.C., January 29–February 2, 1995.   (Abstract).

18   Simmonds P, Balfe P, Peutherer JF, Ludlam CA, Bishop JO, Leigh Brown AJ: Human immunodeficiency virus-infected individuals contain provirus in small numbers of peripheral mononuclear cells and at low copy numbers.   J Virol 1990; 64: 864 – 72.

19   Koyanagi Y, Miles S, Mitsuyasu RT, Merrill JE, Vinters HV, Chen ISY: Dual infection of the central nervous system by AIDS viruses with distinct cellular tropisms.   Science 1987; 236: 819 – 22.

20   Ho DD, McKeating JA, Li XL, et al: Conformational epitope on gp 120 important in CD4 binding and human immunodeficiency virus type 1 neutralization identified by human monoclonal antibody.   J Virol 1991; 65: 489 – 93.

21   Moore JP, Cao Y, Qin L, et al: Primary isolates of human immunodeficiency virus type 1 are relatively resistant to neutralization by monoclonal antibodies to gp120, and their neutralization is not predicted by studies with monometric gp120.   J Virol 1995; 69: 101 – 9.

22   Walker CM, Moody DJ, Stites DP, Levy JA: CD8[+] lymphocytes can control HIV infection in vitro by suppressing virus replication.   Science 1986; 234: 1563 – 6.

23   Walker CM, Thomson-Honnebier GA, Hsueh FC, Erickson AL, Pan L-Z, Levy JA: CD8[+] T cells from HIV-1-infected individuals inhibit acute infection by human and primate immunodeficiency viruses.   Cell Immunol 1991; 137: 420 – 8.

24   Walker CM, Erickson AL, Hsueh FC, Levy JA: Inhibition of human immunodeficiency virus replication in acutely infected CD4[+] cells by CD8[+] cells involves a noncytotoxic mechanism.   J Virol 1991; 65: 5921 – 7.

25   Kannagi M, Chalifoux LV, Lord CI, Letvin NL: Suppression of simian immunodeficiency virus replication in vitro by CD8[+] lymphocytes.   J Immunol 1988; 140: 2237 – 42.

26   Michael NL, Vahey M, Burke DS, Redfield RR: Viral DNA and mRNA expression correlate with the stage of human immunodeficiency virus (HIV) type 1 infection in humans: evidence for viral replication in all stages of HIV disease.   J Virol 1992; 66: 310 – 6.

27   Bagasra O, Hauptman SP, Lischner HW, Sachs M, Pomerantz RJ: Detection of human immunodeficiency virus type 1 provirus in mononuclear cells by in situ polymerase chain reaction.   N Engl J Med 1992; 326: 1385 – 91.

28   Patterson BK, Till M, Otto P, et al: Detection of HIV-1 DNA and messenger RNA in individual cells by PCR-driven in situ hybridization and flow cytometry.   Sience 1993; 260: 976 – 9.

29   Cohen J: Jitters jeopardize AIDS vaccine trials.   Science 1993; 262: 980 – 1.

30   Pantaleo G, Menzo S, Vaccarezza M, et al: Studies in subjects with long-term nonprogressive human immunodeficiency virus infection.   N Engl J Med 1995; 332: 209 – 16.

31   Pantaleo G, Graziosi C, Demarest JF, et al: HIV infection is active and progressive in lymphoid tissue during the clinically latent stage of disease.   Nature 1993; 362: 355 – 8.

32   Embretson J, Zupancic M, Ribas JL, et al: Massive covert infection of helper T lymphocytes and macrophages by HIV during the incubation period of AIDS.   Nature 1993; 362: 359 – 62.

33   Piatak M Jr, Saag MS, Yang LC, et al: High levels of HIV-1 in plasma during all stages of infection determined by competitive PCR.   Science 1993; 259: 1749 – 54.

34   Spira AI, Ho DD. Effect of different donor cells on human immunodeficiency virus type 1 replication and selection in vitro.   J Virol 1995; 69: 422 – 9.

35   Williams LM, Cloyd MW: Polymorphic human gene(s) determines differential susceptibility of CD4 lymphocytes to infection by certain HIV-1 isolates.   Virology 1991; 184: 723 – 8.

36   Lifson AR, Buchbinder SP, Sheppard HW, et al: Long-term human immunodeficiency virus infection in asymptomatic homosexual and bisexual men with normal CD4[+] lymphocyte counts: immunologic and virologic characteristics.   J Infect Dis 1991; 163: 959 – 65.

37   Jassoy C, Harrer T, Rosenthal T, et al: Human immunodeficiency virus type 1-specific cytotoxic T lymphocytes release gamma interferon, tumor necrosis factor alpha (TNF-α), and TNF-β when they encounter their target antigens.   J Virol 1993; 67: 2844 – 52.

38   Huang Y, Zhang L, Ho DD: Characterization of nef sequences in long-term survivors of human immunodeficiency virus type 1 infection.   J Virol 1995; 69: 93 – 100.

39   Kirchhoff F, Greenough TC, Brettler DB, Sullivan JL, Desrosiers RC.   Absence of intact nef sequences in a long-term surviror with nonprogressive HIV-1 infection.   N Engl J Med 1995; 332: 228 – 32.

40   Kestler HW III, Ringler DJ, Mori K, et al: Importance of the nef gene for maintenance of high virus loads and for development of AIDS.   Cell 1991; 65: 651 – 62.

HIV Destroys the Nucleolus: Future Prospect of Molecular and Cellular Biology

Masakazu Hatanaka

Institute for Virus Research, Kyoto University, Kyoto and Institute for Medical Science, Osaka Japan

HIV Destroys the Nucleolus

HIV-1, a causative agent of acquired immunodeficiency syndrome (AIDS), is a complex retrovirus which disrupts human immune systems, and shares many features with non-transforming cytopathic lentiviruses.   Rev has a nucleolar targeting signal (NOS) [46] consisting of an arginine-rich motif in the middle region of Rev (amino acids 35 – 50) [24]. NOS can convey the cytoplasmic large protein to the cell nucleoi when fused in frame [46]. NOS is also proposed to be an RNA binding domain by which Rev interacts with the viral target mRNA, *rev* responsive element (RRE) [34].   Here we report a novel function of the NOS in Rev, that causes cell death.

Rev Deforms Nucleolar Structure

In the course of our immunofluorescence study using COS7 cells, we noticed that Rev induces morphological changes of the nucleoli.   Rev was found to induce nucleolar enlargement and deformity along with the level of Rev accumulation (fig. 1a–l).   Nucleolar damage was monitored by the simultaneous staining with anti-nucleolus antibody and also by the phase contrast microscopy.   Nucleolar enlargement with deformity revealed by Rev staining was accompanied with both sparse staining by anti-nucleoli antibody and increased phase-light regions with denser nucleoplasm.   We classified patterns expressing Rev into three stages by degree of nucleolar damage; stage 1 with intact nucleoli (fig. 1a–c), stage 2 with enlarged nucleoli, fine granular staining by anti-nucleoli antibody, and phase-lightness (fig. 1d–f), and stage 3 with markedly enlarged nucleoli, diffuse minute or scarce staining by anti-nucleoli antibody, and phase-lightness (fig. 1g–l).   Appearance of the stage 1 was seen in nearly 100% of the cells expressing Rev 14 hr after transfection with the Rev expressor, pH2rev.   In contrast, interface cells expressing Rev 66 hr after transfection showed the following distribution in three independent experiments; stage 1, 36%; stage 2, 26%; and stage 3, 38%, on the average.   Cells 48 hr after transfection showed a stage distribution intermediate between the 14 hr and 66 hr patterns (data not shown), suggesting that nucleolar structural changes depended on the degree of Rev accumulation.   On the other hand, Tat driven by the same promoter was found without an exception to have little effect on the nucleolar structure (fig. 1m–o).   pH2rev has no RRE in its own structure.   We, therefore, tested the effect on the nucleoli using pH2rexdL as a control, which is devoid of specific Ab anti nucleoli phase contrast

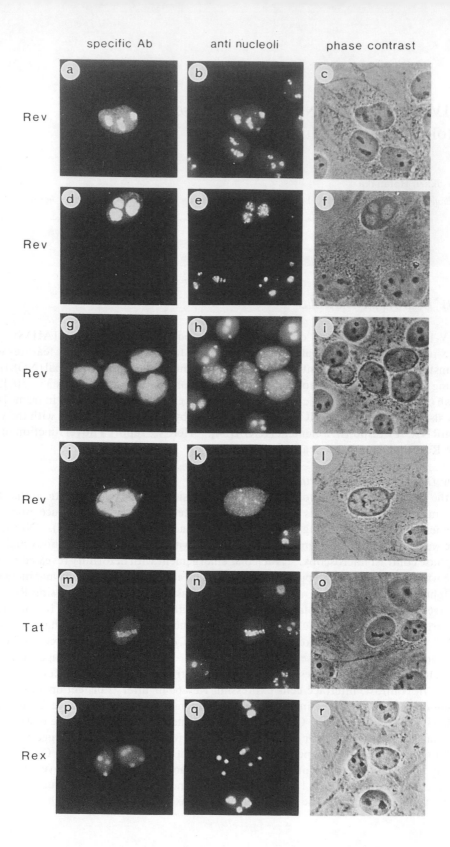

Rev

Rev

Rev

Rev

Tat

Rex

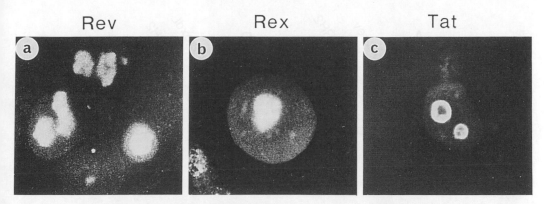

Fig. 2. Indirect immunofluorescence of cells transfected with HIV-1 or HTLV-1 proviral DNA. COS7 cells were transfected with 2.5 μg of pNL432 DNA harboring whole HIV-1 genome in pUC18 (a, c) or 9.6 μg of EcoRI digested λHTLVIC DNA harboring whole HTLV-1 genome in λgtWESλB (b). Cells were fixed 46 hr after transfection immunostained as in *figure 1* and viewed with a confocal laser scanning microscope.

the RXRE. Transfection of this plasma did not alter the nucleolar structure without an exception (fig. 1p–r). Rev expression in COS7 cells driven by the metallothionein promoter caused the similar damage to the nucleoli after metal induction (unpublished data). Transfection of a full-length DNA of HIV-1 [24] also revealed nucleolar deformity with Rev expression by CLSM (fig. 2a). However, that of HTLV-I [23 – 25] showed morphologically intact nucleoli in spite of nucleolar Rex expression (fig. 2b). Tat from the full-length HIV-1 genome was located either in perinucleolar region (fig. 2c) as in Tat alone expression driven by SV40 promoter, or within the deformed nucleoli (data not shown) due to co-expression of Rev. These findings indicate that Rev induces nucleolar deformity regardless in the presence or absence of RRE. Western blot analysis revealed that the expression level of Rev is not higher than that of Rex in COS7/SV40 system (fig. 3). The nucleolar deforming effect is, therefore, considered to be Rev-specific.

rRNAs Accumulate in Nucleoli with Rev

To examine the effect of Rev on the distribution of rRNAs, COS7 cells transfected with pH2rev or pH2rexdL were doubly stained with anti-Rev or anti-Rex antibody, and anti rRNA monoclonal antibody (kindly provided by Dr. J.A. Steitz) derived from an autoimmune MRL mouse. In the cells transfected with pH2rexdL (fig. 4a–c) or pH2rev (fig. 4g–i) 14 hr after transfection, rRNA staining was not affected by the expression of Rev or Rex. Sixty-eight hr after transfection of pH2rev, however, a great deal of rRNAs accumulated in the ballooned nucleoli and concomitantly decreased in teh cytoplasm

Fig. 1. Indirect immunofluorescence of cells transfected with Rev, Tat, or Rex expression vector. COS7 cells were transfected with 2 μg of each plasmid DNA (a–l, pH2rev; m–o, pH2Ftat; p–r, pH2rexdL), fixed 66 hr after trasfection, doubly stained with both FITC (for specific antibodies) and TRITC (for PSS serum), and viewed with a conventional fluorescence microscope. Antibodies used were rabbit antiserum against *N*-terminus of Rev (a, d, g, j), rabbit antiserum against *N*-terminus of Tat (m), rabbit antiserum against *C*-terminus of Rex (p), and PSS serum (b, e, h, k, n, q). Typical patterns of three different degrees of intracellular accumulation of Rev are presented. a, d, and both g and j represent stages 1-3, respectively (see the text). None of the cells highly expressing Tat or Rex showed nucleolar anomaly. Original magnification is ×320 in all photographs.

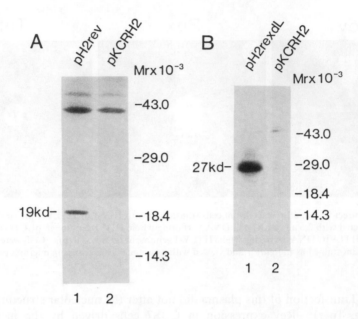

Fig. 3. Western blot analysis of transfected COS7 cells.   Cells on a 10-cm dish were transfected with 5 µg of each expression vector.   Rev and Rex were identified as p19 (A, lane 1) and p27 (B, lane 1), respectively.

(fig. 4j–r), while Rex did not alter the intracellular distribution of rRNAs (fig. 4d–f).   These findings suggest that only accumulated Rev can affect rRNA processing, probably due to rRNA trapping effect by Rev.

Accumulated Rev Blocks rRNA Synthesis

Nucleolar disintegration suggested a dysfunction of ribosome biogenesis in the cells highly expressing Rev.   To examine whether or not Rev affect de novo synthesis of rRNA, we performed pulse labeling of COS7 cells transfected with pH2rev or pH2rexdL using ^{3}H-uridine followed by immunostaining and autoradiography.   Although the cells expressing Rex or Rev 14 hr after transfection were not significantly affected for the uptake of ^{3}H-uridine (fig. 5a–c, g–i), uptake of ^{3}H-uridine was significantly decreased in the cells expressing Rev 70 hr after transfection (fig. 5j–l), compared with the cells expressing Rex (fig. 5d–f).   Transfection itself did not alter the distribution of ^{3}H-uridine compared with non-transfected cells (data not shown).

Fig. 4. Distribution of rRNAs in COS7 cells transfected with Rex or Rev expression vector.   Cells transfected with 2 µg of pH2rexdL (a–f) or pH2rev (g–r) 14 hr or 68 hr after transfection were doubly stained.   a, d, stained with anti-Rex antibody and FITC-conjugated anti-rabbit IgG antibody.   g, j, m, p, anti-Rev antibody and FITC-conjugated anti-rabbit IgG antibody.   b, e, h, k, n, q, anti-rRNA monoclonal antibody Y-10B, and TRITC-conjugated anti-mouse IgG antibody.   c, f, i, l, o, r, viewed by phase contrast microscopy.   Original magnification is ×320 in all photographs.   g–i and j–r represent stage 1 and 3, respectively.   Nucleolar accumulation of rRNAs in the cells expressing high levels of Rev is prominent.   These cells showed concomitantly decreased staining of cytoplasmic rRNAs.

specific Ab anti rRNA phase contrast

Rex 14 hr

Rex 68 hr

Rev 14 hr

Rev 68 hr

Rev 68 hr

Rev 68 hr

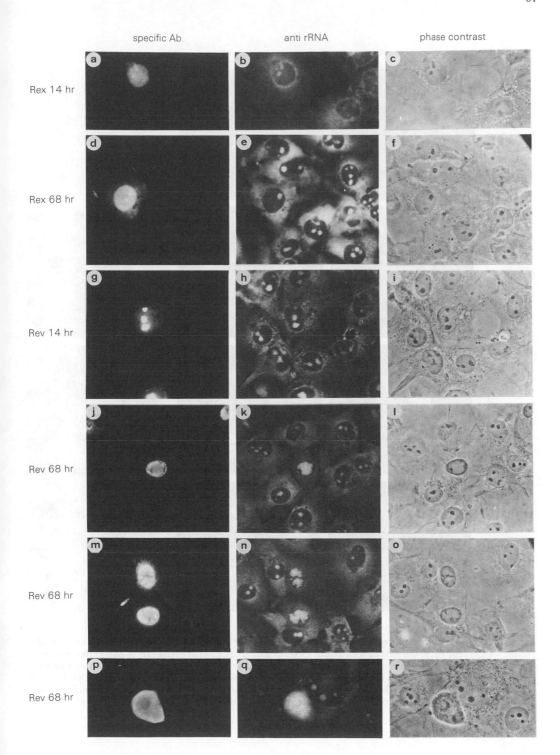

82

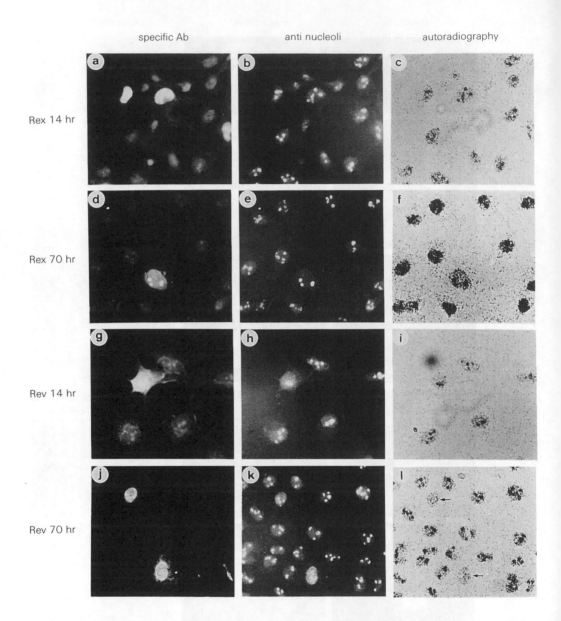

specific Ab   anti nucleoli   autoradiography

Rex 14 hr

Rex 70 hr

Rev 14 hr

Rev 70 hr

Fig. 5. Autoradiography with indirect immunofluorescence of cells transfected with Rex or Rev expression vector. COS7 cells were transfected with 2 μg of DNA of pH2rexdL (a–f) or pH2rev (g–l), pulse labeled with ^{3}H-uridine for 1 hr (a–c, g–i, 14 hr after transfection; d–f, j–l, 70 hr after transfection), immunostained with both FITC (for anti-Rex or anti-Rev) and TRITC (for anti-nucleoli) as in *figure 1*, and autoradiographed. Uptake of ^{3}H-uridine decreased only in the cells expressing Rev 70 hr after transfection (arrows in 1). The other cells showed nucleolar concentration of ^{3}H-uridine, indicating active rRNA synthesis. Original magnification is ×200 in all photographs.

Induced Rev Causes Cell Death by Nucleolar Destruction

Nucleolar disintegration by aberrant accumulation of Rev and rRNAs, and failure of rRNA synthesis may eventually result in cell death.   It has been difficult to stably express high levels of Rev in cells, probably due to toxic effect by Rev.   We, therefore, established inducible stable cell lines expressing high levels of Rev or Rex only in the presence of dexamethasone, pMAMrev, a Rev expressor driven by the mouse mammary tumor virus (MMTV) LTR, or pMAMrex, a Rex expressor driven by the same promoter, was introduced into BHK-21 cells.   Neomycin selection allowed us to establish the cell lines (fig. 6), since the parental vector, pMAM-neo, harbors a neomycin resistance gene.   Then each highly expressing clone of Rev (C147, 73) and Rex (C111) was selected.   When BHK/ Rev (transfectant of pMAMrev) was incubated with dexamethasone for 2 days, the nucleoli were disintegrated and the whole cell was swollen (fig. 6A, Bg–i).   These cells failed to exclude trypan blue (data not shown), indicating cell death.   In constant to Rev, neither BHK/Neo (transfectant of pMAM-neo) nor BHK/Rex (transfectant of pMAMrex) showed significant morphological change (fig. 6A, Ba–f) and excluded trypan blue (data not shown) when induced by dexamethasone.   No toxic effect of Rex is consistent with the results of previous study.   Cell growth curve of cloned BHK cells after induction by dexamethasone revealed the cytotoxicity of Rev (fig. 6C).   The cells of both Rev clones were markedly swollen within 2 days after induction.   To examine the effect of Rev on rRNA metabolism in induced BHK cells, total RNA was extracted from BHK cells, 25 hr after induction with dexamethasone.   As shown in figure 6D, the ratio of nuclear to cytoplasmic rRNAs was significantly elevated in the cells expressing Rev compared with those expressing Neo or Rex.

NOS of Rex Can Not Substitute for NOS of Rev in Nucleolar Damaging Effect

Since NOS of Rev may interact with the nucleolar components we examined whether it has a specific effect on the nucleolar disintegration (fig. 7).   As shown in fig. 8, chimeric Rev, pH2NOXrev whose NOS was substituted by the NOS of Rex [23], did not alter the nucleolar structure (fig. 8d–f); indicating that the NOS of Rev is essential for the nucleolar destruction.   However, chimeric Rex, pH2NOVrex whose NOS was replaced by the NOS of Rev, did not affect the nucleolar structure (fig. 8j–l); suggesting that another region of Rev besides the NOS is also required for the nucleolar damaging effect.   Simple positive charge effect by the 11 contiguous arginine cluster (pH2Argrex) was also shown to be insufficient for the damage of necleoli (fig. 8m–o).

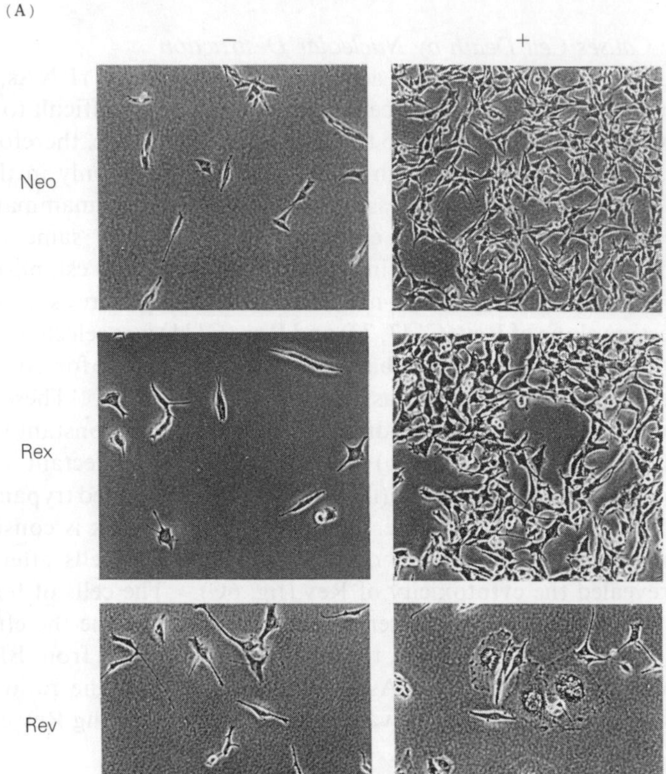

(A)

Fig. 6. Rev-mediated cell death in inducible BHK cells.

(A) Morphological change of BHK cells after Rev expression. Neo = BHK/Neo C143; Rex = BHK/Rex C111; Rev, BHK/Rev C173. − = just before induction; + = 48 hr after induction with 2 μM of dexamethasone. Cells (1×10^5) were plated on a 6 cm dish 16 hr before induction. Morphologically slender cells in induced Rev are spontaneously generated Rev non-expressors. These cells appear at high frequency in the course of passage. Original magnification is ×100 in all photographs.

(B) Indirect immunofluorescence of induced BHK cells. BHK/Neo (a–c), BHK/Rex (d–f), and BHK/Rev (g–i) cells were incubated with 2 μM of dexamethasone for 2 days and immunostained as in *fig. 1a*, incubated with both anti-Rex and anti-Rev antibodies, as a negative control. While Rex expression did not induce a morphological change (d–f), nearly 100% of the cells expressing Rev had disintegrated nucleoli and the whole cell was swollen (g–i). Original magnification is ×320 in all photographs.

(C) Cytotoxic effect of Rev in BHK cells. Cells retaining the ability to exclude trypan blue dye were counted at indicated intervals. Cells (5×10^4, viable) were plated 16 hr before induction (2 μM). Assays were performed in duplicate for each clone, and the average values of each clone were plotted.

(D) Nuclear accumulation of rRNAs in BHK/rev cells. 1×10^6 of BHK/Neo, BHK/Rex, and BHK/Rev cells were plated one day before dexamethasone induction. Cytoplasmic and nuclear RNAs were extracted separately from the same cells 25 hr after induction. One twentieth volume of cytoplasmic RNA and 1/10 volume of nuclear RNA were electrophoresed on 1% agarose gel. rRNAs were visualized by EtBr staining. Lanes 1,4, BHK/Neo cells; lanes 2,5, BHK/Rex cells; lanes 3,6, BHK/Rev cells. The relative ratios of the amount of nuclear to cytoplasmic RNA, compared with that of BHK/Neo cells, were 1.2 in BHK/Rex and 2.9 in BHK/Rev cells, when assessed by optical density. Positions of rRNAs are shown on the right.

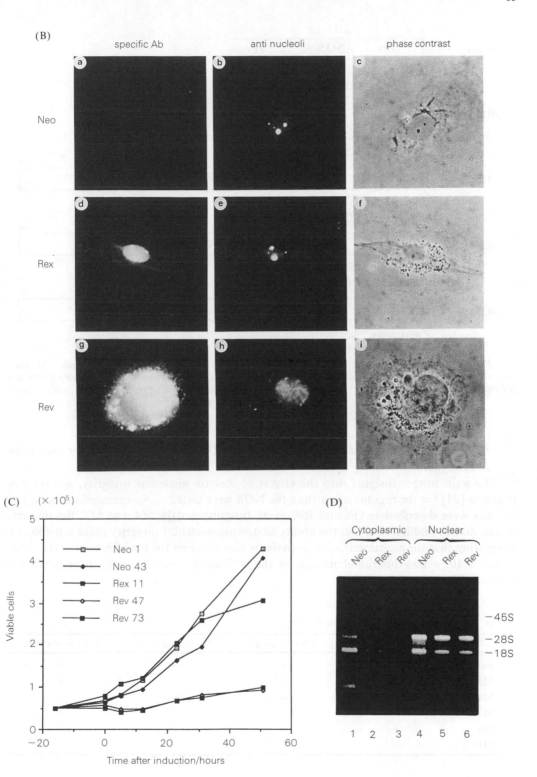

(B)

specific Ab   anti nucleoli   phase contrast

Neo
a   b   c

Rex
d   e   f

Rev
g   h   i

(C)   (× 10⁵)

Neo 1
Neo 43
Rex 11
Rev 47
Rev 73

Viable cells

Time after induction/hours

(D)

Cytoplasmic   Nuclear

Neo Rex Rev   Neo Rex Rev

−45S
−28S
−18S

1   2   3   4   5   6

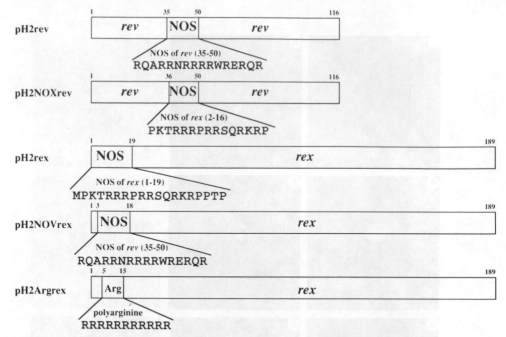

Fig. 7. Structure of the various expression plasmids. NOS = nucleolar targeting signal. All these plasmids have a common parental vector, pKCRH2 consisting of SV40 early promoter, β-globin splice sites, and SV40polyA addition signal.

Both NOS of Rev and the Multimerization Domain are Essential for Nucleolar Disintegration

To gain further insights into the effects of Rev on nucleolar integrity, several Rev mutants [31] for the regions other than the NOS were tested.   As summerized in table 1 (details were described in [Furuta RA, et al, (unpublished)]), M4 and M7, the mutants which do not multimerize, lost the ability to destroy nucleolar integrity (data not shown), suggesting that the multimerization domain, is also required for the effect.   On the other hand, M10, a non-functional mutant at the activation domain, could disintegrate the nucleoli (data shown later).

Table 1. Characteristics of Rev and its mutants

	trans-activation	RNA binding	Multimerization	Nucleolar damage
Rev	+	+	+	+
M3	+	+	+	+
M4	−	+	−	−
M7	−	+	−	−
M8	+	+	+	+
M10	−	+	+	+

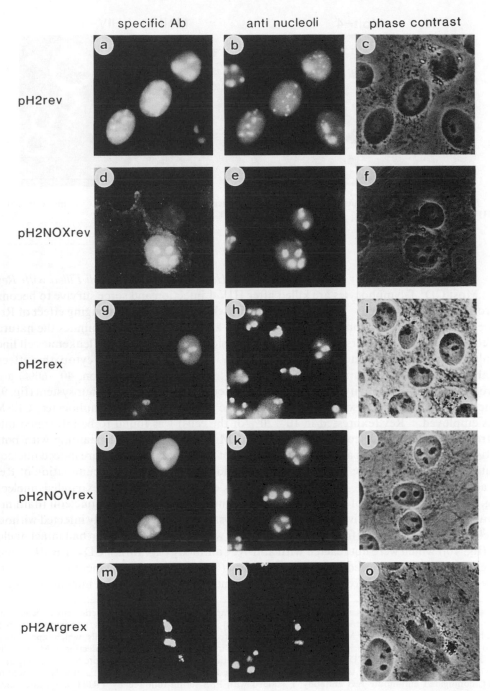

	specific Ab	anti nucleoli	phase contrast
pH2rev	a	b	c
pH2NOXrev	d	e	f
pH2rex	g	h	i
pH2NOVrex	j	k	l
pH2Argrex	m	n	o

Fig. 8. Indirect immunofluorescence of cells transfected with Rev, Rex, or their chimeric mutant expression vectors. COS7 cells were transfected with 2 µg of pH2rev (a–c), pH2NOXrev (d–f), pH2rex (g–i), pH2NOVrex (j–l), and pH2Argrex (m–o), respectively; fixed 66 hr after transfection; doubly stained as in *figure 1*; and viewed with a conventional fluorescence microscope. Only cells expressing wild type Rev had ballooned nucleoli.

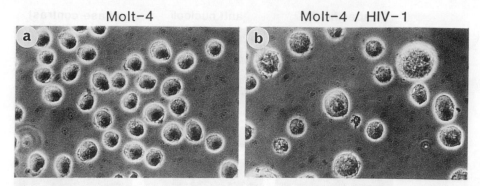

Fig. 9. Phase contrast microscopy of Molt-4 cells acutely infected with HIV-1.   a, mock infection; b, HIV-1 infection (day 7).

T-lymphocytes Acutely Infected with HIV-1 Have Deformed Nucleoli Filled with Rev

Most CD^4 T-lymphocytes are killed after HIV-1 infection and some survive to become chronically infected ones.   It is of interest to see whether nucleolar damaging effect of Rev observed in the transfection into fibroblasts or in an inducible cell line, mimics the natural infection of HIV-1.   At first we tested the expression of Rev in human T leukemic cell line, Molt-4 cells 7 days after in vitro infection of HIV-1, because maximum cytopathic effects (viability, 70 – 80%; syncytia formation, 5 – 10%; Gag or Env expression, 40 – 60%) and reverse transcriptase activity (1×10^7 cpm), are observed on days 7 – 10 in our system (fig. 9). Since conventional microscopy cannot reveal fine inner structure of lymphocytes, CLSM was employed.   Rev (expressed in 10 – 20% of the cells) was found to be infiltrated into extremely deformed necleoli (fig. 10a–e, h) of Molt-4 cells.   Double staining with both anti-Rev and anti-nucleoli antibodies revealed that the fluorescent spots are indeed nucleoli (data not shown).   Figure 10f represents the middle grade nucleolar accumulation of Rev in acutely infected cells.   Virtually all the cells expressing Rev had expanded nucleoli (fig. 10h), whereas most of the other cells hand morphologically intact nucleoli (data not shown).   In contrast surviving cells in the same system became chronically infected without nucleolar damage by Rev (fig. 10g).   Molt-4 cells without HIV-1 infection had intact nucleoli (fig. 10j) which were not reacted with anti-Rev antibody (fig. 10i).   CD4$^+$PBMCs from a healty donor also showed nucleolar deformity (fig. 10k) and enlargement (fig. 10l) with Rev 4 days after in vitro infection of HIV-1.   In contrast to T-lymphocytes, human monocytic

Fig. 10.   Confocal laser scanning microscopic tomographies of human hematopoietic cells infected with HIV-1.   Cells grown in RPMI1640 medium were suspended in PBS, dried on coverslips, and immunostained. a–f, h, acute infection (day 7) of Molt-4 cells; g, persistent infection (day 68) of Molt-4 cells, which represents in vitro growth of surviving cells derived from minor population in acute phase.   i, j, mock infection of Molt-4 cells; k, l, acute infection (day 4) of CD4$^+$ PBMCs; m, mock infection of CD4$^+$ PBMCs; n, acute infection (day 8) of U937 cells; o, mock infection of U937 cells.   a–i, k–m, stained with anti-Rev monoclonal antibody followed by FITC-conjugated anti-mouse IgG antibody; j, stained with PSS serum followed by TRITC-conjugated anti-human igG antibody; n, o, stained with anti-Rev monoclonal antibody followed by TRITC-conjugated anti-mouse IgG antibody.   d and e are extended-focus images consisting of 20 serial confocal images of 0.5 μm intervals. The others are the single image of tomography.   a–c are shown at every six confocal images in the orientation from the bottom (coverslip side) to the top, and constitute a part of d.   h–j, lower power fields (object lens ×60; zoom ratio, ×1.0) compared with the others (object lens, ×60; zoom ratio, ×3.0).

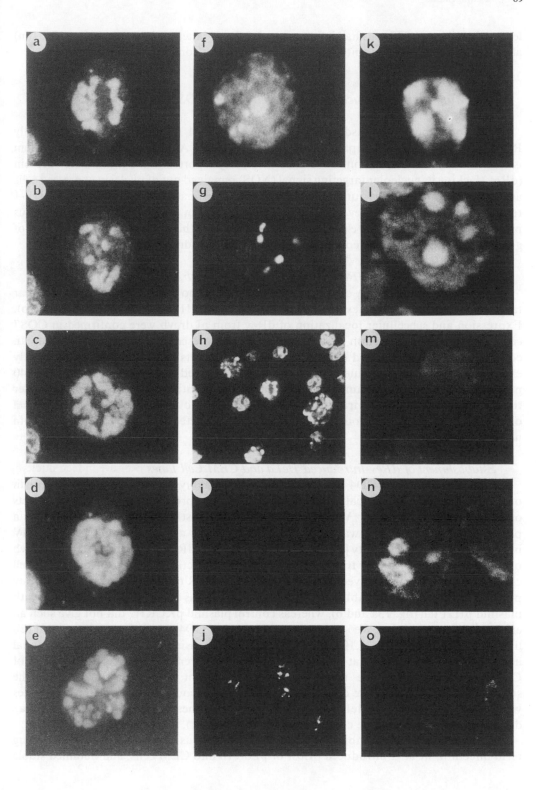

leukemic cell line, U937 cells had intact nucleoli 5 days (data not shown) or 8 days (fig. 10n) after infection of HIV-1 in spite of nucleolar Rev expression [38].

Rev Mutant without Nucleolar Dysfunction for AIDS Therapy

The applications of transdominant mutants of HIV-1 regulatory proteins especially Rev mutant, have been attempted for gene therapy against AIDS, because the Rev protein is essential for viral replication.   We have previously reported that a mutant Rev protein (dRev) lacking its nucleolar targeting signal (NOS) remained out of nuclei in expressed cells and strongly inhibited the function of Rev.   To investigate effects of dRev on HIV-1 replication, we established several dRev expressing human cell lines and examined virus production in these cells.   We demonstrate the efficacy of this mutant for an application of gene therapy against AIDS, comparing it with other transdominant mutants.

Efficient Expression of dRev in COS7 Cells by pLdrevb

We subcloned the cDNA of a Rev mutant with 7 amino acids deletion in its nucleolar targeting signal, named dRev (fig. 11a) [23], into an HIV-1 vector pLbsr (fig. 11b). Expression and subcellular localization of dRev from pLdrevb were confirmed in COS7 cells in transient transfection assay by a immunofluorescence technique (fig. 12).   In contrast to wild type Rev and other transdominant mutants [31], dRev protein efficiently expressed by pLdrevb, remained in cytoplasm of transfected cells like pH2drev with SV40 promoter [23].   We also examined expression and localization of the dRev protein under the control of a cytomegalovirus (CMV) promoter (fig. 11c).   pCdrev gave the high level of expression of the dRev protein in cytoplasm of transfected COS7 and HeLa cells (data not shown).

Establishment of dRev-Introduced HeLa and CEM Cell Lines

First, we established CD4 positive HeLa cell line stably transduced with *drev* gene in order to show subcellular localization of introduced gene products and to examine effects of dRev on virus infection.   We chose HeLa cl.1022 constitutively expressing CD4 as a parental cell line because it was originally established for a focal immuno assay of HIV infectants with high sensitivity [6].   After introduction of dRev expression vector pLdrevb or control plasmid pLbsr by transfection followed by selection with blasticidin S and cell cloning, integration of each vector was confirmed by PCR (data not shown).   The dRev proteins were detected in established cells only when Tat was expressed by transfection with plasmid pH2Ftat, (fig. 13a and b), whereas control plasmid pKCRH2 did not give such an effect (data not shown).   We also analyzed the level of CD4 expression on the cloned cell lines and parental HeLa cl.1022.   FACScan analysis using an anti-CD4 monoclonal antibody, Leu3a, revealed that there is no significant differences in the expression levels of CD4 molecules among the three cell clones (data not shown), assuming that the susceptibility to HIV of these cells could be the same.   Doubling times of three cell lines were as follows, 19.6 hr in HeLa cl.1022, 21.9 hr in cell lines containing pLdrevb (HeLa/dRev) and 23.2 hr in cell line containing pLbsr (HeLa/bsr), respectively.

In order to examine inhibitory effects of dRev on virus production in T-cells in long term infection, we next introduced pLbsr or pLdrevb into CEM cells, and obtained stable

(a)

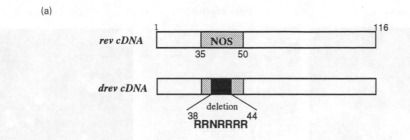

(b)

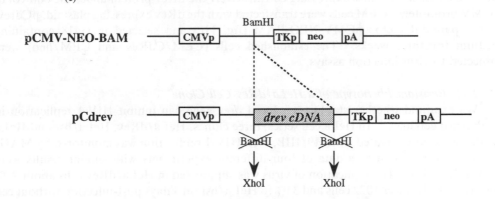

(c)

Fig. 11. (a), structures of cDNAs encoding wild-type Rev and the mutant, dRev. The deduced amino acid sequence of the deletion is shown by single-letter abbreviations. Numbers below hatched box of *rev* and above the delected sequence represent residue numbers counted from the first methionine of Rev.

(b), HIV-1 vector plasmid pLbsr and pLdrevb constructed from a full length proviral clone pNL43 (see materials and methods). The heavy lines represent the RRE in HIV-1 env sequence.

(c), structure of dRev expression vector under the control of CMV promoter. The parental vector pCMV–NEO–BAM contains eukaryotic expression unit with CMV promoter, BamHI cloning site, and selection maker gene. To make pCdrev, an EcoRI fragment of pLdrevb was inserted into cloning site of pCMV–NEO–BAM with XhoI linker. Abbreviations: *bsr* = Blasticidin S-resistant gene; LTR = long terminal repeat; NOS = nucleolar targeting signal; pA = simian virus 40 late polyadenylation signal; SVp=simian virus 40 early promoter; CMVp = cytomegalovirus promoter; TKp = thymidine kinase promoter; *neo* = G418-resistant gene.

anti-Rev   phase contrast   anti-nucleoli

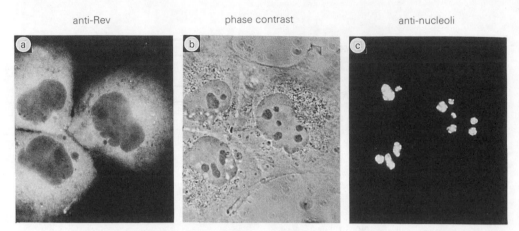

Fig. 12.   Intracellular localization of dRev expressed by pLdrevb.   COS7 cells were transfected with 6 μg of pLdrevb, fixed 48 hr after transfection and stained with both FITC for anti-Rev antiserum (a) and TRITC for serum from a patient with progressive systemic sclerosis (c).   Phase-contrast microscopic view of the same cells (b).

transfectants after selection by blasticidin S and cell cloning.   FACScan analysis also revealed that mean fluorescence intensity given by an anti-CD4 monoclonal antibody were the same among the parental CEM cells, CEM bsr cells (CEM/bsr), CEM dRev mixed population (CEM/dRev mix.), and CEM dRev cloned cells (CEM/dRev cl.) (data not shown).   Doubling time of these cell lines were also almost the same.   In addition, we established CEM cell lines expressing constitutively the dRev protein under the control of a CMV promoter.   CEM cells were transfected with the dRev expressing plasmid, pCdrev, or the parental vector pCMV-NEO-BAM (fig. 11c) and selected in G418 containing medium for three weeks.   The established cells (CEM/CdRev and CEM/neo) were subjected to virus infection assays.

HIV-Resistant Phenotype of a HeLa/dRev Cell Clone

We examind whether stably transduced *drev* gene can inhibit HIV-1 replication in established cell lines.   In HeLa cell series, three clones, HeLa/dRev, HeLa/bsr and HeLa cl.1022 were co-cultivated with H9/IIIB, then HIV-1 replication was monitored by MAGI assay.   The representative data of four different experiments with similar results were shown (fig. 14a).   The replication of virus was suppressed in HeLa/dRev cells about 27% compared to HeLa cl.1022 cells and 35% to HeLa/bsr on 4 days post-infection without cell passage.   Next, we compared the rate of syncytium formation among these cell lines (fig. 14b).   While we observed many syncytia 4 days after infection in control cells, the rate of syncytium formation was very low in HeLa/dRev cells.   Since HIV mediated syncytium formation depends upon the interaction of CD4 and gp120–gp41 complex [22, 29], it reflects the expression of *env* gene induced by the Rev protein, suggesting that dRev efficiently blocked the Rev function of HIV-1 in stably transduced cells.   In order to clarify that dRev conferred such an HIV-1 resistant phenotype on HeLa cells through inhibition of the function of Rev, we examined subcellular localization of viral and anti-viral proteins in the infected HeLa cell.   Rev was localized in nuclei/nucleoli in infected HeLa/bsr, and

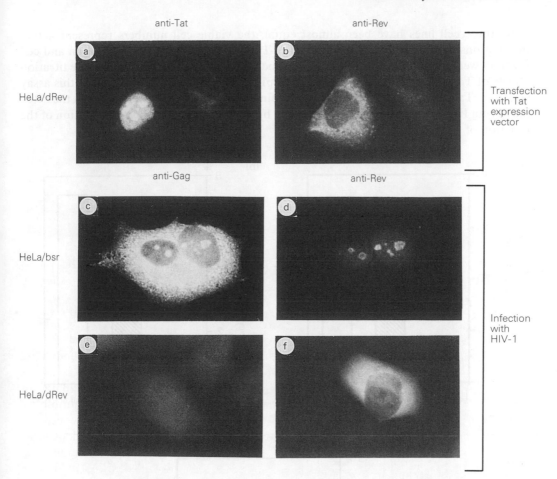

Fig. 13. Tat dependent expression of the dRev proteins in a dRev-introduced cell clone, HeLa/dRev (a and b), and subcellular localization of viral proteins in infected HeLa cells (c–f). The cells of HeLa/dRev were transfected with 4 µg of pH2Ftat, fixed 48 hr after transfection and stained with both TRITC for ant-Tat monoclonal antibody (a) and FITC for anti-Rev antiserum (b). HeLa/dRev and HeLa/bsr were infected with HTLV-IIIB, fixed 48 hr post infection and stained with both TRITC for ant-p24 Gag monoclonal antibody (c and e) and FITC for anti-Rev antiserum (d and f).

viral structural protein, p24 Gag was strongly expressed in all of these cells (fig. 13c and d). These results confirmed that Rev effectively functions in nuclei and induced the synthesis of viral structural proteins.   On the contrary, in HeLa/dRev cells infected with HIV-1, Rev was detected only in cytoplasm, and p24 Gag was not detected in the same cell (fig. 13e and f).   We believe that the cells positively stained in cytoplasm by anti-Rev antibody were infected, because the antibody used here recognize both wild type and mutant Rev and also because the gene expression of both *rev* and *drev* depended on Tat as shown in figures 13a and 13b.   These data indicate that dRev interfered the localization of Rev and that the viral replication was suppressed in these cells.

In addition, many HeLa/dRev cells were alive compared to other control cells on day 6 post infection (fig. 14c).   Since the doubling time and the amount of CD4 expression of these three cell lines have been almost equal, the viable cell numbers represent actual populations escaped from cell death by HIV-1 infection.   Syncytium formation and cell viability were almost the same in HeLa/bsr and HeLa cl.1022, suggesting that the titration effects of Tat and Rev by TAR and RRE of pLbsr vector were not observed in this assay system.   Taking considerations of the above findings together, we concluded that the dRev harboring HeLa cells escaped from cell death by HIV-1 infection through inhibition of the function of Rev.

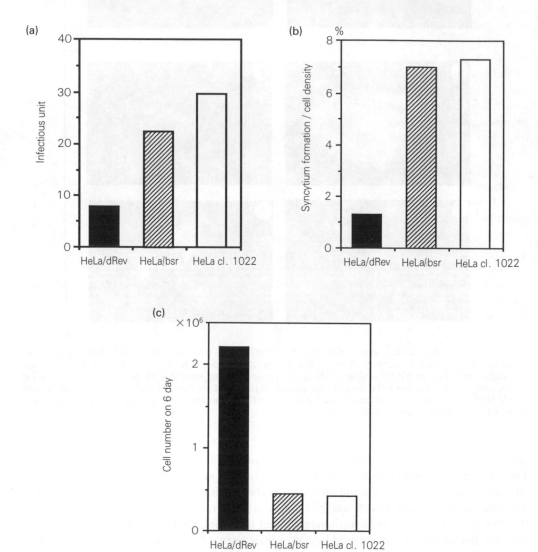

Fig. 14.   Effects of drev gene stably transduced in CD4 positive HeLa cells against infection by HIV-1.   The cloned HeLa dRev cells, HeLa bsr and parental HeLa cl.1022 were co-cultivated with chronically infected H9 cells for 48 hr.   Four days after infection, HeLa cells were assayed for the virus replication that was monitored by MAGI assay (a) (see materials and methods).   The rate of syncytium formation (b) and viable cell numbers counted by trypan blue exclusion (c) are also displayed.

The Inhibitory Effects of dRev on Virus Production in CEM Cells

We established *drev* introduced CEM cells to examine whether dRev does work as an anti-viral molecule in human T-cell line as well as in CD4 positive HeLa cells.   First, we examined effects of dRev under the control of HIV-1 LTR.   Parental CEM cells and stably transduced CEM series (CEM/bsr, CEM/dRev mix., and CEM/dRev cl.) were infected with HTLV-IIIB via cell-free infection at a MOI of 0.001 – 0.05.   Virus production of each cells was quantified by MAGI assay.   Figure 15a shows one of the typical result among five experiments independently performed with various MOIs.   The production of virus in control CEM increased from day 18 post infection.   An increase in the number of infectious unit of CEM/bsr cell was observed on day 20.   Whereas, virus production in both dRev introduced mixed population and cloned cell line has remained very low, though a little increase was observed on days 20 and 24.   This increase could be explained by the insufficient amount of dRev, because dRev was expressed under the control of HIV-1 LTR in these cells.   Therefore, we next performed another infection assay using cells expressing dRev by CMV promoter.   The RT activities of control CEM/neo cells reached the peak on day 12 (fig. 15b).   In CEM/CdRev cells, however, no significant virus production was seen through the experimental period.

In order to confirm that these cells were equally susceptible to HIV-1, we analyzed the viral DNA in the infected cells by a PCR method (fig. 15c).   Forty eight hour post infection, genomic DNAs were prepared from the CMV/CdRev and CMV/neo cells and subjected to semi-quantitative PCR.   Almost same level of HIV-1 specific fragments were amplified from DNA both of CEM/neo and CEM/CdRev.   PCR products of human β-globin gene of CEM/neo and CEM/CdRev cells 48 hr post infection were observed as same, assuming that the DNA of these cells had been amplified eaqualy in this PCR condition, therefore, there was not great difference in the amount of the viral DNA between these cells.   These data clearly demonstrated that the HIV-1 infection to these cells occurred equally.   We therefore, concluded that dRev inhibited the virus production in T-cells as well as in HeLa cells.

dRev is Free from Nucleolar Side-Effects Observed in Another Transdominant Rev Mutant

We have previously found that overexpressed Rev proteins have cytotoxic effects in some cell lines, and these effects were also observed in the cells introduced with Rev mutants including a transdominant mutant [38].   It has been reported that a transdominant mutant Rev M10 was able to block HIV-1 replication in stably transduced cells, and its potential use for gene therapy has been suggested [3, 32].   Cytotoxic effects by dRev, Rev, and RevM10 were examined.   We transfected wild type or mutant Rev expression vectors into COS7 cells, and doubly immunostained with anti-Rev and anti-ribosomal RNA antibodies.   The nucleoli of COS7 cells were deformed and ballooned 48 hr after transfection with wild type Rev or M10 expressor, and ribosomal RNAs disappeared mostly in those cells (fig. 16a–f). These findings are not dependent on cell cycle (Dr. T. Nosaka, personal communication). In contrast, dRev has neither shown nucleolar destructive effects nor an aberrant distribution of rRNA in transduced cells, although the excess amounts of the dRev proteins were expressed (fig. 16g, h, and i) in the same conditions of experiments using Rev and Rev M10.

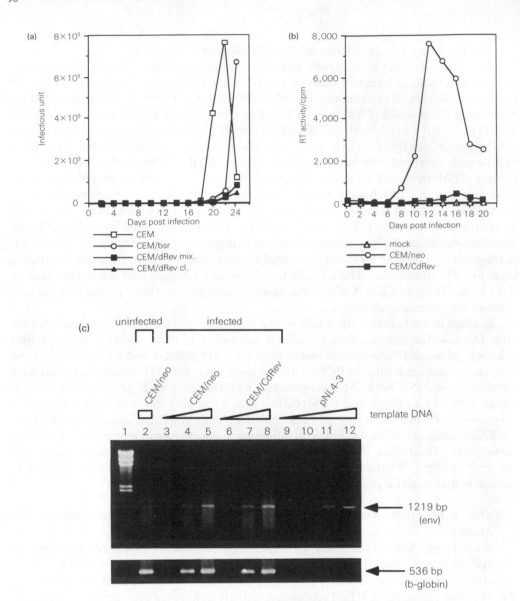

Fig. 15. The inhibitory effect of dRev on the virus production in CEM cells. (a) pLbsr or pLdRevb were stably transduced into CEM cells and HTLV-IIIB was added to 2×10^5 of parental CEM cells and each transfectants (CEM/bsr cell, CEM/dRev mixed population, and CEM/dRev cloned cells) at a MOI=0.001. The titer of culture supernatant was quantitated every other day by MAGI assay. (b) the RT activities of culture supernatant of infected CEM cells containing pCdRev (CEM/CdRev) or pCMV–NEO–BAM (CEM/neo) at a MOI=0.05 were shown. (c) viral DNAs of these cells on day 4 post infection were analyzed by semiquantitative PCR with primer pair to amplify HIV-1 specific DNA (see materials and methods). Upper panel: Ten microliter of PCR reaction mixture was applied to each lane. Lane 1 is a size maker (λ phage DNA digested with HindIII). The amount of DNAs used as a template as follows; lane 2, 25 μl of DNA of uninfected CEM/neo cells (negative control); lane 3–5, 1 μl, 5 μ and 25 μl of infected CEM/neo DNA, respectively; lane 6-8, 1 μl, 5 μl and 25 μl of infected CEM/Cdrev DNA, respectively; lane 9–12, 1pg, 5pg, 25pg and 125pg of pNL4-3 DNA. Lower panel: An internal control PCR was also carried out with primer pair for human β-globin gene. Five microliter of PCR reaction mixtures was applied into each lane which corresponds to template DNAs of upper lane, respectively.

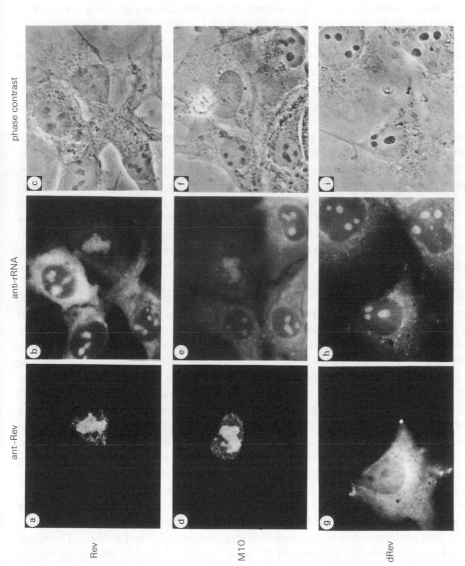

Fig. 16. Distribution of rRNA in COS7 cells transfected with Rev or mutant Rev expression vector. Cells transfected with 5 µg of pH2rev (a–c) or pH2revM10 (d–f) or pH2drev (h–g) were doubly stained 48 hr after transfection. (a), (d) and (h) were stained with rabbit anti-Rev serum and FITC-conjugated anti-rabbit IgG antibody. b, e and i were stained with mouse anti-rRNA monoclonal antibody Y-10B and TRITC conjugated anti-mouse IgG antibody. (c, f) and (g) were viewed by phase-contrast microscopy.

Future Prospect of Molecular and Cellular Biology

In this study, we demonstrated that dRev suppressed HIV-1 production in the several stable transformants with *drev* gene, and clearly show that this suppression was due to interference with Rev localization by dRev in infected HeLa cells, which we have previously reported in co-transfection assay [23].

We introduced *drev* gene into two human cell lines, CD4 positive HeLa cells and CCRF-CEM cells, by two different vectors and found that the virus production by the dRev harboring cells were apparently lower than that by control cells in the all cells tested here. The vector, pLbsr, used in this study was designed as a retroviral vector so that the introduced gene is expressed under the control of HIV-1 LTR, and that the genomic RNAs of the vector is expected to be packaged into a virion in the presence of the Rev and viral structural proteins. Furthermore, mRNA of pLbsr contains two important secondary structural region, TAR and RRE, which are expected to titrate Tat and Rev of HIV. We, however, transduced it into the cells by transfection in this study because packaging devices for HIV vectors are still under development [42, 44]. We measured virus production in culture supernatant from cells expressing *drev* by this vector by MAGI assay, because mRNA transcribed from pLbsr or pLdrevb containing the packaging signal of HIV-1 might be packaged into virion, and so that the amount of p24 and RT activity in culture supernatant of these cells may reflect production of such pseudovirions in addition to wild type ones.

The dRev protein was efficiently expressed in cytoplasm of the transfected COS7 cell from this vector (fig. 12), and the expression of dRev was regulated in stably transduced HeLa cells in a Tat dependent manner (fig. 13a and b). Moreover, dRev was highly expressed and worked as an antiviral molecule when the *drev* introduced HeLa cell was infected with HIV-1 (fig. 13c–f), in which we found the different localization of the functional or unfunctional Rev by immuno-fluorescence. In the infected HeLa/dRev cells, syncytium formation which is one of the typical cytopathic effects observed in HIV-infected cultured cells was suppressed (fig. 14b) and virus production was also suppressed as compared with parental HeLa cl.1022 cells (fig. 14a). A slight inhibition was also seen in HeLa/bsr cells, probably reflecting the titration effects of TAR and RRE against Tat and Rev as discussed above. Furthermore, the number of viable HeLa/dRev cells on day 6 post infection far exceeded than that of the control cells (fig. 14c). Therefore, we concluded that dRev conferred HIV-resistant phenotype on the introduced HeLa cell.

We also performed a cell-free infection study using CEM cells, and found that the virus production was also suppressed in CEM/dRev cells. A delay of the virus production was seen in CEM/bsr probably due to the same effects observed in HeLa/bsr. The virus production was not completely suppressed by dRev in HIV-1 vector system, probably because the expression level of dRev was not sufficient for complete inhibition in this experimental condition. In contrast, almost complete inhibition was observed in CEM/CdRev cells in which *drev* was driven by CMV promoter. Bahner et al. [3] also reported that the retroviral vectors containing transdominant mutant *Rev* gene driven by cytomegalovirus promoter worked more effectively than that by HIV-1 LTR. We believe that Tat dependent expression of anti-HIV molecules may be safe in gene therapy against

AIDS because transduced gene products are not expected to be expressed at a high level without HIV infection and the HIV vector could transfer genes into the HIV target cells in vivo, yet the suppressive effect in this system was not complete.   Further investigation for an more efficacious transmission and expression system of anti-HIV molecules would be necessary.

Although the precise mechanisms of the inhibitory effect of dRev has not been proved yet, it is evident that Rev can not migrate into cell nucleus/nucleous and does not function in the presence of dRev.   Very recently, Duan et al. reported an intracellularly expressed anti-Rev single-chain antibody.   They claimed that the antibody changed the localization of Rev and decreased HIV-1 replication in human cell, which was very similar results to ours [12].   The mechanism how dRev can retain Rev in cytoplasm has not been clarlified.   It is possible that dRev may compete with Rev in cytoplasm for some cellular factors, which carry Rev into nucleus/nucleous.   We, however, presume that dRev may not interact with such molecules, since dRev lacks its nucleolar targeting signal.   Alternatively, dRev may form a hetero-oligomer with Rev, which cannot migrate into nucleus/nucleolus as hypothesized previously [23].   It was reported that an excess amount Rev makes oligomer without RRE and some Rev mutants with substitutions in nuclear targeting signal form a hetero-oligomer with wild type Rev [40].   Multimer formation of Rev with or without RRE, however, remains unsettled.

It is important to mention that dRev works only in cytoplasm of the introduced cell. Until now, a variety of retroviral vectors have been created to inhibit HIV replication, but most of them were designed to work on the events in the nuclei of infected cells, for example, antisense RNA for viral mRNA [30, 35], ribozymes for viral RNAs [39, 45], so-called TAR decoys as competitors of TAR RNA [47] and transdominant mutants of HIV regulatory proteins [3, 28, 32].   Since interactions with cellular components may be necessary for the viral regulatory proteins to function in the nucleus of the infected cell [48], these anti-HIV viral analogues can interact with such cellular factors.   Thus, if large amount of shams of viral products are introduced into cell nuclei as anti HIV reagents, they may affect not only viral replication but also cellular function.   We recently reported that Rev protein has cytotoxic activity with nucleolar dysfunction caused by the failure of ribosomal biosynthesis, and the effect was observed in transfected cells and in T cells acutely infected with HIV-1 but not in chronically infected cells [38].   These observations indicated that the high expression of Rev may be lethal to cells.   Here, we also demonstrated that a highly expressed transdominant mutant RevM10 induced nucleolar ballooning and deformity with aberrant accumulation of rRNAs like wild type Rev in transfection experiments (fig. 16).   Although, these phenomena could be explained by the excess amount of expression, dRev did not show such effects at the same level of expression.   To sum up, dRev remains in cytoplasm, inhibits viral replication effectively, and does not affect nuclear events directly.   Malim et al. showed that transduced RevM10 gene produced effective blockade against HIV-1 in CEM cells without remarkable side-effects on some T cell functions using selected clones of transduced cells [32].   Also similar results have been shown by Bahner et al., and they discussed that it is important to check the toxicity of these gene on normal cellular function [3].   We think that much should be done to examine toxicity of transduced gene products in various conditions.

Our data reported previously [23, 38] and here suggest that it is possible that dRev protein blocks cell death caused by HIV-1 through two pathways.   One is an inhibitory effect on viral protein production, including *env* gene product, which induced cell death (reviewed in 16, 21).   The other is that dRev is able to retains Rev in cytoplasm to prevent Rev from nucleolar accumulation which may cause nucleolar dysfunction occasionally leading cell to death.   Taking considerations of the above aspects together, we may reasonably conclude that dRev is a good candidate for gene therapy against AIDS.

Acknowledgments

The work presented in my lecture was performed by the following people:
Drs. Furuta RA, Nosaka T, Miyazaki Y, Kubota S, Sakurai M, Ariumi Y, Maki M, Hattori T: *Institute for Virus Research, Kyoto University*
Drs. Takamatsu T, Fujita S: *Kyoto Prefectural University of Medicine*
Drs. Sano K, Nakai M: *Osaka Medical College*
and
Dr. Sato A: Shionogi Institute for Medical Science.
We thank Dr. Cullen BR for anti-Rev antiserum and various *rev* mutant; Dr. Adachi A for pSE; Dr. Steiz JA for anti-rRNA monoclonal antibody; Dr. Chesebro B for HeLa cl.1022 cells, Dr. Gallo RC for HTLV-IIIB; Dr. Oroszlan S for devices of MAGI assay. We thank Dr. Sano K, *Diagnostic Research and Development Department, ASAHI Chemical Industry* CO., for help in measurement of the RT activity, and also thank Dr. Kondo A, Imada K, Sakaida H for help in FACS analysis.
This work was supported in part by grants from the Life Insurance Association of Japan and from the Ministry of Education, Science and Culture of Japan.

References

1   Adachi A, Gendelman HE, Koenig S, Folks T, Willey R, Rabson A, Martin MA: J Virol 1986; 59: 284.
2   Aldovini A, Young RA: J. Virol 1990; 64: 1920.
3   Bahner I, Chen Z, Yu XJ, Hao QL, Guatelli JC, Kohn DB: J Virol 1993; 67: 3199.
4   Baker SJ, Markowitz S, Fearon ER, Willson JKV, Vogelstein B: Science 1990; 249.
5   Chang DD, Sharp PA: Cell 1989; 59: 789.
6   Chesebro B, Wehrly K, Metcalf J, Griffin DE: J Infect Disease 1990; 163: 64.
7   Cook KS, Fisk GJ, Hauber J, Usman N, Daly TJ, Rusche JR: Nucleic Acid Res 1991; 19: 1577.
8   Cullen BR: Methods Enzymol 1987; 152: 684.
9   Cullen BR: J Virol 1991; 65: 1053.
10   Cullen BR: FASEB J 1991; 5: 2361.
11   Cullen BR, Green WG: Cell 1989; 58: 423.
12   Duan L, Bagasara O, Laughlin MA, Oakes JW, Pomerantz RJ: Proc Natl Acad Sci USA 1994; 91: 5075.
13   Endo S, Kubota S, Siomi H, Adachi A, Oroszlan S, Maki M, Hatanaka M: Virus Genes 1989; 3: 99.
14   Gendelman HE, Phelps W, Feigenbaum L, Ostrove JM, Adachi A, Howley PM, Khoury G, Ginsberg HS, Martin MA: Proc Natl Acad Sci USA 1986; 83: 9759.
15   Green MR: AIDS Res 1993; 3: 41.
16   Haseltine WA: FASEB J 1991; 5: 2349.
17   Hattori T, Sagawa K, Matsushita S, Koito A, Suto H, Matsuoka M, Yokoyama M, Takatsuki K: Jpn. J. Cancer Res 1987; 78: 235.
18   Hope TJ, McDonald D, Low J, Parslow TG: J Virol 1990; 64: 5360.
19   Izumi M, Miyazawa H, Kamakura T, Yamaguchi I, Endo T, Hanaoka F: Exp. Cell Res 1991; 197: 229.
20   Kimpton J, Emerman M: J. Virol 1992; 66: 2232.
21   Koga Y, Sasaai M, Yoshida H, Wigzell H, Kimura G, Nomoto K: J Immunol 1990; 144: 94.

22 Kowalski M, Potz J, Basiripour L, Dorfman T, Goh WC, Terwilliger E, Dayton A, Rosen C, Haseltine WA, Sodroski J: Science 1987; 237: 1351.
23 Kubota S, Furuta R, Maki M, Hatanaka M: J Virol 1992; 66: 2510.
24 Kubota S, Siomi H, Satoh T, Endo S, Maki M, Hatanaka M: Biochem Biophys Res Commun 1989; 162: 963.
25 Lee MH, Sano K, Morales FE, Imagawa DT: J Clinical Microbiol 1987; 25: 1717.
26 Lee TC, Sullenger BA, Gallardo HF, Ungers GE, Gilboa E: New Biologist 1992; 4: 66.
27 Lever A, Gottlinger H, Haseltine W, Sodroski J: J Virol 1989; 63: 4085.
28 Liem SE, Ramezani A, Li X, Joshi S: Human Gene Therapy 1993; 4: 625.
29 Lifson JD, Finberg MB, Reyes GR, Rabin L, Banapour B, Chakrabarti S, Moss B, Wong-Staal F, Steiner KS, Engleman EG: Nature (London) 1986; 323: 725.
30 Lisziewicz GJ, Sun D, Zon G, Daefler S, Wong-Staal F, Gallo RC, Klotman ME: J Virol 1993; 67: 6882.
31 Malim MH, Bohnlein S, Hauber J, Cullen BR: Cell 1989; 58: 205.
32 Malim MH, Freimuth WW, Liu J, Boyle TJ, Lyerly HK, Cullen BR, Nabel GJ: J Exp Med 1992; 176: 1197.
33 Malim MH, McCarn DF, Tiley LS, Cullen BR: J Virol 1991; 65: 4248.
34 Malim MH, Tiley LS, McCarn DF, Rusche JR, Hauber J, Cullen BR: Cell 1990; 60: 675.
35 Matsukura M, Zon G, Shinozuka K, Robert-Guroff M, Shimada T, Stein CA, Mitsuya H, Wong-Staal F, Cohen JS, Broder S: Proc Natl Sci USA 1989; 86: 4244.
36 Mishina M, Kurosaki T, Tobimatsu T, Morimoto Y, Noda M, Yamamoto T, Terao M, Lindstrom J, Takahashi T, Kuno M, Numa S: Nature (London) 1984; 307: 604.
37 Nosaka T, Siomi H, Adachi Y, Ishibashi M, Kubota S, Maki M, Hatanaka M: Proc Natl Acad Sci USA 1989; 86: 9798.
38 Nosaka T, Takamatsu T, Miyazaki Y, Sano K, Sato A, Kubota S, Sakurai M, Ariumi Y, Nakai M, Fujita S, Hatanaka M, Exp Cell Res 1993; 209: 89.
39 Ohkawa J, Yuyama N, Takebe Y, Nishikawa S, Taira K: Proc Natl Acad Sci USA 1993; 90: 11302.
40 Olsen HS, Cochrane AW, Dillon PJ, Nalin CM, Rosen CA: Genes Dev 1990; 4: 1357.
41 Perkins A, Cochrane A, Ruben S, Rosen C, J AIDS 1989; 2: 256.
42 Poznansky M, Lever A, Bergeron L, Hasltine W, Sodroski J: J. Virol 1991; 65: 532.
43 Queen C, Baltimore D: Cell 1983; 33: 741.
44 Richardson JH, Child LA, Lever AML, J Virol 1993; 67: 3997.
45 Sarver N, Cantin EM, Chang PS, Zaia JA, Lande PA, Stephens DA, Rossi JJ: Science 1990; 247: 1222.
46 Siomi H, Shida HS, Nam SH, Nosaka T, Maki M, Hatanaka M: Cell 1988; 55: 197.
47 Sullenger BA, Gallardo HF, Ungers GE, Gilboa E, Cell, 1990; 63: 601.
48 Trono D, Baltimore D: EMBO J 1990; 9: 4155.
49 Zapp ML, Hope TJ, Parslow TG, Green MR: Proc Natl Acad Sci USA 1991; 88: 7734.

Lentivirus Pathogenesis:
New Insights from New Technologies

Ashley T. Haase

Department of Microbiology, University of Minnesota, Minneapolis, MN, USA

The Natural Histories of Lentivirus Infections and Central Issues in Pathogenesis

Lentivirus infections in animals and humans progress through three stages of acute infection, persistent infection, and symptomatic reinfection (fig. 1).   In the first few weeks of infection, lentiviruses from visna-maedi in sheep to human immunodeficiency virus (HIV) in humans invade and replicate locally, spread via the lymphatics and blood stream, and multiply at secondary sites, primarily in the organs constituting the macrophage phagocytic system and lymphoid tissues (LT).   In HIV infection, this acute stage is accompanied in the majority of cases by flu-like symptoms, fever, pharyngitis and rashes and resolves with a virus-specific immune response.   The appearance of virus-specific antibodies and cytotoxic T lymphocytes (CTLs) also coincides with a dramatic decrease in circulating virus but, in contrast to other acute infections, infected cells persist despite the immune response.   Because there are relatively few symptoms or physical signs of disease in the course of the persistent infection, it has not been generally recognized until recently that this is stage of very active viral replication and host response to contain infection and repair the ongoing damage to the immune and other systems.   Eventually, however, over several years the cumulative pathological toll of lentivirus infection is manifest in the late symptomatic stages of infection to which the infected individual usually succumbs [1].

The central features then that distinguish lentivirus infections are the persistence of virus in the face of the host's immune response and the eventual disease that results after an incubation period measured in years.   In this article, I will focus on the role of covert infection in the persistence of lentiviruses, and the mechanisms and dynamics of immune depletion in HIV infection suggested by new single-cell technologies that we devised such as in situ PCR [2] that directly reveal the number and types of cells that harbor lentiviruses in the tissues of infected individuals.

Covert Infection and Persistence

I hypothesized many years ago that lentiviruses persist because they can establish covert infections in which the initial steps of the viral life cycle through formation of the provirus are completed but viral gene expression is so restricted that there is insufficient synthesis and

104

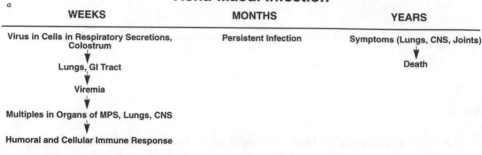

Natural Histories

Visna-Maedi Infection

a

WEEKS	MONTHS	YEARS

Virus in Cells in Respiratory Secretions, Colostrum
↓
Lungs, GI Tract
↓
Viremia
↓
Multiples in Organs of MPS, Lungs, CNS
↓
Humoral and Cellular Immune Response

Persistent Infection

Symptoms (Lungs, CNS, Joints)
↓
Death

b

HIV Infection

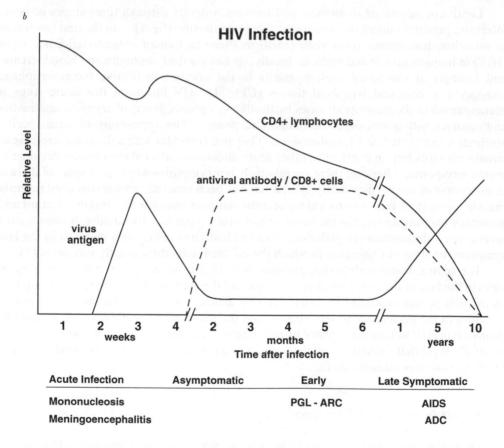

Relative Level

CD4+ lymphocytes

antiviral antibody / CD8+ cells

virus antigen

1	2	3	4	2	3	4	5	6	1	5	10

weeks   months   years

Time after infection

Acute Infection	Asymptomatic	Early	Late Symptomatic
Mononucleosis		PGL - ARC	AIDS
Meningoencephalitis			ADC

Fig. 1. Natural histories of lentiviral infections. Animal lentiviruses like Visna-Maedi and human lentiviruses (HIV) cause slow infections that progress through acute, persistent, and late symptomatic stages. Reproduced from [1] with permission.

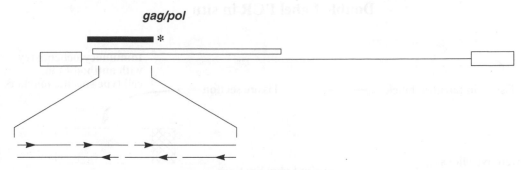

Fig. 2. Amplification and detection of the *gag/* region of the HIV genome using a multiple primer set.   The *gag/pol* region (▭) of the HIV previous with flanking long terminal repeats (□—□) and radioactive probe (■*) to detect the amplified product from are above and the MPS (→, ←) and products are shown below the provirus.   The primers are positioned such that the small products generated overlap and can base pair during the annealing step of the PCR.   In this way, the small products that are amplified most efficiently transiently form intermediates of sufficient size to be retained inside the cell.   At later stages of the PCR, these intermediates are extended to form covalently lonked stable products retained within the cell.

presentation of antigen for detection and destruction of the cell by host defenses [3].   It is only within the past few years that we have been able to show that there are latently infected cells in tissues that harbor a single copy of lentiviral DNA and few if any detectable transcripts or other evidence of viral gene expression.   The formal proof of the existence of these cells had to await development of methods with requisite sensitivity to detect 10 kb or 10^{-18} gm of viral nucleic acid in a cell.

In situ PCR

We devised in situ PCR to be able to detect latently infected cells.   As figure 2 illustrates, we use a set of multiple primers that generate overlapping segments of about 200 bases at the 5′ end of the HIV genome.   The overlaps can base pair during the annealing step of the PCR so that the size of the product is much greater than the individual segment. In this way, we solved the problem of the antithetical requirements of in situ PCR: only small DNA products are synthesized efficiently in fixed cells in tissues and only large products are efficiently retained [2, 4].

We also subsequently developed methods for in situ PCR applicable to fixed and paraffin-embedded tissues that can be combined with immunohistochemistry (fig. 3).   By reaching the tissue sections first with antibodies such as those that identify the CD4+ subset of T lymphocytes, we can identify and later enumerate cells of a particular type in which the subsequent in situ amplification and detection demonstrate viral DNA [5].

How and Where HIV Hides

With these methodologies in hand we could search for covertly infected cells and we chose to concentrate this search on LT which, from the natural history of lentiviral

Double Label PCR in situ

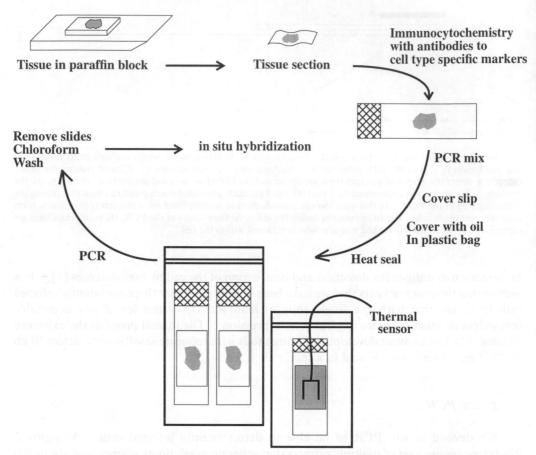

Fig. 3. Schematic representation of double-label PCR.   After tissue sections have been cut from fixed and embedded material and adhered to slides.   The sections are reacted with antibodies to cell-type-specific markers, e.g., CD4 and stained immunocytochemically.   The sections are then covered with the PCR reaction mixture containing the MPS, coverslipped, and placed in a bag with mineral oil, to prevent evaporation during thermocycling.   The thermal sensor is similarly placed in a bag with mineral oil.   After thermocycling, the slides are removed and washed with CHCl₃ and buffered saline.   The amplified product is detected by in situ hybridization with the radiolabelled probe shown in *figure 2*.   Modified from ref. 15 and reprinted by permission.

infections and other evidence [6 – 9] was the likely reservoir.   We examined LT from a variety of sites, deep and superficial lymph nodes, gut-associated LT, tonsils and spleen; and from earlier stages of infection, with no evidence of opportunistic infections; and the later symptomatic stage [5].

Even in the earlier stages of infection, and at all sites, there was evidence of HIV DNA in large numbers of cells.   In lymph nodes, most of the infected cells were scored with the double-label in situ PCR as CD4+ T lymphocytes in the follicular mantle and paracortical areas (fig. 4) with a smaller number in the germinal centers of secondary follicles.   There were also monocytes and macrophages with demonstrable HIV DNA in the lymph nodes

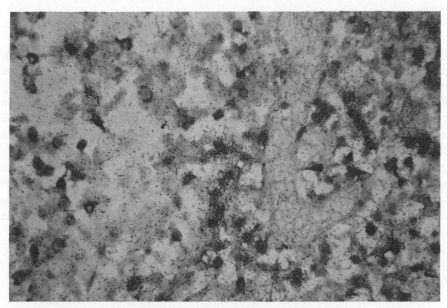

Fig. 4. HIV-infected CD4⁺ lymphocytes in a lymph node identified by double-label in situ PCR. After double-label PCR in situ, hybridization and radioautography, the section was stained and photographed in epipolarized and transillumination. Under these conditions, collections of silver grains representing the signal from cells whose nuclei contain HIV DNA impart a green appearance to the nuclei. CD4⁺ cells have been stained brown. The large numbers of cells in the paracortical region of this lymph node with green nuclei and brown cytoplasm are CD4⁺ T lymphocytes with HIV DNA. Reproduced with permission from ref. 16.

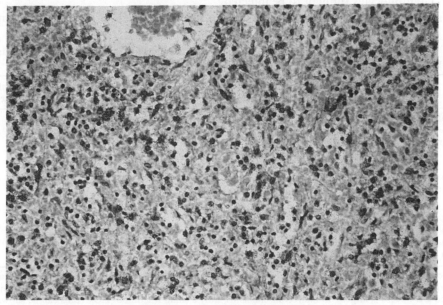

Fig. 5. HIV-infected macrophages in spleen identified by in situ PCR. The cells with green nuclei are fixed tissue macrophages in the red pulp of the spleen, identified by their morphology and anatomical location following in situ PCR. Reproduced with permission from ref. 5.

but by far the largest number of macrophages with viral DNA were the fixed tissue macrophages in the venous sinuses of the red pulp of the spleen (fig. 5).

To assess viral gene expression in the infected $CD4^+$ T lymphocytes and macrophages, we hybridized subjacent sections to a radiolabelled HIV-specific probe to detect viral RNA in situ.   As we had found in studies of animal lentiviral infections [10] about ninety percent of the cells with HIV DNA had no RNA detectable by this method (fig. 6a), with sensitivities in the range of a few copies of viral transcripts per cell [11].   About one percent of the cells with viral DNA had viral transcripts estimated to be as abundant as productively infected cells (fig. 6b).

In situ PCR and hybridization thus reveals a large reservoir of cells with the predicted characteristics to account for persistence, cells with the HIV provirus but no detectable viral RNA.   This analysis not only provided formal and direct experimental proof of how HIV-infected cells might elude host defenses but also where the covertly infected cells reside in LT.

The Mechanism and Dynamics of Immune Depletion

The new single-cell technologies, moreover, shed light on the mechanism and dynamics of immune depletion.   Initially, accounting for the loss of $CD4^+$ T lymphocytes in HIV infection appeared to be straightforward since the virus infected and killed these cells in vitro.   Direct mechanisms, however, fell out of fashion when HIV RNA could only be detected in a small fraction of the lymphocytes in the blood stream and LT [12].   The new theories (table 1) all involved indirect mechanisms consonant with the small fraction of $CD4^+$ T lymphocytes thought to be infected.

From the fresh perspective provided by in situ PCR much, if not all, of the immune

Table 1.   Theories on the mechanisms of immune depletion in HIV infection and predicted numbers of infected $CD4$ lymphocytes

Theory	Predicted number of infected $CD4^+$ lymphocytes
1. Infection of a large fraction of $CD4^+$ lymphocytes and/or progenitors. Cells killed pari passu with activation of viral gene expression, either directly or indirectly by elimination by host defenses.	Large
2. Productive infection of a small fraction of $CD4^+$ cells. Viral antigens shed, bind to uninfected cells which then die as a result of: a) syncytium formation b) host defenses c) superantigen elimination d) apoptosis	Small

Indirect mechanisms of immune depletion.   Viral replication in $CD4^+$ T cells, or recognition and elimination of cells with viral antigens by the immune system is responsible for the loss of cells.   The predicted number of infected $CD4^+$ cells is large.   In indirect mechanisms, only a small fraction of $CD4^+$ cells can be shown to be infected and other mechanisms must be invoked to account for loss.   The in situ PCR analyses provide evidence in favor of direct mechanisms.

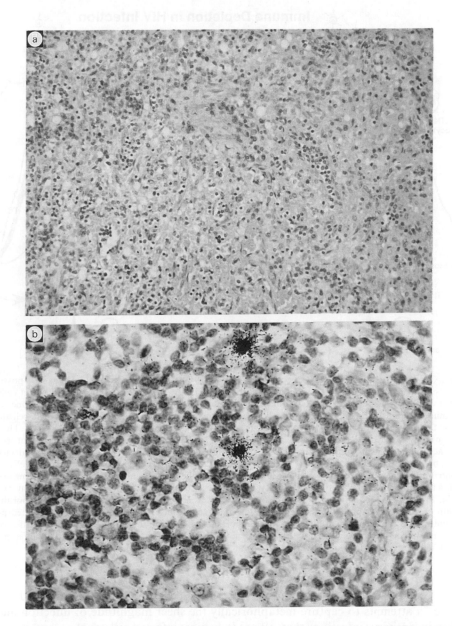

Fig. 6. HIV gene expression in LT. Subjacent sections subsequent to those used to detect HIV DNA (*fig. 4, 5*) were hybridized in situ with a radiolabelled probe to detect all classes of unspliced and spliced HIV RNAs. There was little evidence of viral gene expression in the fixed tissue macrophages of the red pulp of the spleen (*fig. 6a*) and only a small fraction of the cells with HIV DNA had viral RNA (*fig. 6b*). Two cells with signal equivalent to high levels of HIV RNAs in productive infections are shown *figure 6b*. The radioautograph was photographed conventionally so that the silver grains appear black.

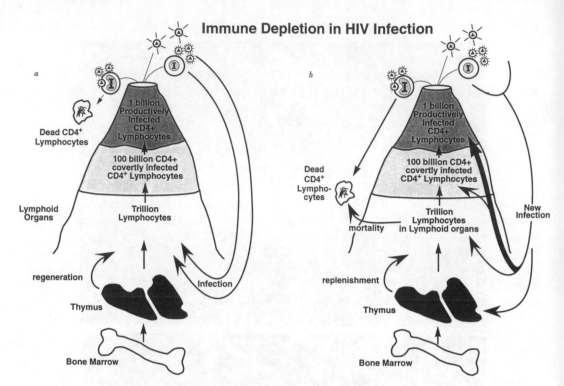

Fig. 7. Volcano model of HIV infection. The double-label PCR in situ method makes it possible to directly estimate how many CD4$^+$ lymphocytes harbor HIV DNA. In situ hybridization to detect cells with abundant viral RNA makes it possible to estimate the fraction with high levels of expression. If the bone marrow and thymus maintain a total of about a trillion lymphocytes in the adult the estimates from the single-cell analyses of LT are that about 100 billion CD4$^-$ T lymphocytes contain viral DNA but little if any viral RNA. This is the pool of covertly infected cells that provide a mechanism to elude host defenses and the reservoir that feeds the ongoing active infections. The latter are estimated to be about one percent or 1 billion productively infected cells (🔬). The virus (☼) and infected cells (🔬*) perpetuate the infections process (↓) by infecting other cells. They also contribute to immune depletion as they die or are killed by the host's immune system. The decline in CD4$^+$ T cells is a function of this loss, ordinary mortality, and regeneration of T cells from bone marrow and thymus. In *figure 7a*, the pool of productively infected cells is depicted as arising from the covertly infected pool through activation of viral gene expression accompanying an immune response. The model in *figure 7b* incorporates recent findings on the dynamics of infection that supports the conclusion that most of the actively infected cells represent new infections (thicker ❬) with rapid turnover and regeneration of the productively infected cells. Modified and reproduced from ref. 1 with permission.

depletion can be accounted for by infection of CD4$^+$ cells. The volcano model [1] shown in figure 7a attempts to capture metaphorically the sheer magnitude of infection and the paradox in lentivirus infections that, although in most infected cells viral gene expression is dormant, viral genes are expressed in a small fraction of the population. A small fraction of a large number, however, is still a large number, of the order of a billion or more cells with levels of viral gene expression comparable to productive infections. If these cells are killed as a consequence of viral replication or because they are now recognized as infected and eliminated by immune surveillance mechanisms, there will be a war of attrition in the immune system whose length and outcome will depend on the capacity of the marrow and thymus to replate CD4$^+$ T lymphocytes.

The volcano model in figure 7(*a*) is a snapshot of infection at one point in time.   The model shown in figure 7(*b*) incorporates recent studies with antiviral drugs that support the conclusion that most actively infected cells represent new infections rather than transitions from latent to productive infections [13, 14].   These kinetic analyses lead to similar estimates of steady state concentrations of a billion productively infected CD4$^+$ lymphocytes that are rapidly lost and replaced, consistent with the view that immune depletion is a direct consequence of viral infection.

Summary

Single-cell molecular technologies have been developed over the years to answer enduring and basic questions in viral pathogenesis: In the course of viral infections, where does a virus go and how does it get there?   If infection is persistent, why do host defenses fail to eradicate virus and virus-infected cells?   If infection is associated with disease, what are the mechanisms of injury and death of cells? [15]   In this article I have described some advances in our understanding of the persistence of lentiviruses and the mechanisms of immune depletion in HIV infections based on in situ methods to detect viral nucleic acids in cells in tissue sections.   These analyses of HIV infection in vivo reveal a vast reservoir of covertly infected cells in LT to perpetuate infection and a smaller but still large pool of productively infected cells whose death cumulatively results in immune depletion.   While the magnitude of the problem of containing HIV infection is evident from these studies, it is quite possible that a shift in the balance between active and dormant infections could significantly alter outcome.   The continuing development of antiviral agents will hopefully prove this to be the case.

References

1   Hasse AT: The role of active and covert infections in lentivirus pathogenesis.   Ann NY Acad Sci 1994; 724: 75 – 86.
2   Haase AT, Retzel E, Staskus K: Amplification and detection of lentiviral DNA inside cells.   Proc Natl Acad Sci USA 1990; 87: 4971 – 4975.
3   Haase AT, The slow infection caused by visna virus.   Curr Top Microbiol Immunol 1975; 72: 101 – 156.
4   Embretson JE, Staskus KA, Retzel EF, Haase AT, Bitterman P: PCR amplification of viral DNA and viral host cell mRNAs in situ, In: Mullis KB Ferré F, Gibbs RA (eds.), The Polymerase Chain Reaction, Birkhäuser, Boston, 1994, pp 55 – 64.
5   Embretson J, Zupancic M, Ribas JL, Burke A, Rácz P, Tenner-Rácz K, Haase AT: Massive covert infection of helper T lymphocytes and macrophages by human immunodeficiency virus during the incubation period of AIDS.   Nature 1993; 362: 359 – 362.
6   Armstrong JA, Horne R: Follicular dendritic cells and virus-like particles in AIDS-related lymphadenopathy.   Lancet 1984; ii: 370 – 372.
7   Tenner-Rácz K, Rácz P, Schmidt H, Dietrich M, Kern P, Louie A, Gartner S, Popovic M: Immunohistochemical, electron microscopic and in situ hybridization evidence for the involvement of lymphatics in the spread of HIV-1.   AIDS 1988; 2: 299 – 309.
8   Pantaleo G, Graziosi C, Butini L, Pizzo PA, Schnittman SM, Kotler DP, Fauci AS: Lymphoid organs function as major reservoirs for human immunodeficiency virus.   Proc Natl Acad Sci USA 1991; 88: 9838 – 9842.
9   Fox CH, Tenner-Rácz K, Rácz P, Firpo A, Pizzo PA, Fauci AS: Lymphoid germinal centers are reservoirs of human immunodeficiency virus type 1 RNA.   J Infect Dis 1991; 164: 1051 – 1057.
10   Staskus KA, Couch L, Bitterman P, Retzel EF, Zupancic M, List J, Haase AT: In situ amplification of visna

virus DNA in tissue sections reveals a reservoir of latently infected cells.   Microb Pathog 1991; 11: 67 – 76.

11   Haase AT, Analysis of viral infections by in situ hybridization.   In Valentino K, Roberts J, Barchas J (eds.), In situ hybridization—applications to neurobiology.   Symposium Monograph, Oxford Uniersity Press, Fairlawn, New Yersey, 1987, pp 197 – 219.

12   Harper ME, Marselle LM, Gallo RC, Wong-Staal F: Detection of lymphocytes expressing human T-lymphotropic virus type III in lymph nodes and peripheral blood from infected individuals by in situ hybridization.   Proc Natl Acad Sci USA 1986; 83: 772 – 776.

13   Ho DD, Neumann AU, Perelson As, Chen W, Leonard JM, Markowitz M: 1995; Rapid turnover of plasma virions and CD4 lymphocytes in HIV-1 infection.   Nature 1995; 373: 123 – 126.

14   Wei X, Ghosh SK, Taylor ME, Johnson VA, Emini EA, Deutsch P, Lifson JD, Bonhoeffer S, Nowak MA, Hahn BH, Saag MS, Shaw GM: Viral dynamics in human immunodeficiency virus type 1 infection.   Nature 1995; 373: 117 – 122.

15   Haase AT: Methods in viral pathogenesis: tissues and organs.   In: Nathanson N (ed.), Viral Pathogenesis, Raven Press, in preparation.

16   Adolph KW (ed.) Molecular virology techniques, Part A. Vol 4 of Methods in Molecular Genetics. Academic Press, San Diego, 1994.

Human Papillomavirus and Immunosuppression

Eggert Stockfleth, Lutz Gissmann

Department of Obstetrics and Gynecology, Loyola University Chicago, Cancer Center, Maywood, IL. USA

Introduction

Human papillomaviruses (HPVs) are epitheliotropic agents infecting either mucosal surfaces or the skin.   Currently, almost 70 different types have been reported, 30 of them infecting the anogenital tract.   It is now generally accepted that infection with particular types of HPV such as HPV 8, HPV 16 and HPV 18 are the most important events in development of several cancers like skin cancer and cervical cancer.   The great majority of these tumors carry integrated HPV DNA sequences and constitutively express two early viral genes, E6 and E7.

Immunosuppression, whether hereditary, iatrogenic, or acquired, permits the virus or the infected cells to escape immunosurveillance, leading to development and persistence of premalignant lesions and the development of cancer.   For many years, it has been appreciated that there is an increased risk to develop HPV-associated cancers among individuals suffering from epidermodysplasia verruciformis, renal transplant recipients, Hodgkin's disease or HIV-induced immunosuppression.   Human papillomaviruses are unusual among other viruses, because they cannot be propagated in vitro and in most instances are present in tiny quantities in lesions in vivo.   Advances in recombinant DNA technology made genomic clones of all different HPV types available, and expression of their individual genes can be achieved in a variety of prokaryotic and eukaryotic systems such as *Escherichia coli*, baculovirus, yeast and vaccinia.   These techniques made it possible to study the role of HPV in different human cancers.

Immune Response to Human Papillomavirus Infections

Humoral Immune Response

Most studies worldwide deal almost exclusively with the characterization of the humoral immune response to the HPV types 6, 8, 11, 16 and 18.   The majority of the published data contains information on the presence of IgG and IgA class antibodies in patients sera.   Different assay systems were used such as Western blot, ELISA (enzyme linked immunosorbent assay) and RIPA (radioimmunoprecipitation assay).   Initial studies on the humoral immune response against genital papillomaviruses were performed

113

using fusion proteins expressed in *E. coli* in Western Blot assays [1, 2]. Subsequently, the ELISA technique was employed, taking advantage of either synthetic peptides or complete viral proteins. Another method measuring HPV specific antibodies directed against conformational epitopes was introduced by Müller et al. [3], who used viral proteins produced by in vitro transcription/translation for radioimmunoprecipitation.

Human antibodies against late viral capsid proteins like L1 or L2 [4], of HPV 6 and HPV 11, respectively, were found to be predominant in patients afflicted with condylomata acuminata or in sera of patients with recurrent respiratory papillomatosis [5 – 7]. The biological function of these antibodies is still unclear because in the latter case they obviously cannot prevent recurrence of the disease. However, it has been shown that sera of patients containing high antibody titers against intact HPV 11 particles are able to neutralize reinfection as assayed in the athymic mouse xenograft system [8]. Since the first report in 1989 [3], the correlation of specific antibodies to HPV early protein E7 in sera of patients with HPV 16 or HPV 18 positive cervical cancer is now well established in the literature [9, 12]. A similar association does exist for HPV early protein E6 (and possibly also for E2 and E4) specific antibodies [12]. Depending on the test system employed, antibodies to E6 and E7 are present in 15% to 70% in sera of cervical cancer patients but only 1.4% to 15% in age-matched controls [1, 3, 10]. Similar results were obtained for HPV 16E4, HPV 16E6 and for HPV 18E7 [3, 9, 11, 12]. In spite of the fact that the antibodies to the early HPV proteins possibly can be considered as a marker of cervical cancer, the biological processes leading to this immune response are far from being understood. The E6 and E7 gene expression is regulated by the degree of cellular differentiation in the infected epithelium. In HPV positive malignant lesions of the cervix, transcripts for the E6 and E7 proteins are present in all epithelial layers [13]. The specific antibody response in these patients can be explained by the long term exposure of the immune system to these proteins. The antibody titers were shown to rise with tumor progression and seem to decrease following tumor therapy [61]. The available data point to an immunogenicity of the virus-infected epithelium and thus may represent a target for immunosurveillance mechanisms. However, it is still unknown, whether antibodies to early viral proteins are only markers for infection or if their presence can influence the outcome of the disease.

Cell Mediated Immunity

It is well established that cell mediated immunity (CMI) plays an important role in human host defense against persistent viral infections such as herpes viruses and hepatitis B [71]. The growth and progression of HPV-associated, potentially malignant anogential lesion seems to be controlled by local immunosurveillance mechanisms, i.e. tumor cell-recognition and -elimination by specific cytotoxic T lymphocytes [14] and natural killer cells [15]. Also the reduced expression of major histocompatibility complex class I molecules (MHC-I), frequently observed in cervical carcinomas, may be important for tumor progression [16, 79]. It is as yet unknown whether certain HPV proteins play a role in MHC-I down-regulation, or whether cellular mutations lead to this phenotype. In rabbits, a strong linkage between skin wart regression and aDR alpha Eco RI fragment of the rabbit papillomavirus and an extended relative risk of malignant transformation comparable with aDQ alpha Pvu fragment was discovered. This indicates a genetic control of wart evolution genes in the class II region of the MHC complex [23].   In contrast to normal keratinocytes cervical cancer cells are HLA class II positive and thus may function as antigen presenting cells contributing to immunological reactions.   Langerhans' cells generally work as antigen presenting cells to stimulate CD4$^+$ helper T cells.   In epithelium of high grade CIN (cervical intraepithelial neoplasia) lesions (CIN II/III) but not in low grade lesions, Langerhans' cells occur in only small numbers and are characterized by a modified morphology and distribution [25, 26], pointing to a reduced capability to trigger T helper cell mechanisms.

HPV Infection and Immunodeficiency

Information about the ability of the host immune system to control HPV infections are based on the increased prevalence of HPV-associated premalignant and malignant lesions in patients suffering from Epidermodysplasia verruciformis (EV) and Hodgkin's disease (HD) as well as in allograft recipients [80].

Initial reports on the association between HPV infection and immunodeficiency dealt with HPV 5 or HPV 8 and the development of squamous cell skin cancer in patients with Epidermodysplasia verruciformis [Lewandowsky and Lutz 1932].   EV is an uncommon disease with extensive polymorphous, HPV induced warts, that in about 30% of all the cases and within 25 years convert to malignancies.   Two forms have been described: (i) a benign form with mostly plane papillomas in which HPV 3 is present, and (ii) a potentially progressive malignant form in which mostly HPV 5 and HPV 8 [27], were demonstrated. X-rays and most likely ultraviolet (UV-B) irradiation can induce malignant transformation and therefore should not be used therapeutically [28, 29].   Since the first study on EV associated HPVs in 1978 [30] more than 20 specific HPVs have been discovered, but only a few of them, predominantly HPV 5 and HPV 8 have been found to be associated with carcinomas originating from benign lesions.   EV patients have depressed cell-mediated immunity (CMI), very likely resulting in a failure to identify EV associated HPVs and, therefore, to eliminate the lesions that persist throughout lifetime.   This failure is due to the noticeable inhibition of natural killer (NK) cell activity [15], and of cytotoxic T-cells toward their specific targets [81].   The nature of the particular defect of antigen presentation and/or recognition is still far from being understood.   EV-associated HPV antigens, like other viral antigens, may still be presented in the context of both MHC class I and class II molecules, either by specialized antigen presenting cells (APC) or by 'non-specialist' cells, i.e., HPV-infected keratinocytes.   In EV the role of APC appears to be preserved [31, 81]. There are several examples showing that virus-infected or tumor cells can act as APC when exposed to various cytokines, e.g., tumor necrosis factor-α (TNF-α), interleukin 2 (IL-2), etc., [82] although antigen presentation by 'non-specialist' cells without the necessary costimulatory signals could lead to the induction of immunotolerance.   Ultraviolet B (UV-B) can induce both, nonspecific immunosuppression, by generation of immunosuppressive cytokines, and specific immunotolerance through alteration of antigen presentation.

EV-associated HPVs like HPV 5, 8, 14, 17, 20 and 47, are also considered to play an important part in the pathogenesis of certain skin cancers in renal transplant recipients [32]. Today, renal transplantation is a well established procedure, with many patients surviving more than twenty years.   They request lifelong immunosuppressive treatment with azathioprine and corticosteroids preventing graft-rejection.   Opportunistic infections due to immunosuppression is one of the main problems in these patients.   The modification in cell-mediated immunity brought about by continued immunosuppressive therapy is thought to be a factor contributing to an increased incidence of anogenital cancers, lymphomas and skin tumors [83].   The numbers of patients developing cutaneous carcinomas reaches up to 40% ten years after transplantation [33, 34] and it is obvious that the probability of developing viral warts increases with the duration of immunosuppression. In 1989 Barr et al. reported a 20% prevalence of viral warts in a group of recipients with a graft life of lower than five years, but a 77% prevalence in those with a graft life of five to twenty-two years [35].   The carcinomas often are squamous cell carcinomas (SSC), that are generally preceded by virus (HPV) induced warts and premalignant keratosis. Bowen's disease, keratocanthomas and basal cell carcinomas have also been described [34, 36].   Remarkably, sometimes unsuspicious looking 'warty' lesions exhibit histological changes of SSC [37].   The majority of the keratotic skin lesions and cancers are associated with sun exposure of the skin.   Nevertheless, recent data suggested that HPV, along with immunosuppressive treatment and ultraviolet (UV) irradiation, is an important etiologic factor for the development of carcinomas [35]. It appears that a continued immunosuppression is important for maintenance of HPV-related disease in these patients; when the immunosuppressive drugs are removed following graft rejection most warts will regress immediately [84].   Bavinck et al. assume that exposure to sunlight before the age of 30 contributes more significantly to the risk of skin cancer but not to keratotic skin lesions in renal transplant recipients, than exposure after the age of 30 [85].   In a study reported from Australia, 25% of renal recipients surviving 9.5 years and 50% of those surviving 20 years developed skin cancer.   In contrast, Barr et al. recorded that only 2% of patients in Scotland with a graft life up to five years and 13% of recipients with a graft life of 5 to 22 years were affected.   It seems to be possible that ultraviolet irradiation induces a local immunosuppression.   These effects would be more prominent in light skinned subjects and may promote HPV proliferation and tumor promotion [83].   This might explain the favorite localization of such lesions on sun-exposed skin areas [36].

The majority of EV-associated SCCs contain HPV 5 or HPV 8 DNA in an episomal form, with chromosomal integration being a rare event [38].   In vitro studies demonstrated that HPV 8 E6 but not the E7 gene has transforming activity [39].   This is in contrast to HPV types 16 and 18 whose genomes are frequently integrated into the host chromosomes. In cervical squamous cancers E6 and E7 are expressed consistently [40], and of both genes seem to be required for malignant transformation.   So far, the detection of HPV DNA in cutaneous SCC of renal transplant recipients has been controversial, with EV-associated types and a variety of common cutaneous and genital HPV types being identified in some but not all studies [35, 41 – 44].   The recent identification of new HPV types in skin cancers of immunosuppressed patients further expands the range of HPV-linked human malignancies and permited new approaches to the study of the pathogenesis of skin cancers in these patients [86].

Little is known about humoral immune-responses to HPV in recipients with and without skin cancer.   Jochmus-Kudielka et al. described in 1992, that anti-HPV 16 E4 and E7 antibody-positivity was elevated in renal transplant recipients as compared to age-matched controls, but the antibody positivity did not correlate with the duration of immunosuppression.   They assumed that anti-HPV 16 E4 and E7 antibodies are in fact unlikely to be effective in preventing the disease. However, these antibodies might be useful as markers for HPV 16 infection and viral replication in lesions of immunosuppressed patients [45]. Analysis of colpohistology showed that the prevalence of HPV was twice as high in graft recipients as compared to a non-immunosuppressed control group [46]. Intraepithelial neoplasia (CIN) occured more frequently in renal transplant recipients, during drug-induced immunosuppression, but there was no clear-cut relation to the detection of HPV.

Bavinck et al. investigated the prevalence of antibodies to the early (E) protein E7 and the major capsid late (L) protein L1 of HPV 8 in renal transplant recipients. In addition, they studied the association of HLA class II molecules with these antibodies [39, 47 – 49]. Sera from patients with or without skin cancer were screened for the presence of IgG and IgM antibodies to HPV 8 E7 and L1. Individuals who had IgM antibodies but no IgG antibodies to L1 of HPV 8 (patients with no apparent class switch from IgM to IgG) had skin cancer in 50% of all cases, while patients positive for IgG antibodies developed skin cancer in only 18%. A strong linkage between lack of class switching and HLA–DR7 was discovered. It was postulated that HLA–DR7 is associated with an impaired presentation of late antigens of HPV 8 to CD4 positive regulatory T lymphocytes during infection. Future experiments will verify this hypothesis and demonstrate which peptides are implicated.

Hodgkin's disease (HD) is characterized by the presence of a small population of transformed cells, the Reed-Sternberg cells, and a higher number of reactive cells including lymphocytes, eosinophils, histiocytes, and plasma cells. The etiology of HD is still unknown but recent data provide strong evidence that Epstein-Barr Virus (EBV) is associated with this disease. The reactive cell population in HD consists of predominantly CD4$^+$ helper T cells but lacks CD8$^+$ cytotoxic T cells and natural killer cells. Insufficient HLA class I expression could be a possible mechanism to prevent on CD8$^+$ cytotoxic immune response within these patients [87]. In contrast, the humoral immune response seems to be unaffected even during treatment with radio- and chemotherapy [88].

Patients suffering from HD have an increased risk of developing HPV-associated lesions. Sixhundred sixty-six women having a gynecological examination showed indication of condylomata, dysplasia or carcinoma of the cervix or anogenital region in a significantly higher percentage than in published results from Papanicolaou screening services [50]. The cellular immunosuppression seems to be responsible for the high frequency of HPV-associated lesions. Little is known about humoral responses to HPV in HD with or without genital or skin disorders. Steeger et al. (1990) [89] described an increase of HPV 8 E7 and L1 antibodies in HD patients. Stockfleth also detected a high level of antibodies against HPV 16 E6 and E7 tested by ELISA and RIPA [91]. Usually, 15 years after radiotherapy 13% of HD patients develop a secondary malignant tumor with increasing risk after this time. They have a higher probability for developing lymphomas, carcinomas of the head, neck, breast, lung, stomach etc. [90]. Stockfleth further reported a high percentage of prae- and malignant skin disorders like keratoacanthoma, basal cell carcinoma and dysplastic melanocytic naevi in these patients. Out of 50 patients, 62% showed HPV-associated skin lesions especially verrucae, Morbus Bowen and Erythroplasia of Queyrat. Meanwhile, results from different studies established that patients with HD should be monitored cautiously for HPV infections of the skin and neoplasm of the lower anogenital tract [91].

An increased frequency of HPV-DNA in exfoliated cervical cells of otherwise healthy women during pregnancy was described but this data was not confirmed by others [52, 53]. An explanation for this observation could be a temporary immunosuppression of women during pregnancy, that would be responsible for the increased incidence of genital warts and CIN lesions in pregnant women [53].

HPV and HIV

Women infected with HIV have an at least 10-fold increased risk of active HPV infection and a 12-fold increased risk of cervical dysplasia as compared to healthy uninfected women [54]. In addition, cervical disease in such patients is abnormally aggressive. HPV is more likely to be detected in symptomatic HIV infected women than in either asymptomatic HIV positive or HIV negative women [55, 56]. In HIV-negative patients the chance of recurrent CIN is associated with increased severity of the CIN lesions, whereas in HIV positive patients, recurrence is related to the degree of immunosuppression. The immunosuppressive effects of HIV infection can be monitored by measuring the concentration of circulating $CD4^+$ lymphocytes. Women with $CD4^+$ cell counts below $200/mm^3$ area of a significantly increased risk for genital HPV infection and premalignant cervical disease than HIV-infected women with higher $CD4^+$ counts [57]. The severity of HPV-associated CIN has also been correlated to the degree of immunosuppression in women with AIDS [58]. In contrast, studies asymptomatic HIV-infected women have revealed, that the association of HIV with HPV and cervical disease is independent of the degree of immunosuppression [59]. One possible explanation for these contrasting observations could be that peripheral $CD4^+$ levels do not reliably mirror local immunosurveillance. The cervix harbors an effective mucosal immune system contributing to humoral and cellular immune response. HIV can be isolated from the vaginal secretions of women with AIDS as well of asymptomatic women infected with HIV. Both groups have HIV-induced IgA antibodies in vaginal secretions [93]. HIV positive women furthermore have lymphocytic infiltrates in their cervical epithelium including $CD4^+$ T-helper cells, $CD8^+$ T-cytotoxic cells, phagocytic $CD4^+$Langerhans' cells, and cells that express HLA–DR antigens [94]. Subepithelial $CD4^+$ and $CD8^+$ lymphocytes are also present in HPV-infected cervix, and their relative numbers change with the severity of the CIN [60]. The numbers of Langerhans' cells are rather decreased within cervical HPV lesions [25]. Cervical epithelial cells in HPV-infected women express HLA-DR antigen [97], demonstrating their competence for antigen presentation.

Women infected with HIV are also more likely to be infected with multiple HPV genotypes [96] indicating that decreased immunosurveillance in HIV-seropositive women permits more rapid HPV replication and increases viral load in the cervix.

Recent studies describing a direct interaction between HIV and HPV showed that the regulatory tat protein of HIV enhances trans-activation of the HPV 16 upstream regulatory region (URR) [65]. Cotransfection of *tat1* and the HPV transcriptional regulatory gene E2 into a cervical carcinoma cell line (SiHa), or cocultivation with HIV-1-infected cells, results in enhanced transactivation of the URR. This observation suggest that, besides intercellular interactions, direct intracellular interactions between these two viruses are possible and that the increased rate of HPV-associated cervical disease in asymptomatic

HIV-seropositive women may result from molecular interactions, of HPV and HIV molecules [65].   This observation however needs further clarification, especially since HIV and HPV do not infect the same target cells.

It also seems to be conceivable, that women infected with HPV are more likely to get infected with HIV and disturbance of the epithelium barrier may enhance HIV transmission and HPV-associated lesions.   In several studies, comparison of results obtained from cervical screening with those from colposcopy or colposcopically directed biopsies demonstrated, that the Papanicolaou test (PAP) alone does not reliably detect abnormalities of the lower genital tract as well as neoplasms in women with HIV infection. Future studies are required to verify, whether the time point of acquisition of HPV and HIV effects the onset and progression of cervical disease.

A likely association of HIV infection and the incidence of genital warts in homosexual men was recognized early in the AIDS epidemic [66, 98].   Revalence occurrence of HPV-associated penile and anal warts are two fold increased in HIV-seropositive as compared to seronegative men [99].   There are common features in the etiology of cervical- and anal cancer.   The endocervical and anal canal both descend from the cloagenic membrane, and their epithelial structures are comparable [67].   It is conceivable, that the anal mucosa supports the development and progression of HPV-associated pre- and malignant lesions, similar to those found in the cervix.   Anal intraepithelial neoplasia (AIN) was shown to be associated with a history of anal warts, frequent unprotected anal intercourse, presence of HPV and low $CD4^+/CD8^+$ ratio [66].   Before the beginning of the AIDS epidemic, the most common manifestation of anal HPV infection was anal condylomata acuminata, which is very rarrely associated with the development of anal cancer.   Anal carcinoma has been an uncommon tumor occuring in women and patients above the age of 50.   With increasing numbers of HIV infected persons, the spectrum of HPV-associated disease of the anus has changed.   Studies from the United States demonstrated a high prevalence of anal intraepithelial neoplasia in HIV-positive homosexual and bisexual patients, particularly in those with advanced HIV infection and anal condylomata acuminata [68].   As in cervical cancer, HPV 16 and HPV 18 have been found in most AIN [69, 70, 103].   Breese et al. found in STD clinic, that when samples are taken repeatedly every six months, HPV detection is increased over time in HIV-positive but not in HIV-negative men.   Repeated evaluation detects anorectal HPV infection in 51% of HIV-negative men, 77% of asymptomatic HIV-positive men, and 94% with AIDS-related complex (ARC) [100]. Bernard et al. investigated the relation of human papillomavirus and herpes simplex virus (HSV) infection in penile and anal lesions of HIV-immunocompromised men.   Their results showed that HIV infection enhances expression of mostly high-risk HPV-types associated with the immunosuppression as measured by the $CD4^+$ cell count, but also enhances HSV infection [72, 104].   There may be two major reasons accounting for the increased risk of development of HPV-associated anogenital cancer in patients suffering from HIV infection.   First, these patients have also a high incidence of other forms of cancer, like lymphomas, Kaposi's sarcoma, melanomas, adenosarcoma of breast etc. [73], suggesting decreased tumor immunity.   Secondly, risk factors for acquiring a HIV infection, like promiscuity, are the same for acquiring a HPV infection [70].   Patients suffering from HIV have a variety of abnormalities in cell-mediated immunity, like functional defects in $CD4^+$ cells [74], defects in IL-2 response, and insufficient immune-response to agents different than HIV [101].

HPV are also associated with certain oral lesions, like warts, condylomata, and focal epithelial hyperplasia. HPV 6, 11, 13, 16, 18 and 32 are chiefly correlated with these lesions. HIV-positive patients appear to be predisposed to oral infection with unusual HPV types. Greenspan et al. detected HPV 7 in oral lesions of HIV-positive patients, which is generally associated with butcher's warts of the hands and had not been described in oral cavity [77].

In summary, a number of studies argue that HPV-associated diseases are very common among HIV-infected individuals. To date, the incidence of HPV-related cancer is increasing in these patients. HPV-associated cancer can take years to develop and HIV-positive patients frequently die earlier of other causes, like opportunistic infections or more aggressive tumors. Accordingly, when these patients live longer due to improvements in medical therapy, it is feasible that the incidence of HPV-associated cancer will further increase. For that reason, it is indicated to monitor these patients cautiously for HPV-associated pre- and malignant cancer.

Acknowledgments

We thank Prof. Dr. H. Adldinger and Dr. A. M. Kaufmann for their support and for helpful discussions.

E.S. is a fellow of the 'Jung-Stiftung für Wissenschaft and Forschung', Hamburg, Germany.

References

1   Jochmus-Kudielka I, Schneider A, Braun R, et al: J Natl Cancer Inst 1989; 81: 1698 – 1704.
2   Kochel HG, Monazahian M, Sievert K, et al: Int J Cancer 1991; 48/5: 682 – 688.
3   Muller M, Viscidi RP, Sun Y, et al: Virology 1992; 187/2: 508 – 514.
4   Galloway DA, Jenison SA: Mol Biol Med 1990; 7/1: 59 – 72.
5   Suchankova A, Ritter O, Hirsch I, et al: Acta Virol (Praha) 1990; 34/5: 433 – 442.
6   Bonnez W, Da-Rin C, Rose RC, Reichman RC: J Gen Virol 1991; 72/Pt 6: 1343 – 1344.
7   Bonnez W, Kashima HK, Leventhal B, et al: Virology 1992; 188/1: 384 – 387.
8   Christensen ND, Kreider JW, Shah KV, Rando RF: J Gen Virol 1992; 73/Pt 5: 1261 – 1267.
9   Kanda T, Onda T, Zanma S, et al: Virology 1992; 190/2: 724 – 732.
10 Mann VM, de-Lao SL, Brenes M, et al: Cancer Res 1990; 50/24: 7815 – 7819.
11 Bleul C, Muller M, Frank R, et al: J Clin Microbiol 1991; 29/8: 1579 – 1588.
12 Nindl I, Benitez-Bribiesca L, Berumen J, Farmanara N, et al: Arch Viol 1994; 137: 341 – 353.
13 Durst M, Glitz D, Schneider A, zur-Hausen H: Virology 1992; 189/1: 132 – 140.
14 Chen L, Mizuno MT, Singhal MC, et al: J Immunol 1992; 148/8: 2617 – 2621.
15 Malejczyk J, Majewski S, Jablonska S, Rogozinski TT, Orth G: Int J Cancer 1989; 43/2: 209 – 21.
16 Cromme FV, Meijer CJ, Snijders PJ, et al: Br J Cancer 1993; 67/6: 1372 – 380.
17 Phelps WC, Yee CL, Muenger K, Howley PM: Cell 1988; 53/4: 539 – 547.
18 Couturier J, Sastre-Garau X, Schneider-Maunoury S, Labib A, Orth G: J Virol 1991; 65/8: 4534 – 4538.
19 Scheffner M, Werness BA, Huibregtse JM, Levine AJ, Howley PM: Cell 1990; 63/6: 1129 – 1136.
20 Huibregtse JM, Scheffner M, Howley PM: Mol Cell Biol 1993; 13/8: 4918 – 4927.
21 Werness BA, Levine AJ, Howley PM: Science 1990; 248/4951: 76 – 79.
22 Crook T, Tidy JA, Vousden KH: Cell 1991; 67/3: 547 – 556.
23 Han R, Breitburd F, Marche PN, Orth G: Nature 1992; 356/6364: 66 – 68.
24 Glew SS, Duggan-Keen M, Cabrera T, Stern PL: Cancer Res 1992; 52/14: 4009 – 4016.
25 Viac J, Guerin-Reverchon I, Chardonnet Y, Bremond A: Immunobiology 1990; 180: 328 – 338.
26 Hughes RG, Norval M, Howie SE: J Clin Pathol 1988; 41/3: 253 – 259.

27   Orth G: Ciba Found Symp 1986; 120/157: 157 – 174.
28   Androphy EJ, Dvoretzky I, Lowy DR: Arch Dermatol 1985; 121/7: 864 – 868.
29   Lutzner MA: J Am Acad Dermatol 1984; 11/5 Pt 1: 891 – 893.
30   Orth G, Jablonska S, Favre M, Croissant O, Jatzabek-Chotzelska M, Rzesa G: Proc Natl Acad Sci USA 1978; 75/3: 1537 – 1541.
31   Haftek M, Jablonska S, Orth G: Dermatologica 1985; 170/5: 213 – 220.
32   Stark LA, Arends MJ, McLaren KM, et al: Br J Cancer 1994; 69: 222 – 229.
33   Euvrard S, Chardonnet Y, Dureau G, Hermier C, Thivolet J: Arch Dermatol 1991; 127/4: 559 – 564.
34   Euvrard S, Chardonnet Y, Pouteil-Noble CP, Kanitakis J, Thivolet J, Touraine JL: Transplant Proc 1993; 25/1 Pt 2: 1392 – 1393.
35   Barr BB, Benton EC, McLaren K, et al: Lancet 1989; 1/8630: 124 – 129.
36   Bavinck JNB, Gissmann L, Class FHJ, et al: Journal of Immunology 1993; 151: 1579 – 1586.
37   Blessing K, McLaren KM, Benton EC, et al: Histopathology 1989; 14/2: 129 – 139.
38   Yabe Y, Tanimura Y, Sakai A, Hitsumoto T, Nohara N: Int J Cancer 1989; 43/6: 1022 – 1028.
39   Iftner T, Bierfelder S, Csapo Z, Pfister H: J Virol 1988; 62/10: 3655 – 3661.
40   Gissmann L: Curr Opin Genet Dev 1992; 2/1: 97 – 102.
41   Lutzner M, Croissant O, Ducasse MF, Kreis H, Crosnier J, Orth G: J Invest Dermatol 1980; 75/4: 353 – 356.
42   Andre P, Orth G, Evenou P, Guillaume JC, Avril MF: J Am Acad Dermatol 1990; 22/1: 131 – 132.
43   Dyall-Smith D, Trowell H, Dyall-Smith ML: Int J Dermatol 1991; 30/11: 785 – 789.
44   Soler C, Chardonnet Y, Euvrard S, Chignol MC, Thivolet J: Dermatology 1992; 184/4: 248 – 253.
45   Jochmus-Kudielka I, Bavinck JN, Claas FH, Schneider A, Van der Woude FJ, Gissmann L: Journal of Investigative Dermatology 1992; 98: 389 – 390.
46   Busnach G, Civati G, Brando B, et al: Transplant Proc 1993; 25/1 Pt 2: 1389 – 1390.
47   Nishikawa T, Yamashita T, Yamada T, Kobayashi H, Ohkawara A, Fujinaga K: Jpn J Cancer Res 1991; 82/ 12: 1340 – 1343.
48   Steger G, Jarzabek-Chorzelska M, Jablonska S, Pfister H: J Invest Dermatol 1988; 91/1: 76 – 81.
49   Steger G, Olszewsky M, Stockfleth E, Pfister H: J Virol 1990; 64/9 4399 – 4406.
50   Katz RL, Veanattukalathil S, Weiss KM: Acad Cytol 1987; 31/6: 845 – 854.
51   Rando RF, Lindheim S, Hasty L, Sedlacek TV, Woodland M, Eder C: Am J Obstet Gynecol 1989; 161/1: 50 – 55.
52   Schneider A, Hotz M, Gissmann L: Int J Cancer 1987; 40/2: 198 – 201.
53   Byrne MA, Taylor-Robinson D, Munday PE, Harris JR: Aids 1989; 3/6: 379 – 382.
54   Laga M, Icenogle JP, Marsella R, et al: Int J Cancer 1992; 50/1: 45 – 48.
55   Vermund SH, Kelly KF, Klein RS, et al: Am J Obstet Gynecol 1991; 165/2: 392 – 400.
56   Feingold AR, Vermund SH, Burk RD, et al: J Acquir Immune Defic Syndr 1990; 3/9: 896 – 903.
57   Johnson JC, Burnett AF, Willet GD, Young MA, Doniger J: Obstet Gynecol 1992; 79/3: 321 – 327.
58   Nasseri M, Gage JR, Lorincz A, Wettstein FO, Virology 1991; 184/1: 131 – 140.
59   Kreiss JK, Kiviat NB, Plummer FA, et al: Sex Transm Dis 1992; 19/1: 54 – 59.
60   Powell WS, McKenzie HJ: J Reprod Med 1992; 37/6: 525 – 528.
61   Gross Fisher S, Benitez-Bribiesca L, Nindl I, Stockfleth E, et al: Lancet 1995; submitted.
62   ter-Meulen J, Schweigler AC, Eberhardt HC, et al: Int J Cancer 1993; 53, 257 – 259.
63   Vermund SH, Schiffman MH, Goldberg GL, Ritter DB, Weltman A, Burk RD: Am J Obstet Gynecol 1989; 160/2: 304 – 308.
64   Brandsma J, Burk RD, Lancaster WD, Pfister H, Schiffman MH: Int J Canter 1989; 43/2: 260 – 262.
65   Vernon SD, Hart CE, Reeves WC, Icenogle JP: Virus Res 1993; 27/2: 133 – 145.
66   Frazer IH, Medley G, Crapper RM, Brown TC, Mackay IR: Lancet 1986; 2/8508: 657 – 660.
67   Melbye M, Palefsky J, Gonzales J, et al: Int J Cancer 1990; 46/2: 203 – 206.
68   Palefsky JM, Gonzales J, Greenblatt RM, Ahn DK, Hollander H: JAMA 1990; 263/21: 2911 – 2916.
69   Beckmann AM, Daling JR, Sherman KJ, et al: Int J Cancer 1989; 43/6: 1042 – 1049.
70   Palefsky JM, Holly EA, Gonzales J, Berline J, Ahn DK, Greenspan JS: Cancer Res 1991; 51/3: 1014 – 1019.
71   Wildy P, Gell PG: British Med Bulletin 1985; 41(1): 86 – 91.
72   Maden C, Beckmann AM, Thomas DB, et al: Am J Epidemiol 1992; 135/10: 1093 – 1102.
73   Spina M, Tirelli U: Curr Opin Oncol 1992; 4: 907 – 910.
74   Stein DS, Timpone JG, Gradon JD, Kagan JM, Schnittman SM: Clinical Infectious Diseases 1993; 17: 749 – 771.
75   Nickoloff BJ, Huang YQ, Li JJ, Friedman-Kien AE: Lancet 1992; 339/8792: 548 – 549.
76   Kaaya EE, Voevodin A, Szalecki P, et al: J Acquir Immune Defic Syndr 1993; 6/8: 964 – 965.
77   Greenspan D, De Villiers EM, Greenspan JS, de Souza YG, zur Hausen H: J Oral Pathol 1988; 17/: 9 – 10.
78   Adler-Storthz K, Ficarra G, Woods KV, Gaglioti D, DiPietro M, Shillitoe EJ: J Oral Pathol Med 1992; 21/ 4: 164 – 170.
79   Connor ME, Stern PL: Int J Cancer 1990; 46(6): 1029 – 34.

80   Benton C, Shahidullah H, Hunter J: Papillomavirus Report 1992; 3(2): 23 – 26.
81   Cooper KD, Androphy EJ, Lowy D, Katz SI: J Invest Dermatol 1990; 94: 769 – 776.
82   Murray N, McMichael A: Curr Opin Immunol 1991; 4(4): 401 – 7.
83   Streilein JW: New Engl J Med 1991; 325(12): 884 – 7.
84   Benton C, Shahidullah H, Hunter J: Papillomavirus Report 1992; 3(2): 769 – 776.
85   Bavinck JN, Gissmann L, Claas FHJ, Van Der Woude, et al: J of Immunol 1993; 151: 1579 – 1586.
86   Shamanin V, Glover M, Rausch C, Proby C, et al: Cancer Research 1994; 54: 4610 – 4613.
87   Poppema S, Visser L: Amer J Patho 1994; 145(1): 37 – 41.
88   Minor C: Ann Intern Med 1979; 90: 887 – 892.
89   Steger G, Olszewsky M, Stockfleth E, Pfister H: J Virol 1990; 64: 4399 – 4406.
90   Van Leeuween FE, Somers R, Taal BG, van Harde P, et al: J Clin Oncol 1989; 7(8): 1046 – 58.
91   Stockfleth E, Gissmann L: 1995; (unpublished data).
92   Gissmann L, 1995; (unpublished data).
93   Archibald DW, Witt DJ, Craven DE, Vogt MW, et al: J Infec Dis 1987; 156(1): 240 – 1.
94   Pomerantz RJ, de la Monte SM, Donegan ST, Rota TR, et al: Ann In Med 1988; 108(3): 321 – 7.
95   Fais S, Delle Fratte F, Mancini F, Cioni V, et al: J Clin Path 1991; 44(4): 290 – 2.
96   Maiman M, Fruchter RG, Serur E, Remy JC, et al: Gynecol Oncol 1990; 38(3): 377 – 82.
97   Maiman M, Tarricone N, Vieira J, Suarez J, et al: Obstet & Gynecol 1991; 78(1): 84 – 8.
98   Kent C, Samuel M, Winkelstein W: JAMA 1987; 258(23): 3385 – 6.
99   Rüdlinger R: Schweizerische Rundschau für Medizin Praxis 1988; 77(44): 1202 – 7.
100   Breese P: Papillomavirus workshp Seattle, 1991.
101   Krowka J, Stites D, Mills J, Hollander H, et al: Clin & Experin Immunol 1988; 72(2): 179 – 85.
102   Holmberg SD: Cancer Detec & Prev 1990; 14(3): 331 – 6.
103   Stockfleth E: Thieme Verlag Siegenthaler/Haas, A Delicate Balance 1994; Band 6: 225 – 259.
104   Bernard C, Mougin C, Madoz L, Drobacheff C, et al: Int J Cancer 1992; 52: 731 – 737.

HIV Variability and its Implications
for Epidemiology, Natural History and Pathogenesis

Carla Kuiken, Vladimir Lukashov, Marion Cornelissen, Jaap Goudsmit

Human Retrovirus Laboratory, University of Amsterdam, Academic Medical Center, 1105AZ Amsterdam, the Netherlands

Introduction

The external envelope protein gp120 of HIV contains variable domains alternating with conserved domains. The hypervariable V3 region can be used as a handle to study the evolutionary behavior of HIV-1. The V3 region changes in such a way that, with the knowledge that has been accumulated in over ten years of study, can be considered 'systematic'. This paper contains studies of two types: small-scale studies of the evolution of the virus in a small number of patients; and large-scale, 'population-wide' studies of the molecular epidemiology of HIV-1. The two types overlap. The Dutch situation, and in particular the presence of two large and several smaller cohorts of people infected with HIV-1, or at high risk for such an infection, forms a unique opportunity for study. The organization structure that supports these cohorts, consisting of three equally important partner institutes, with each a different scientific specialty, guarantees that the data and materials gathered in the cohorts are used to their maximum effect. The present work is also largely a result of this invaluable resource.

The molecular epidemiology of the epidemic in the Amsterdam cohorts of homosexuals and IV drug users is the subject of the first studies described. The virus that is found in a large number of seroconverting individuals is described, providing an overview of circulating virus variants in Amsterdam. This study is also the first to describe a systematic difference between the virus found in the two different risk groups. The distinction between the V3 regions found in homosexuals and IV drug users is further explored. Two other HIV-1 genes, *vpr* and *vpu*, are studied and the distinction appears to be present only in *vpr*, suggesting that there may be more to it than a simple epidemiological effect.

Two studies concern the evolution of different virus variants within patients. Rather than direct sequences, which comprise a 'master' sequence or a consensus of the variants that are present in the patient, these studies are based on clonal sequences, which each represent a single HIV-1 variant. The study in which the emergence of virus with very different V3 regions was described, contingently upon the emergence of the syncytium-inducing property in vitro, in cultured and (later) in uncultured patient material, has formed the basis for the later work in which the V3 region was found to play a causative role in the formation of syncytia [1,2]. Syncytium induction was subsequently shown to be associated with rapid progression to AIDS [3,4].   Sequences from the serum and CSF of patients with and without AIDS dementia complex were studied in an attempt to uncover differences between the viruses causing ADC and viruses not causing ADC.   The attempt was not very successful, and the study focuses on the method used rather than the result. Other studies did find sometimes dramatic differences [5]; it is clear from this discrepancy that sampling effects can easily lead to inconsistent results.

Subsequently, the development of the V3 region in time is analyzed, both within persons and on a population-wide scale.   It is shown that the V3 region generally does not change beyond recognition in the study period of 5 years.   The variation at any time in the population after 5 years of infection is shown to be comparable to that in the group that has seroconverted very recently, but larger than it was in the long-term infected group when they seroconverted five years earlier.   This indicates that any selection during transmission does not have an appreciable effect on the population variation in V3.   Next, the variation in V3 is analyzed with respect to the speed of progression to AIDS, and it appears that rapid progression is associated with a lower evolution rate of the V3 region.

But firstly some technological choices to ensure the avoidance of artificial selection biases have to be clarified: the amplification and sequencing strategy, the choice for particular sequence analyses and the preference for the V3 domain.

Technical Remarks Concerning V3 Sequencing

Sequencing Molecular Clones Derived from RT-PCR Products vs from Limiting Dilutions of RNAs

Sequence analysis is a relatively new discipline which arose with the possibility to determine genetic sequences, decennia ago.   A number of efficient sequence analysis tools were developed in the mean time, but the discipline has undergone a revolutionary change with the arrival of PCR technology.   This technological development has resulted in a change in the typical data set from a few (usually long) sequences to several tens or even hundreds of usually short ones.

Two different approaches to PCR amplification followed by sequence analysis were used to study the influence of the errors introduced by the *taq* polymerase during PCR.   In the first method the products obtained after amplification were cloned in a AT cloning system and multiple clones were analyzed.   In the second method [6] single cDNA molecules were isolated by dilution before being amplified and directly sequenced.   In this case errors introduced by the *taq* polymerase during PCR do not cause problems.   Even in the most extreme case, in which one single cDNA/DNA molecule is added, and a *taq* error occurs in the first PCR cycle only 25% of the final PCR product would display the mutation, since the two original strands and one of the two copies generated in the PCR would still be correct.   In the case the obtained sequences showed ambiguities this could be due to *taq* errors or multiple input cDNA and therefore these sequences were discarded from the analysis.

RNA was isolated from an AIDS patient with both NSI and SI virus variants.   Sixteen individual clones, obtained after cloning were sequenced directly [7] and compared with 12 sequences obtained from sufficiently diluted cDNA to ensure that each nucleotide sequence was derived from one copy of cDNA.   No difference was obtained between the

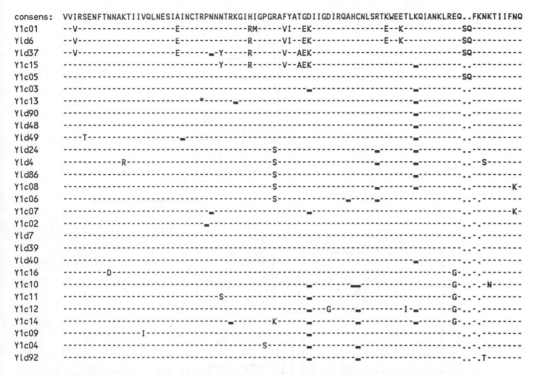

Fig. 1. Consensus in amino acids of SI (Y) virus populations of a single individual [79], following the limiting dilution technique (Y1d#) vs the clonal sequencing techniques (Y1c#). Dots were introduced to make the alignments; dashes are identical amino acids; ■■ represent silent mutations; * represents a stop codon.

consensus sequence derived from 16 clonal sequences and the one derived from 12 direct sequences of single molecules (fig. 1).   It was noted that the clonal sequences showed more random nucleotide substitutions, which were not observed in the diluted cDNA sequencing method.

Phylogenetic analysis using the MEGA program (neighbor-joining) showed no difference between the two sequence data sets, since sequences derived by either method were intermixed.   Two monophyletic groups were, however, observed.   This difference was not due to the sequencing method used, but depended on the phenomena that NSI and SI variants represent different populations (fig. 2) [8].   The ratio NSI versus SI sequences obtained by different sequencing method was virtually identical.   The limited dilution sequencing method is rather time-consuming and the comparison with the clonal sequencing method showed no real differences.   This eliminates the need to analyze multiple single cDNA molecules for most sorts of epidemiological studies.   Although in special studies like transmission from mother to child the need for the latter method still exists.

Techniques for Sequence Analysis
Many traditional sequence analysis techniques are unsuited for large numbers of sequences.   Most phylogenetic analysis algorithms are almost unusable with more than

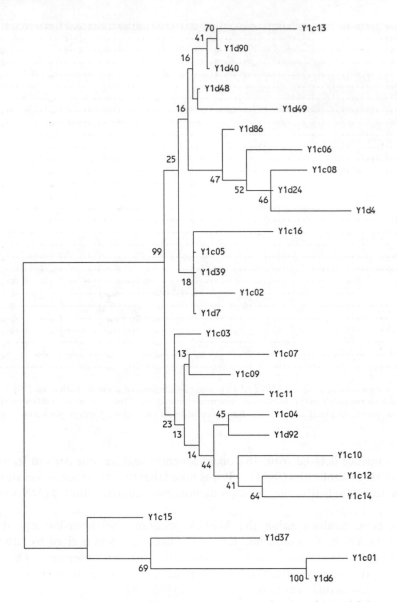

Fig. 2. Phylogenetic analysis with the MEGA program using the neighbor-joining method.

30 sequences, even on very powerful computers. The same is true for the statistical geometry [9, 10] and split decomposition [11] techniques. Recently, the Neighbor-joining algorithm was presented [12] which can comfortably handle a few hundred sequences and is not much inferior to the acknowledged master of the field, maximum-likelihood analysis [13]. An adaptation of this latter algorithm is now available in the program FastDnaml [14], which can handle around 50 – 100 sequences.

In the social sciences, many analytical tools exist which can be used with several hundreds of observations and variables.   By defining each position in an alignment as a variable, and each sequence as an observation, several of these can be used quite fruitfully for sequence analysis, as is shown by Kuiken et al. [15].   However, this introduces new problems, for instance that of multiple testing (see below).   Furthermore, many problems remain for which the social science instruments provide no ready-made solutions. Permutation studies, which have become feasible in the last decade, may be used to address these problems.   In these studies, a statistic of interest is defined and its value is calculated for the dataset that is being studied, as well as for a large number of random data rearrangements (called permutations).   If the value found for the real data is more extreme than most of those found in the permutations, the value is regarded as 'significant'.   In part, problems associated with assessing 'significance' are caused by the 'multiple test problem', the fact that many hypotheses are tested at the same time, often implicitly.   Sequence comparison often implies testing the same hypothesis for all positions in the sequence.   The basis of any statistical test is the probability that a statistic of this size is found when in fact the null hypothesis is true, i.e. the effect we are looking for is absent.   When the test is repeated often, the probability of finding a high value for the test statistic due to chance fluctuation increases.   It is possible to correct the descriptive level for this increase, but to do this correction the number of tests must be known.   In sequence analysis, this number depends on how many positions are free to vary, which can only be guessed at.   Thus, the significance of a test result cannot be determined accurately.   In spite of this drawback, however, important, questions can be at least provisionally answered using these techniques, which therefore may well gain importance in sequence analysis.

Is V3 a Region Representative for the Whole Envelope?

Because the V3 region is involved in many biological functins of the virus, and thus is under many different selective pressures, it is not surprising that it does not show the same evolutionary patterns as other regions of the HIV-1 genome.   Studies of other regions, e.g. [16], suggest this behavior is not unique to V3, so it is doubtful if any 'representative' region can be found.   The relationship between the evolution of V3 and other regions and genes has not been studied extensively, but genes that are compared, like *vpr*, *vpu* and the V3 region, appear to evolve very independently; only a slight association could be found between the distance between two samples in one gene and that in another.   Although this may be a consequence of the fact that the sequences are rather short, it might also stem from frequent recombination in this population.   Other studies show that recombination in HIV-2 [17] as well as between different HIV-1 subtypes [18, 19] can occur, but no estimate has been made about the frequency of recombination and its importance in generating viral diversity.   Between-subtype recombination is relatively easy to detect when two genes from an isolate are sequenced and turn out to have very different phylogenetic relations. Recombination between more similar variants will only show up in detailed studies [16, 20–24]; an added complication is that in epidemics of recent origin, all virus variants are relatively similar, making it difficult to establish with certainty that sections have been exchanged.   It might turn out that recombination plays a much bigger role in the Amsterdam epidemic than was assumed until now.

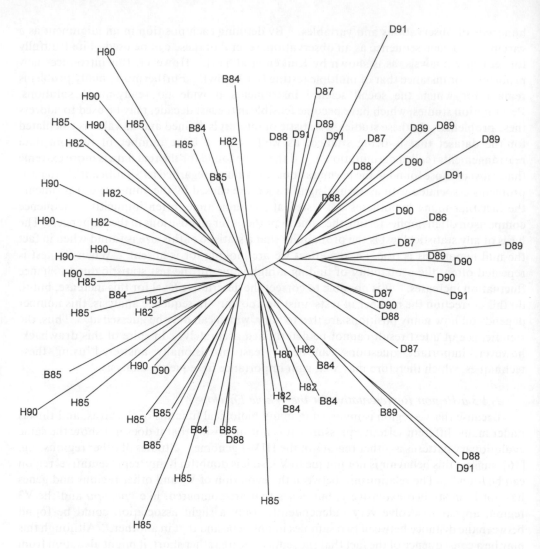

Fig. 3. Dendrogram produced on the basis of all 74 nucleotide sequences. The dendrogram was calculated by the neighbor-joining method and drawn with the DRAWTREE program. Sequence names have been replaced by symbols for legibility. Letters H, D and B indicate sequences from homosexuals, DUs, and hemophiliacs respectively; the number indicates the year of sampling.

Molecular Epidemiology of HIV-1 Using the V3 Domain as Yard Stick

The epidemic in Amsterdam, judging from V3 sequence data, is a good example of a young, expanding epidemic in a naïve population. The phylogenetic tree has a definite star shape, suggesting a hypothetical common ancestor in the middle, with the actual sequences grouped almost equidistantly around it (fig. 3). There is some association between the sampling year and the length of the branches, but it is not strong, indicating that more factors than chronological time influence the distance from the taxa to the center of the tree. When the recently discovered dynamics of the HIV infection [25 – 27] are taken into account, it is perhaps surprising that any association is found at all; with a turnover of millions to billions of virus particles per day in an infected person, the macroscopic distances between isolates from different years could be much more chaotic than they are.

In the Amsterdam cohorts of homosexuals and drug users, thus far only subtype B sequences have been found, although other subtypes can be found among Dutch infected people, namely in those who have become infected through sexual contact with someone from an AIDS-endemic region.   Furthermore, it appears that the Dutch epidemic in the cohorts is stable around the subtype B consensus: sequences from late seroconversions have almost the same consensus as those from people who have become infected 10 years before, in the early stages of the epidemic.   The average difference between the early samples and the subtype B consensus is 3.9%: For the subtypes A and C – E consensus, they range from 17% to 21%.   The 1991 and 1992 sequences differ 6.41% from subtype B, and 18% to 22% from the other subtypes.

Risk Group-Related Variation in HIV-1 Genes

An unexpected finding is the distinction between virus obtained from homosexuals and IV drug users.   The origin of this distinction is as yet uncertain.   As is shown in figure 4, the distribution of differences in the *vpu* gene is suggestive of a non-random pattern, but this in itself only suggests, but does not prove that there is a functional difference between the variants from the two risk groups.   The Amsterdam IVDU variant is also found in drug users from Germany, Scotland and Italy [28].   The similarity of the IVDU variant to an isolate from an upstate New York patient whose risk group is unknown, HIV-1-BAL, in both regions available for comparison (*vpu* and V3) indicates that it is not a unique European maverick.   In several datasets from the United States, the variant also occurs and (from the very scant available evidence) appears to be loosely associated with risk group [29].   However, this still does not exclude the possibility of a founder effect that subsequently spread across the Atlantic.   It seems unlikely that any data can totally disprove a founder effect, but some can render it highly improbable, like a strong continuation of the pattern that suggests itself: a distinction that is well-conserved in some genes and absent in others.   Mutagenesis experiments may solve the dilemma, but here the remarks made earlier about the problems associated with mimicking in vivo circumstances in in vitro experiments apply: both negative and affirmative results may still be caused by one of the myriad differences between the test tube and the infected person.

A biological difference between the variants might be related to the different transmission modes.   It seems likely that virus that is injected directly into the bloodstream is subject to less constraints, since it arrives immediately in the environment it was derived from, while in sexual transmission the virus has to pass a mucosal barrier.   Thus, it would be expected that the constraints are stronger on the homosexual variant, and consequently that this forms a minority selected from the total pool.   In the Los Alamos repository [30], it is the drug user variant that forms a minority, but an explanation for this can be found in the fact that in the Western world, the homosexual community has historically been the focus of most HIV research, as its members are easy to reach, highly motivated and

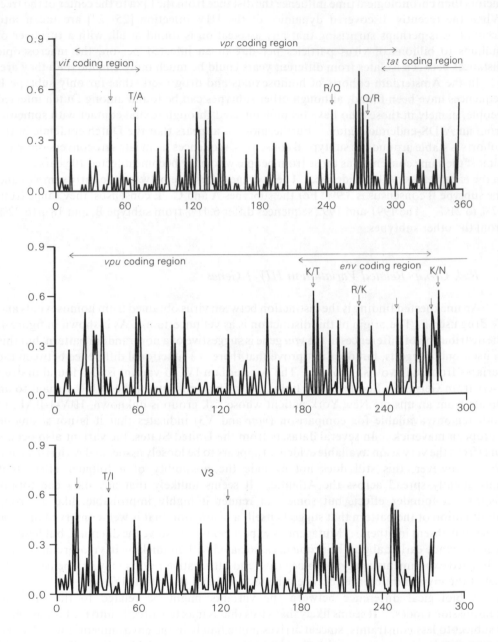

Fig. 4. Location of the discriminating position in the three regions (data from the Dutch samples; V3 data are based on the comparison set). Variability of each position was calculated by summing the number of pairwise differences over all sequences, and dividing by the number of comparisons. Vertical arrows indicate positions that showed significant differences between the risk groups. Changes are silent unless the corresponding amino acid changers are indicated. Amino acid changes in the *vpu* sequence are based on the *env* reading frame. Horizontal arrows indicated the *vpr* and *vpu* sections that encode other genes.

cooperative.   As a consequence, samples from IV drug users are relatively rare, especially in the United States.

Another possible explanation of the homosexual/drug user distinction could lie in host characteristics.   It is not unlikely that the immune system of drug users and homosexual show differences that are caused by the different life styles.   The number and type of other frequent infections presumably also differ.   An overview was published recently of studies of possible differences in immunological parameters between drug users and the 'normal' population [31].   Direct comparisons in this respect of drug users and homosexuals, as far as could be assessed, have not been made.

V3 Genotype vs Phenotype: the Link Between Population-Wide and Individual Variation

The evolution of the human immunodeficiency virus type 1 can be described at many different levels, from intra-individual to world-wide.   At each higher level, complexities of the lower levels are necessarily disregarded to some extent.   The complexities of viral evolution within one person are manifold [8,32].   There is ample evidence that samples from different tissues from one person and one time point will contain different variants [16,33–43], although the differences are small and the variants can still be seen to be closely related [40,44].   Similarly, consecutive samples from the same tissue of a patient also yield different variants [8,44–48].   The differences represent part random (sampling) variation, and part tissue- or environment-specific variation.   Separating one from the other is a major challenge in sequence analysis.

An example of a successful attempt at unravelling the relations between genotype and phenotype is the discovery that the capacity of HIV-1 to induce syncytia in PBMC can be predicted quite accurately on the basis of two amino acids in V3 [1,8,49,50].   The MT2 assay is used to assess the SI phenotype in vitro because of its ease of use and high (but not perfect) association with syncytium inducing capacity in PBMC [51].   At the clonal level, the association is very strong.   Predictions based on direct sequences are less accurate. Six out of 138 seroconversion samples analyzed had a predicted SI phenotype based on direct V3 sequences [data not shown].   One of these turned out to have an NSI phenotype in the MT2 assay.   This predicted-SI/MT2-NSI combination has been reported once before [50] and may be explained by the fact that the virus variant in question is not MT2-tropic.   Of the late samples, only one (of 45) had a predicted SI phenotype, while eight others had an SI phenotype in the MT2 assay, but an NSI sequence.   This discrepancy is probably caused by the presence of a minority of SI virions in the sample.   These SI virions do not show up in the direct sequence, since they form a small subset of the total, but they outgrow the NSI virions in a PBMC culture and cause syncytia in the MT2 assay.   The phenomenon where the dominant V3 variant in a cocultivation experiment was different from the one found in uncultured patient PBMC, but appeared to be predictive of the major variant found in the patient material several months later, is related to this: cocultivation selected the SI virus variant that was already present, but took much longer to outgrow the NSI variant in the patient (fig. 5).   This phenomenon was recently confirmed in a study by Spira and Ho [52].

In contrast to that of the NSI/SI phenotype, the genetic basis for the ability of the virus

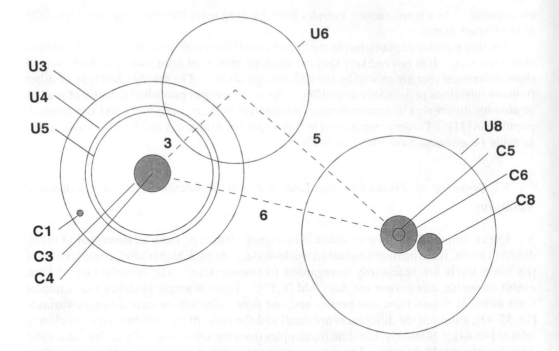

Fig. 5. Two-dimensional representation of the changes in the sequence populations of patient H479, based on the multidimensional scaling of the matrix of Hamming distances between nucleotide consensus sequences. Distances between the circle centers represent these Hamming distances. Thus, the difference between cultured samples 3 (C3 and 6 (C6) is 6 nucleotides, while between uncultured samples 5 and 6, it is 3 nucleotides. The radius of each circle is proportional to the mean Hamming distance between the clones and the consensus sequence of each sample. The circles were added to the figure manually. Hatched circles represent cultured material (C) and open circles represent uncultured patient material (U). Samples 1–4 (C1–4) are showing in culture the NSI phenotype, samples 5–8 (C5–8) the SI phenotype.

to infect macrophages has remained elusive, although it has been shown that this property depends at least partially on V3 [53–58]. The analyses in which differences in V3 populations in serum and CSF are analyzed with the aid of a resampling technique [32] form one attempt in a long series using various types of material and various methods [34,40,41,59]. Most studies report some differences between the sequences compared (although this may be the result of publication bias, the fact that studies with no positive results often are not published), but as often, the results cannot be confirmed by the next study. Subtle differences in the materials and methods used maket it difficult to compare results of the studies. To date, although a large number of sequence elements that are of influence have been described [60], it is still not known what exactly determines macrophage tropism in HIV-1.

In the analysis of HIV-1 sequence data, one of the challenges is to separate the influence of functional constraints and pressures from that of epidemiological factors and sampling effects [29,32]. The distinction between V3 sequences from dementia and non-dementia AIDS patients was very subtle [32]. An effort was made to assess the statistical significance of the results, but still no guarantee exists that the differences can be reproduced in other datasets.   In a very similar study by Power et al. [5], a different result was obtained. One amino acid was seen with almost perfect consistency in patients who developed AIDS dementia complex, but never in the non-demented group.   Unfortunately, this amino acid is found very frequently in the general, non-demented population, so this results is almost certainly due to a sampling effect.   In this case, the data were so consistent that no statistical analysis would have provided a safeguard; only comparison with extraneous datasets shows that the result is anomalous.

The population dynamics of HIV are many times more complex than was assumed at the start of these studies, around five years ago.   Estimates of the amount of virus particles and the turnover rate of virions and infected lymphocytes (at least in symptomatic patients) surpass the expectations by orders of magnitude [25–27].   There were indications of the size of the viral reservoir even before these studies were done.   When effective antiviral drugs are administered to patients, resistant virus variants may be found within a week after start of the medication, as was discovered in the case of 3TC [61].   It appears that, when the need arise, specific mutants are waiting to produce progeny almost immediately.   The number of infected lymphocytes in a patient has recently been estimated to lie between 5×10^6 and 5×10^{10} cells, depending on the disease stage [62].   On the basis of in vitro experiments with HIV-1 reverse transcriptase, it is estimated that on average, one mutation is introduced into the viral genome in each replication round [63–66].   Not all infected lymphocytes produce virus, but when we take into account that macrophages and several other cell types can also be infected with HIV, it is clear that an enormous reservoir of HIV variants is available to generate the necessary mutations.   Any two samples from the same patient yield different variants, and it is not yet known which part of this variation is random and which part is systematic.   The potential of the virus to respond to changes in the environment (new antibody populations, introduction of anti-retroviral drugs) is enormous, as illustrated by the almost immediate appearance of (drug- or neutralization) resistant mutants.

Even so, the virus is not omnipotent.   As is shown by Coffin [67], relative fitness has a very large influence on the relative abundance of different mutants; a mutant that has a very slight fitness disadvantage is reduced to forming a tiny minority of the population, and consequently does not have a very high multiplication rate.   If several individually deleterious mutations must be combined to attain a fitness advantage (like increased drug resistance), this combination may still be almost impossible to reach.   The first deleterious mutation reduces the fitness, and therefore the mutant cannot reach a high frequency in the population.   Thus, the absolute rate at which 'second-generation' mutants are generated from this first-generation mutant is much lower, and it takes much longer before the second mutation is introduced.   This second mutation, if it is again deleterious, slows the mutants down even more, and it may now form such a small minority that it is threatened with extinction; the introduction of the third mutation becomes very difficult indeed.

Evolution of the V3 Region within a Host

We have evaluated differences between seroconversion samples and samples taken later in infection.   It has been shown many times that shortly after transmission, the quasispecies present in the recipient is much narrower (contains much less variation) than

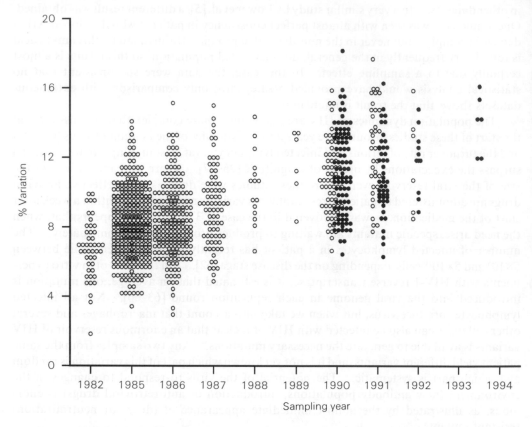

Fig. 6.   Variation in the V3 region of seroconversion (○) and follow-up (●) samples from the homosexual population.   Depicted are pairwise Hamming distances (expressed as percentage of the sequence length) between sequences from the sampling year.   Late sequences from 1993 (3) and 1994 (1) were pooled.

that of the donor [7,68–74].   Furthermore, the variant that forms the majority in the new host, is usually a minor one in the donor.   It is generally accepted that some form of selection takes place in the recipient.   Three models have been proposed by Zhu et al. [74]: small inoculum (this means that a chance process determines which variant, if any, establishes the infection); selection at the point of entry (the winning variant is the one best able to cross the barriers) and replication speed (many virions reach an infectable cell, but only the fastest-replicating one is found frequently, and the others remain an invisible minority).   The three models are not incompatible: it may be (indeed, it seems likely) that all three factors play a role in determining the type and strength of selection: both the number of infectious virions and/or productively cells present in the inoculum, the type of barrier that has to be passed (in particular in sexual and vertical transmissions), and the replication capacity of the variants that succeed in reaching the new host, can limit the efficiency of infection.   Empirical evidence exists for a role for all three.   There are some studies that suggest that not all HIV-1 V3 variants are suitable for transmission to a new host [75–77], indicating selection at the point of entry; there are indications that infection

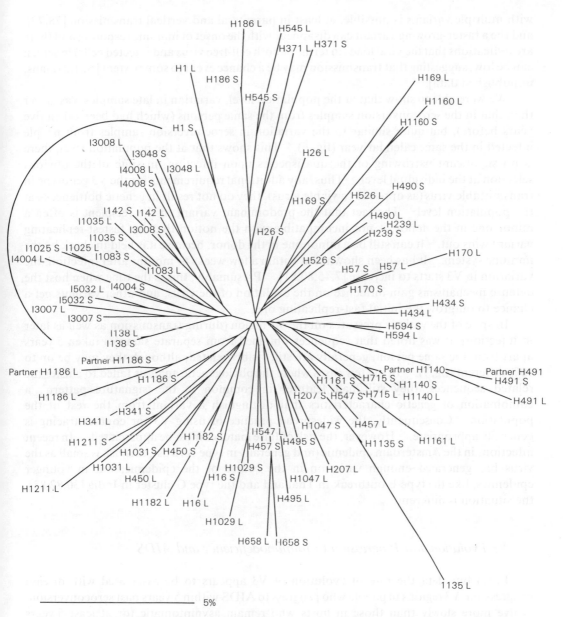

Fig. 7. Neighbor-joining tree of all 45 pairs of seroconversion and late samples. Sequences from known related infections are in all cases related to the sequences on the same branch of the tree. Codes I, H: intravenous drug user, homosexual; S, L: seroconversion sample, late sample.

with multiple variants is possible, at least in parenteral and vertical transmission [78,79], and the a faster-growing variant can disappear with the onset of immune response; and there are indications that the viral load (in terms of both cell-free virus and infected cells) in semen can be low, suggesting that transmission may be a chance event to some extent [S. Jurriaans, unpublished data].

We were able to show that at the population level, variation in late samples was larger than that in the seroconversion samples from the same persons (which had been taken five years before), but quite similar to the variation in seroconversion samples from people infected in the same calendar year (fig. 6). This shows that at the population level, there is no significant narrowing of the quasispecies upon infection, in spite of the obvious selection at the individual level. Thus, any additional requirements for the V3 genotype in transmittable virus (as opposed to viable virus), they do not result in genetic bottlenecks at the population level. The fact that the predominant variant in the recipient is often a minor one in the donor, is not incompatible with the notion that the fastest-replicating variant wins out. It can still be a minor one in the donor, because it is held in check by the immune system. It has been shown that within a few weeks to months after infection, the variation in V3 starts to increase [7,45,80,81]. Presumably, this is the time when host the defense mechanisms gain influence on the evolution of the virus, and other variants get a chance to outgrow the initial fast-replicating one.

In spite of the various pressures on the V3 region (during transmission as well as later in infection), it was noted that sequences obtained from separate samples taken 5 years apart from the same person, generally are still visibly related, although they may be up to 10% different (fig. 7). In the few cases where the phylogenetic analysis failed to cluster the related sequences, they still had features in common in the 'signature pattern', a combination of genetic characteristics that distinguish a variant from the rest of the population. Consequently, the widespread practice of using V3 for contact tracing is generally appropriate. However, the risk of false matches must be appreciated. In recent infections in the Amsterdam epidemic (and generally in type B virus), this risk is small as the virus has generated enough variation in the course of the epidemic; but in younger epidemics, like the type E outbreak in Thailand and the type C cluster in India [30,82,83], the situation is different.

V3 Evolution and Progression to Immunodeficiency and AIDS

From our data the rate of evolution of V3 appears to be associated with disease progression: V3 regions in people who progress to AIDS within 5 years past seroconversion, evolve more slowly than those in hosts who remain asymptomatic for at least 5 years (fig. 8). This can be explained in two ways. Either the immune system is more vigilant in slow progressors, leading to the necessity (for the virus) to produce more diverse variants to stay ahead of this pressure (the 'host influence' model) or the virus infecting the rapid progressors is inherently more pathogenic (or more closely related to pathogenic variants), so that collapse of the immune system begins after only a small number of V3 varians have been generated (the 'viral factors' model). The fact that the 5-year evolution rate was found to be lower also in people who develop immunodeficiency later (fig. 9), but at the 5 year time point still have a normal CD4 count, lends support to the second model.

(a)

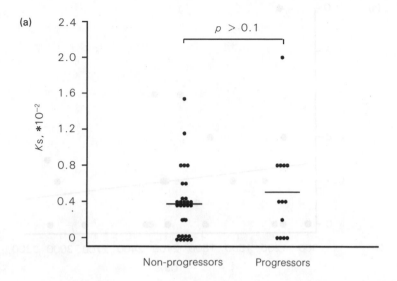

(b)

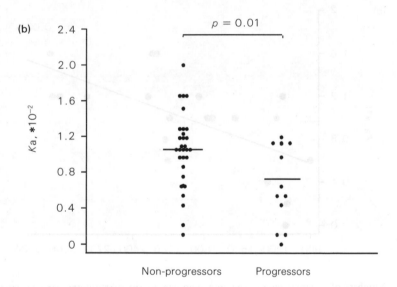

Fig. 8. Numbers of synonymous (a) and non-synonymous (b) nucleotide substitutions per site per year in the V3 region.

138

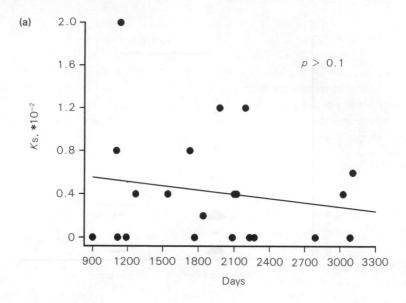

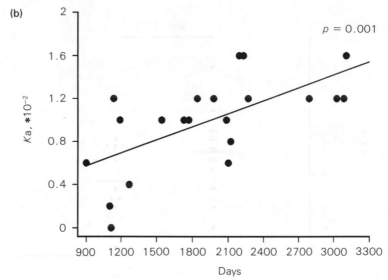

Fig. 9. Numbers of synonymous (a) and non-synonymous (b) substitutions per site per year and the duration of immunocompetent period in HIV-1 infection. Statistics for (b)-correlation. 64, R squared. 41.

Intermediate samples will be analyzed to resolve this question.

The transition from the asymptomatic to the symptomatic phase is a logical starting point in intra-individual studies. Localized genomic changes may contribute significantly to the pathogenesis of HIV, like *nef* deletions in longterm asymptomatic individuals [84]. Still, non-silent mutations accumulate at a significantly lower rate in progressors compared to non-progressors, suggesting two conclusions:

(1)   length of the immunocompetent period determines the rate of non-silent mutations in the V3 region;

(2)   the accumulation of non-silent mutations in the V3 region contribute little to progression to immunodeficiency and AIDS.

HIV Quasispecies in Equilibrium at Population Level and Selected Variation at Within-Person Level

In view of the tremendous virion and lymphocyte turnover, combined with a high mutation rate, the most surprising finding of the sequence analysis studies presented here and elsewhere may not be the extent of variation in HIV, but rather its relative constancy in spite of these driving forces. The potential for change towards a fitter genotype (and phenotype) appears not to be a limiting factor for evolution under natural circumstances: if a mutation is beneficial, the virus will probably come up with it very quickly. Even so, our data show that both at the population level and at the within-individual level, the amount of variation is limited, and less than we know to be possible from studies of virus from other sources (persons or geographical regions). At the population level, the quasispecies expands but centers around the same consensus for ten years. At this level, the HIV quasispecies appears to be in equilibrium [85]. At the individual level, the quasispecies appears to be moving, although slowly. It remains to be decided if this movement is real or a sampling artefact: it may be that a succession of within-person consensus sequences change erratically, gaining and losing mutations depending on very temporary (and possibly random) circumstances. What we are looking at is 'seleccted variation' [67]: at the within-person level, the quasispecies is in equilibrium only until an environmental change forces it to adapt. One of the most important questions that must be answered in the molecular evolution of HIV is how the mutants are selected; what determines when and where the viral population reaches its equilibrium, and when and how it is disturbed.

References

1   De Jong JJ, Goudsmit J, Keulen W, Klaver B, Krone WJA, Tersmette M, De Ronde A: J Virol 1992; 66: 757.
2   De Jong JJ, De Ronde A, Keulen W, Tersmette M, Goudsmit J: J Virol 1992; 66: 6777.
3   Koot M, Keet IPM, Vos AHV, Goede de REY, Roos MTL, Coutinho RA, Miedema F, Schellekens PTA, Tersmette M: Ann Int Med 1993; 118: 681.
4   Richman DD, Bozzette SA: JID 1994; 169: 968.
5   Power C, McArthur JC, Johnson RT, Griffin DE, Glass JD, Perryman S Chesebro B: J Virol 1994; 68: 4643.
6   Simmonds P, Balfe P, Peutherer JF, Ludlam CA, Bishop JO, Leigh Brown AJ: J Virol 1990; 64, 864.
7   Mulder-Kampinga GA, Kuiken CL, Dekker J, Scherpbier HJ, Boer K, Goudsmit J: J Gen Virol 1993; 74: 1747.

8   Kuiken CL, De Jong JJ, Baan E, Keulen W, Tersmette M, Goudsmit J: J Virol 1992; 66: 4622.
9   Eigen M, Winkler-Oswatitsch R, Dress A: Proc Natl Acad Sci USA 1988; 85: 5913.
10 Nieselt-Struwe K: Doctoral Dissertation, University of Bielefeld 1992.
11 Bandelt HJ, Dress AWM: Adv Math 1992; 94: 47.
12 Saitou N, Nei M: Mol Biol Evol 1987; 4: 406.
13 Felsenstein J: J Mol Evol 1981; 17: 368.
14 Olsen GJ, Matsuda H, Hagstrom R, Overbeek R: CABIOS 1994; 10: 41.
15 Kuiken CL, Nieselt-Struwe K, Weiller GF, Goudsmit J: In: Methods in Molecular Genetics Vol 4. Molecular Virology, Orlando, Academic Press 1994: p100.
16 Pedroza Martins L, Chenciner N, Åsjö B, Meyerhans A, Wain-Hobson S: J Virol 1991; 65: 4502.
17 Gao F, Yue L, White AT, Pappas PG, Barchue J, Hanson AP, Greene BM, Sharp PM, Shaw GM, Hahn BH: Nature 1992; 358: 495.
18 Li WH, Tanimura M, Sharp PM: Mol Biol Evol 1988; 5: 313.
19 Sabino EC, Shpaer EG, Morgado MG, Korber BTM, Diaz RS, Bongertz V, Cavalcante V, Galvao-Castro B, Mullins JI, Mayer A: J Virol 1994; 68: 6340.
20 Clavel F, Hoggan MD, Willey RL, Strebel K, Martin MA, Repaske R: J Virol 1989; 63: 1455.
21 Delassus S, Cheynier R, Wain-Hobson S: J Virol 1991; 65(1): 225.
22 Vartanian JP, Meyerhans A, Åsjö B, Wain-Hobson S: J Virol 1991; 65: 1779.
23 Howell RM, Fitzgibbon JE, Noe M, Ren Z, Gocke DJ, Schwartzer TA, Dubin DT: AIDS Res Human Retroviruses 1991; 7: 869.
24 Groenink M, Andeweg A, Fouchier RAM, Broersen S, Van der Jagt RCM, Schuitemaker H, De Goede R, Bosch ML, Huisman HG, Tersmette M: J Virol 1992; 66: 6175.
25 Coffin JM: Science 1995; 267: 483.
26 Ho DD, Neumann AU, Perelson AS, Chen W, Leonard JM, Markowitz M: Nature 1995; 373: 123.
27 Wei X, Ghosh SK, Johnson VA, Emini EA, Deutsch P, Lifson JD, Bonhoeffer S, Nowak MA, Hahn BH, Saag MS, Shaw GM: Nature 1995; 373: 117.
28 Kuiken CL, Goudsmit J: AIDS Res Human Retroviruses 1994; 10: 319.
29 Kuiken CL, Cornelissen MTE, Gibbs AJ, Zorgdrager F, Hartman S, Goudsmit J: 1995; Submitted.
30 Myers G, Korber B, Wain-Hobson S, Smith RF, Pavlakis GN: Human Retroviruses and AIDS 1993, Theoretical Biology and Biophysics, Los Alamos, 1993.
31 Mientjes GHC: Studies on the natural course of HIV infection among injecting drug users 1994; Thesis.
32 Kuiken CL, Goudsmit J, Weiller GF, Armstrong JS, Hartman S, Portegies P, Dekker J, Cornelissen MTE: J Gen Virol 1995; 76: 175.
33 Pang S, Vinters HV, Akashi T, O'Brien WA, Chen ISY: J AIDS 1991; 4: 1082.
34 Steuler H, Storch-Hagenlocher B, Wildemann B: AIDS Res Human Retroviruses 1992; 8: 53.
35 Nielsen C, Pedersen C, Lundgren JD, Gerstoft J: AIDS 1993; 7: 1035.
36 Epstein LG, Kuiken CL, Blumberg BM, Hartman S, Sharer LR, Clement M, Goudsmit J: Virol 1991; 180: 583.
37 Martins L Pedroza, Chenciner N, Wain-Hobson S: Virol 1992; 191: 837.
38 Korber BTM, Farber RM, Wolpert DH, Lapedes AS: Proc Natl Acad Sci USA 1993; 90: 2176.
39 Sala M, Zambruno G, Vartanian J-P, Marconi A, Bertazzoni U, Wain-Hobson S: J Virol 1994; 68: 5280.
40 Keys B, Karis J, Fadeel B, Valentin A, Norkrans G, Hagberg L, Chiodi F: Virol 1993; 196: 475.
41 Korber BTM, Kunstman K, Furtado M, McEvilly MM, Patterson B, Levy R, Wolinsky S: J Virol 1994; 68: 7467.
42 Delassus S, Cheynier R, Wain-Hobson S: J Virol 1992; 66: 5642.
43 Itescu S, Simonelli PF, Winchester RJ, Ginsberg HS: Proc Natl Acad Sci USA 1994; 91: 11378.
44 Kuiken CL, Lukashov VV, Leunissen JAM, Goudsmit J: 1995; Submitted
45 Wolfs TFW, Zwart G, Bakker M, Valk M. Kuiken CL, Goudsmit J: Virol 1992; 185: 195.
46 Holmes EC, Zang LQ, Simmonds P, Ludlam CA, Leigh Brown AJ: Proc Natl Acad Sci USA 1992; 89: 4835.
47 Simmonds P, Zhang LQ, McOmish F, Balfe P, Ludlam CA, Brown AJ Leigh: J Virol 1991; 65: 6266.
48 Lukashov VV, Kuiken CL, Goudsmit J: 1994; Submitted.
49 Fouchier RAM, Groenink M, Kootstra NA, Tersmette M, Huisman HG, Miedema F, Schuitemaker H: J Virol 1992; 66, 3183.
50 De Wolf F, Hogervorst E, Goudsmit J, Fenyö E-M, Rübsamen-Waigmann H, Holmes H, Galvao-Castro B, Karita E, Wasi C, Sempala SDK, Baan E, Zorgdrager F, Lukashov VV, Osmanov S, Kuiken CL, Cornelissen MTE: the WHO network on HIV-1 isolation and characterization; AIDS Res Human Retroviruses 1994; 10: 1387.
51 Koot M, Vos AHV, Keet RPM, Goede de REY, Dercksen MW, Terpstra FG, Coutinho RA, Miedema F, Tersmette M: AIDS 1992; 6: 49.
52 Spira A, Ho DD: J Virol 1995; 69: 422.

53 Westervelt P, Trowbridge DB, Epstein LG, Blumberg BM, Li Y, Hahn BH, Shaw GM, Price RW, Ratner L: J Virol 1992; 66(4), 2577.
54 Hwang SS, Boyle TJ, Lyerly HK, Cullen BR: Science 1991; 253: 71.
55 Shioda T, Levy JA, Cheng-Mayer C: Proc Natl Acad Sci USA 1992; 89: 9434.
56 Cann AJ, Churcher MJ, Boyd M, O'Brien W, Zhao JQ, Zack J, Chen ISY: J Virol 1992; 66: 305.
57 O'Brien WA, Koyanagi Y, Namazie A, Zhao J-Q, Diagne A, Idler K, Zack JA, Chen ISY: Nature 1990; 348: 69.
58 Shioda T, Oka S, Ida S, Nokihara K, Toriyoshi H, Mori S, Takabe Y, Kimura S, Shimada K, Nagai Y: J Virol 1994; 68: 7689.
59 Westervelt P, Henkel T, Trowbridge DB, Orenstein JM, Heuser J, Gendelman HE, Ratner L: J Virol 1992; 66: 3925.
60 Malykh A, Reitz M, Louie A, Hall L, Lori F: Virol 1995; 206: 646.
61 Schuurman R, Nijhuis M, Leeuwen van R, Schipper P, Collis P, Danner SA, Mulder J, Loveday C, Christofferson C, Kwok S, Sninsky J, Boucher CAB: J Infect Dis 1995; in press.
62 Wain-Hobson S: In: The Evolutionary Biology of Viruses. New York, Raven Press, 1994; p185.
63 Bebenek K, Abbotts J, Roberts JD, Wilson SH, Kunkel TA, J Biol Chem 1989; 264: 16948.
64 Preston BD, Poiesz BJ, Loeb LA: Science 1988; 242: 1168.
65 Roberts JD, Bebenek K, Kunkel TA: Science 1988; 242: 1171.
66 Takeuchi Y, Nagumo T, Hoshino H: J Virol 1992; 62: 3900.
67 Coffin JM: Current Topics in Microbiology and Immunology 1992; 176: 143.
68 Delwart EL, Sheppard HW, Walker BD, Goudsmit J, Mullings JI: J Virol 1994; 68: 6672.
69 McNearney T, Hornickova Z, Kloster B, Birdwell A, Storch GA, Polmar SH, Arens M, Ratner L: Ped Res 1993; 33: 36.
70 Scarlatti G, Leitner T, Halapi E, Wahlberg J, Marchisio P, Clerici-Schoeller MA, Wigzell H, Fenyö E-M, Albert J, Uhlen M, Rossi P: Proc Natl Acad Sci USA 1993; 90: 1721.
71 Wolinsky SM, Wike CM, Korber B, Hutto C, Parks WP, Rosenblum LL, Kunstman KJ, Furtado MR, Munoz J: Science 1992; 255: 1134.
72 Burger H, Gibbs RA, Nguyen P-N, Flaherty K, Gulla J, Belman A, Weiser B: Vaccines 1990; 255.
73 Wolfs TFW, Zwart G, Bakker M, Goudsmit J: Virol 1992; 189: 103.
74 Zhu T, Mo H, Wang N, Nam DS, Cao Y, Koup RA, Ho DD: Science 1993; 261: 1179.
75 McNearney T, Hornickova Z, Markham R, Birdwell A, Arens M, Saah A, Ratner L: Proc. Natl. Acad. Sci. USA 1992; 89: 10247.
76 Zhang LQ, MacKenzie P, Cleland A, Holmes EC, Brown, AJ Leigh, Simmonds P: J Virol 1993; 67: 3345.
77 Shpaer EG, Delwart EL, Kuiken CL, Goudsmit J, Bachmann MH, Mullins JI: AIDS Res Human Retroviruses 1994; 10: 1679.
78 Lamers SL, Sleasman JW, She JX, Barrie KA, Pomeroy SM, Barrett DJ, Goodenow MM: J Clin Invest 1994; 93: 380.
79 Cornelissen MTE, Mulder-Kampinga GA, Veenstra J, Zorgdrager F, Kuiken CL, Hartman S, Dekker J, Van der Hoek L, Sol C, Coutinho RA, Goudsmit J: J Virol 1995; 69: 1810.
80 Pang S, Shlesinger Y, Daar ES, Moudgil T, Ho DD, Chen ISY: AIDS 1992; 6: 453.
81 Lamers S, Sleasman JW, She JX, Barrie KA, Pomeroy SM, Barrett DJ, Goodenow MM: J Virol 1993; 67: 3951.
82 Tsuchie H, Maniar JK, Yoshihara N, Imai M, Kurimura T, Kitamura T: Jpn J Med Sci Biol 1993; 46: 95.
83 Pfützner A, Dietrich U, Eichel von U, Briesen von H, Brede HD, Maniar JK, Rübsamen-Waigmann H: J AIDS 1992; 5: 972.
84 Kirchhoff F, Greenough TC, Brettler DB, Sullivan JL, Desrosiers RC: New Engl J Med 1995; 332: 228.
85 Domingo E, Holland JJ: In: The evolutionary biology of viruses, New York, Raven Press, 1994.

Vaccine and Therapy

The Role of Prophylaxis in HIV Disease

Paul A. Volberding

University of California San Francisco, CA, USA

The ability to prevent opportunistic infectious complications of HIV disease with the use of prophylactic antibiotics is an important element in overall patient care. Prophylaxis is most appropriate for infections causing mortality or serious morbidity which are relatively common, predictable, and for which effective treatments exist.   Infections which meet these criteria include *Pneumocystis carinii* pneumonia, toxoplasma encephalitis, cryptococcol meningitis, herpes simplex virus, *Mycobacterium avium*-intracellulare, and potentially a *Cytomegalovirus retinitis*.   For these infections, prophylactic antibiotics are either available or are in advanced stages of development.   Prophylaxis of *Pneumocystis carrinii* pneumonia is successful and prolongs overall survival.   For other infections, the clinical benefits are somewhat less certain.   Fluconazole can for example, prevent *Cryptococcol meningitis*, but in at least one trial, this was not associated with reduced overall mortality.   As populations of HIV-infected individuals progress to more advanced disease stages, prophylaxis will become an increasingly important concern.   Effective strategies of opportunistic infection prophylaxis should be developed which broaden our ability to prevent these complicating infections.   Because of this long-term use of multiple medications, clinicians must address the growing risk for adverse drug interactions and toxicities.   Summaries of currently recommended prophylactic strategies will be reviewed.

The Dilemma of Developing and Testing AIDS Vaccines

Dani P. Bolognesi

Duke University Medical Center, Durham, NC, USA

Introduction

On June 17, 1994 the National Institute of Allergy and Infectious Diseases AIDS Research Advisory Committee recommended to the Institute that it continue but not expand the current vaccine trials with the two recombinant gp120 subunit vaccines furthest along in development and proceed with expanded clinical trial evaluation only when more compelling information becomes available with these or other candidates. To some, particularly vaccine developers, this action was viewed as a major setback given the extensive efforts and resources that have been expended for developing and testing these products. The valuable scientific and practical information that could emerge from the trials, even if the vaccines were partly successful, is now further from reach. To others, who felt that testing products with questionable promise for efficacy consituted a risky and unjustifiably costly undertaking that would ultimately have a negative impact on present and future vaccine trials, the recommendations of this body were more satisfying. Between these two extremes lies a sizable gulf of uncertainty as to what the best way to proceed might be.

These events illustrate the hurdles that HIV vaccines must face in order to move to large-scale trials. They also highlight the continuing struggle to establish standards that a vaccine must meet that are acceptable to scientists, vaccine developers, government officials, and representatives of the communities affected by such trials. Why these are such difficult issues and what needs to be achieved in order to maintain the momentum toward an effective vaccine against HIV will be the focus of this discussion.

General Principles of Vaccine Development Against Viruses

From the standpoint of vaccine development, it is becoming more and more apparent that HIV is like no other virus. Key features that have led to successful vaccines with other viruses appear to be missing and are replaced by ones that are not conducive to vaccine development. First and foremost is the issue of natural immunity, or the spontaneous resolution of the infection and disease caused by a virus as a consequence of an effective immune response mounted by the host. This signals that the pathogen harbors targets

147

against which successful immune defenses can be mounted.   Correlates of immunity (or protection) can be derived and used to guide vaccine development.   The ability of host defenses to effectively clear the pathogen is also important for another reason, namely that it provides the rationale for developing live attenuated forms of the organism as vaccines. Like the pathogen itself, these would be eliminated after the establishment of protective immunity, thus providing an important measure of safety.   Indeed, the most successful vaccines are live attenuated forms, although whole inactivated preparations have also been effective.   Moreover, development of vaccines against such viruses has not had to deal with features such as variablilty, latency and immunopathogenicity that have prevented successful vaccines with other viruses (e.g. viruses of the common cold, members of the herpesvirus family) and are the trademarks of HIV.

In the absence of natural immunity, one must confront several serious obstacles: 1) correlates of immunity become difficult to establish, 2) the rationale for live attenuated or even whole inactivated vaccines is weakened because of concerns for safety, 3) the specter that all immune responses to the pathogen may not necessarily be salutary must be resolved, and 4) the need to better understand virulence and how to overcome it becomes paramount. Thus, empiricism that historically has been so dominant in vaccine development against viruses gives way to a concerted effort to understand the fine details of infection and pathogenesis and how this is balanced with the ensuing host responses.

Animal Models for HIV Vaccine Development

When faced with such obstacles, vaccine developers have sometimes turned to animal models.   However, once again HIV presents a major barrier, since animal models have been unable to provide uniform guiding principles or correlates for protection easily translatable to humans.   This is largely due to the fact that the requirements for protection in various animal models have been rather uneven.   The differences between the models and the vaccine outcomes may reflect the respective virulence of the virus in a particular host (fig. 1).   Acute disease models induced by strains such as the SIVmac251 isolate are refractory to most vaccination attempts with the exception of live attenuated viruses and, to a lesser extent, whole inactivated virus approaches [5].   On the other hand, a more moderate but nonetheless lethal disease course occurs in pigtailed macaques infected with SIVmne, and vaccine approaches that are not successful with acute disease models do show efficacy in this model [12].   Possibly even less stringent are criteria for vaccine success in models such as HIV-2 infections in macaques and HIV-1 infections in chimpanzees, neither of which produces disease.   This may reflect the measure of host control on the virus or some form of natural immunity; the more effective this is, the more likely that a vaccine will be efficacious.   The virulence of the challenge virus itself and its ability to expand and establish high levels of viremia is a related factor, since in models like SIVmne the virus loads can be between 10- and 100-fold lower than in animals infected with SIVmac251.

In aggregate, these observations may be related to the question of natural immunity cited earlier, in that even degrees of host control that fall short of complete clearance of the virus appear to be important.   The overriding issue to be resolved is which, if any, of these models are the most representative of HIV infection and disease in humans and how best to use them.   Perhaps each one represents a segment of the overall spectrum of HIV infection

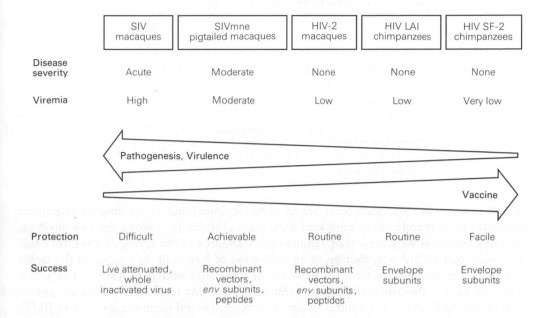

SIV macaques	SIVmne pigtailed macaques	HIV-2 macaques	HIV LAI chimpanzees	HIV SF-2 chimpanzees
Disease severity Acute	Moderate	None	None	None
Viremia High	Moderate	Low	Low	Very low

Pathogenesis, Virulence

Vaccine

| **Protection** Difficult | Achievable | Routine | Routine | Facile |
| **Success** Live attenuated, whole inactivated virus | Recombinant vectors, *env* subunits, peptides | Recombinant vectors, *env* subunits, peptides | Envelope subunits | Envelope subunits |

Fig. 1.   Relative vaccine efficacy in non-human primates infected with SIV, HIV-2, and HIV-1 suggests viral pathogenesis/virulence correlates inversely with ease of vaccination.

in people defined now as rapid (SIVmac251), intermediate (SIVmne), and long-term non-progressors (chimpanzees/HIV-1).   It is, therefore, likely that animal models have and will continue to be an indispensable component for vaccine development against HIV, and a better understanding of the lessons they teach us will make their value even greater.

Pre-Clinical and Clinical Studies with Envelope Subunit Vaccine Candidates

These issues and uncertainties notwithstanding vaccine developers initially focused on vaccine approaches based on the virus envelope.   Several independent studies had demonstrated that recombinant envelope products were effective in preventing HIV infection in chimpanzees and that antibodies were the best correlate of protection (for review see 3). The hypothesis that threshold levels of neutralizing antibodies might protect people against HIV infection became plausible, and a number of clinical trials were initiated to evaluate the safety and immunogenicity of envelope-based candidate vaccines.   The best performance was achieved by two recombinant gp120 vaccines prepared in mammalian cells.   In terms of magnitude, breadth, and duration of the neutralizing antibody responses to several laboratory strains, the results in humans surpassed even those achieved in the chimpanzee model (for review see 24).   In both low- and high-risk volunteers, these vaccines also proved to be very well tolerated [24].

It was at this point that the question arose of proceeding to larger trials in high-risk volunteers to evaluate efficacy.   Guidelines as to the features a vaccine would have to

Table 1.   Guidelines for entry into efficacy trials

	Spring 1993
Primate protection studies	√
Safety in Phase I/II	√
Immunogenicity	
• Vaccine strain	√
• Circulating strains in target population	?

√ = Meets criteria;   √√ = Exceeds criteria;   ? = Not determined; X = Fails to meet criteria.

exhibit in order to enter such trials began to be fashioned, but in the absence of defined correlates of immunity these were kept very general (table 1). When the two envelope vaccine candidates were measured against such standards in the spring of 1993, they had essentially met all but one, that being an indication of how well they matched the target viruses in the population virologically, immunologically, and genetically. The initial approach used to determine this was to evaluate their ability to induce antibodies capable of neutralizing fresh patient isolates by use of peripheral blood mononuclear cells (PBMC) as targets (fig. 2). Although quite effective in their ability to induce neutralizing antibodies to HIV isolates that were adapted to T-cell lines, which actually overlapped with those found in HIV-infected individuals, the immune responses elicited by these vaccines have failed to neutralize fresh patient isolates on PBMCs [10,14]. A flurry of studies ensued to determine whether this was an assay problem or whether it reflected a fundamental difference between primary and laboratory isolates. The outcome of these and continuing efforts points heavily away from this being an assay problem, a point that will be revisited later.

In the meantime, a new challenge virus for chimpanzees that had been propagated only on PBMC became available and made it possible to determine if the absence of in vitro neutralization correlated with lack of protection in vivo [19]. The results were quite surprising in that protection was achieved with both gp120 products despite the absence of singnificant levels of neutralizing antibodies to the challenge virus [7,20]. A possible explanation of why protection is easily achieved against this virus in these and other studies reflects a point made earlier (fig. 1) about the relationship between virulence and vaccine efficacy. The virus load in HIV-SF-2-challenged chimpanzees is considerably lower than with HIV LA1, where a threshold of neutralizing antibodies is a requirement for protection. As the relative significance of the neutralization results and the protection studies was being debated, another important set of information became available, namely, detection of infections in volunteers participating in both Phase I and Phase II vaccine trials with these products [2].

How each of these developments affected the perception of the suitability of these vaccines for expanded clinical testing is illustrated in table 2. In the spring of 1993, the two envelope candidates appeared to be on their way to meeting all of the requirements; but by the fall of 1993 they fell somewhat short on measures of breadth of activity as determined by neutralization of primary isolates. In the spring of 1994 the chimpanzee data became

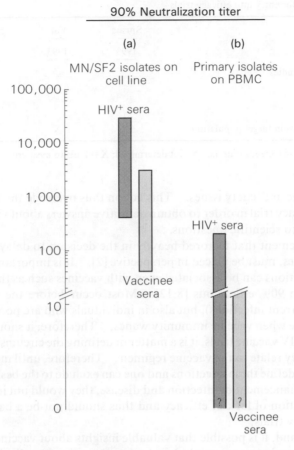

Fig. 2. Neutralization of laboratory strains versus primary isolates. The bars indicate the range of neutralization titers of sera from HIV-1 infected individuals and uninfected volunteers who have been vaccinated with MN and SF-2 envelope glycoproteins on:
a) laboratory isolates grown on T-cell lines (MN, SF-2) and
b) primary isolates (panel of 10) representative of clade B (origin of MN and SF-2) passaged only on peripheral blood mononuclear cells (PBMC).
Note that sensitivity of primary isolates to neutralization is much lower with both HIV+ sera and sera from vaccines, but while a fraction of sera from HIV-1-infected individuals can still neutralize some of the isolates, none of the vaccinee sera tested register positive readings. The minimum positive reading in our assay systems is a titer of 1 : 10.

available casting considerable doubt on the significance of the in vitro neutralization and leading many observers to turn toward further clinical studies for definitive answers. However, by the summer of 1994 the issue of infections in vaccinees emerged and decreased confidence in the potential efficacy of these vaccines. This perception also exacerbated concerns that an increase in risk behavior may occur as a result of participation in such a trial, which could place volunteers at a higher risk for HIV infection. Such concerns for safety, coupled with the desire to preserve precious human and material resources for future trials, led to the recommendation not to go forward until more could be learned about the

Table 2.   Guidelines for entry into efficacy trials

	Spring 1993	Fall 1993	Spring 1994	Summer 1994
Primate protection studies	√	√	√√	√√
Safety in Phase I/II	√	√	√	?
Immunogenicity				
• Vaccine strain	√	√	√	√
• Circulating strains in target population	?	X	X	X

√ = Meets criteria; √√ = Exceeds criteria; ? = Not determined; X = Fails to meet criteria.

unresloved scientific and safety issues.   This action thus overrode the recognized value of performing an efficacy trial in order to obtain definitive answers about vaccine performance as well as answers to scientific questions.

However, one element that factored heavily in the decision to delay the trials, namely, infections in vaccines, must be placed in perspective [2].   It is important to remember that breakthrough infections can be associated even with vaccines such as those for hepatitis B, that are more than 90% efficacious [8,12].   Most occur before the vaccine regimen is completed (intercurrent infections), but also in individuals who are poor responders to the vaccine or with time when vaccine immunity wanes.   Therefore, it should be no surprise if they are found in HIV vaccine trials, it is a matter of defining the circumstances surrounding the infections as they relate to the vaccine regimen.   Therefore, until more is known about the conditions that define these infections and one can exclude to the best of one's ability the phenomenon of enhancement of infection and disease, they would not in and of themselves represent an indication of lack of efficacy and thus should not be a barrier for entry of a vaccine into efficacy trials.

On the other hand, it is possible that valuable insights about vaccine efficacy as well as HIV infection and pathogenesis might be obtained by careful studies of these infections. For instance, how vaccine failure is related to the immunization schedule or the responder status of the vaccinee could be determined.   Does a vaccine fail against certain but not other isolates ?   Does vaccination influence the course of infection and disease progression in individuals who become infected ?   And lastly, can such information be used to help guide decisions as to when a vaccine is ready for efficacy trial testing ?

The Debacle of Primary Isolate Neutralization

Returning to the question of the primary isolate neutralization dilemma, the problem, as mentioned earlier, is not likely to lie with the assay.   This is because a number of human monoclonal antibodies as well as a limited number of sera from acutely infected individuals and long-term non-progressors who have been studied thus far effectively neutralize such isolates.   Examples of monoclonal antibodies to both gp120 and gp41 that have impressive neutralization potency on field isolates come from studies in several laboratories.   As originally shown by Fenyo and colleagues [1] and more recently in studies from Ho's group [13], polyclonal sera derived within a six month window after acute infection effectively neutralize autologous primary isolates, a property that appears to be lost in time as the virus diversifies. However, there are also examples of polyclonal sera from a subset of long-term non-progressors that exhibit broad and effective neutralization of panels of field isolates [11]. In all of these instances the immune reponse has recognized sites that are shared by the complex virus populations that comprise primary isolates. To date, as noted earlier, immunization with gp120 or gp160 has not produced antibodies with this capability.

One explanation might be that these are all instances where the immune system is exposed to the dynamics of virus infection, replication, and diversification, as opposed to immune responses to static molecules. We also now know from studies in several laboratories including our own that the envelope of the virus exists in the form of an oligomer, as opposed to a monomer as in the case of the gp120 vaccines (for review, see 15). Moreover, subsequent to binding to the CD4 receptor, this complex, which is held together by the gp41 transmembrane protein, undergoes dramatic conformational changes that trigger the processes of fusion and entry into the cell (fig. 3). These changes involve intermolecular interactions between gp120 and gp41 as well as intramolecular rearrangements within each molecule, particularly gp41, as it forms a membrane attack complex. This is a process that is common to many fusogenic viruses, the prototype being the influenza virus, as brought to light by elegant studies of Carr and Kim[4], and our model for HIV derives in part from that example. The immune system may thus 'see' these transitional forms and mount responses to what otherwise might be inaccessible (hidden) epitopes. Defining such target epitopes, which are essential for the virus and probably represent conserved domains shared by most or all HIV species, may contribute to the design of more effective vaccines.

There is indeed new evidence from several laboratories that the envelope of primary isolates is configured differently from that of T-cell line adapted viruses in that it shields certain targets for neutralization both by recombinant CD4 and antibodies [18,21]. This has prompted suggestions that envelope vaccines based on primary isolates and exhibiting an oligomeric form of the envelope may be more effective for induction of neutralizing antibodies to field isolates. However, results of studies in animal models and in humans indicate that the development of antibodies that effectively cross-neutralize primary isolates is not only rare, but occurs only after long-term exposure to the infecting virus. It is thus difficult to envision how immunization with nonreplicating oligomeric envelope would overcome this problem. Actual experiments in which synthetic envelope oligomers have been used to immunize animals have indeed not produced neutralizing antibodies effective against primary isolates (T. Matthews, P. Berman, and B. Moss, personal communication). Therefore, other strategies will be necessary to devise immunogens with such properties. Encouraging in this regard are approaches based on identifying target epitopes of human monoclonal antibodies that effectively neutralize primary isolates and reconfiguring these as effective immunogens.

Discussion

In summary, we have witnessed unexpected developments and perhaps learned valuable lessons as the first wave of vaccines approached the all important milestone of efficacy trial testing. These vaccines were based on the hypothesis that neutralizing

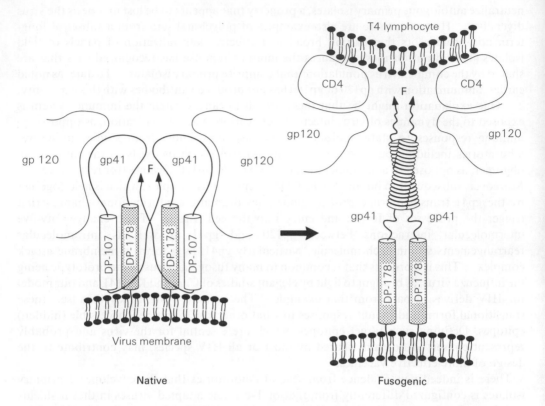

Fig. 3. Model for a structural transition in the HIV-1 TM protein leading to an active fusogenic attack complex. A model is proposed which indicates a structural transition from a native oligomer to a fusogenic state following a trigger event (possibly gp120 binding to CD4). Features include: 1) the native state is held together by noncovalent protein-protein interactions to form the heterodimer of gp120/41 and other interactions, principally through gp41 interactive sites (DP178 and DP107), to form homo-oligomers on the virus surface of the gp120/41 complexes; 2) shielding of the hydrophobic fusogenic peptide at the *N*-terminus (F) in the native state; and 3) the leucine zipper domain (DP107) exists as a homo-oligomer coiled-coil only in the fusogenic state. When triggered, the fusion complex is generated through formation of coiled-coil interactions in homologous DP107 domains, resulting in an extended α-helix similar to the model for influenza. This conformational change positions the fusion peptide for interaction with the cell membrane.

antibodies could represent a correlate of protection. For the present, the definitive clinical studies to answer this question have been put on hold until more information becomes available. There are other hypotheses such as cellular immunity or mucosal immunity that could either stand alone or, as is much more appealing to many, be combined through imaginative vaccine approaches in order to elicit a more comprehensive immunity. These are currently in development and could be ready for large-scale trials over the next several years (table 3). They include complex recombinant pox vectors that, in addition to the envelope, include other structural as well as regulatory gene products of the virus and have proven capable of inducing both neutralizing antibodies and CTL. The added benefit of immunity at mucosal sites can be achieved with other viral and bacterial vectors such as adenovirus, poliovirus, mengovirus, and salmonella. Other approaches include vaccina-

Table 3.   HIV vaccine candidates in development[1]

Second Generation (being considered for clinical trials)

- Complex pox vectors (vaccinia, avipox) consisting of multiple HIV gene products (*gag, pol, env, nef*)
- VLP[2]
- Pseudovirions[3]
- Peptide cocktails (including oral formulations)

Third Generation (in research)

- Live attenuated viruses
- Whole inactivated viruses
- Naked DNA
- Viral vectors (adenovirus, poliovirus, mengovirus, rhinovirus)
- Bacterial vectors (BCG, Salmonella, Shigella)
- Chimeric proteins[4]

---

1. For review see [24].
2. Nucleic acid free, non-infectious virus-like particles (VLP) that self-assemble in yeast, insect, and mammalian expression systems involving *env, gag,* and *pol* gene products of HIV.
3. Nonreplicating multiply mutated HIV.
4. Immunogenic protein sequences from other organisms coupled to HIV proteins or peptidees.

tion with DNA and the live attenuated virus vaccines.   The latter, spearheaded by Desrosiers [6], is thus far the most successful vaccine strategy and now a major research topic to determine if it can be made safe and what mechanism is responsible for its superior efficacy.

Thus, despite substantial efforts to develop a vaccine against HIV, it is evident that many important questions still remain unanswered.   Continued efforts are needed to understand basic features of HIV infection and pathogenesis, to improve animal models, and to identify correlates of protection.   In addition to searching for correlates of immunity in cases of vaccine breakthrough infections or in long-term non-progressors, one must also consider the significance of a growing number of instances in which protection against HIV infection occurs without recognizable correlates of immunity.   For instance, there are the examples with the SF-2 challenge virus in chimpanzees, where protection occurs in the absence of neutralizing antibodies even against laboratory strains [9,16].   Similarly, studies with several different vaccine approaches against HIV-2 reveal little or no neutralizing antibodies or CTL at the time of challenge, and yet protection against infection is achieved [23].   Finally, from studies in cohort HIV exposed non seroconverters [25] and in monkeys exposed to low dose rectal challenges [17], one again finds indications of possible protection in the absence of classical immune correlates.

What are these situations telling us about host control of virus replication and pathogenesis?   Are there host defense mechanisms that are not easily detectable as classical effector mechanisms (e.g., neutralizing antibodies and CTL) that when supplemented with vaccination, can effectively block infection?   Investigation of these and related examples of protection in the absence of identifiable correlates would seem worthwhile, and such studies may eventually show that even the measurable correlates that are familiar to us may be only markers but not the actual mechanism of protection.

To conclude, the biomedical establishment cannot become passive or discouraged over the recent developments.   It has little alternative but to redouble its efforts and be prepared to maintain a long-term solid commitment until an effective vaccine against this devastating pathogen is achieved.   This commitment must not only emphasize basic research, but also support properly justified preclinical and clinical studies of a more empirical nature that have historically proven so valuable in vaccine development.   Regardless of how much progress one can achieve scientifically, it will never be enough to guarantee that a vaccine will or will not succeed; that requires well-designed clinical trials which in turn will identify the elusive correlates of protection that can guide development of improved vaccines.

In any event, it is now evident that a great deal of momentum is required to drive an HIV vaccine to the all-important milestone of an efficacy trial.   Badly needed are acceptable guidelines designed to best forecast the likelihood that vaccine candidates will prove efficacious.   In the absence of immune correlates, more emphasis might be placed on vaccine efficacy in several animal models with varying degrees of virus virulence and disease.   Similarly, appropriately designed Phase II studies in individuals at risk for HIV infection may help to guide entry into large definitive efficacy trials.   Thus, whereas the recent experience has been a trying one for the vaccine field, one can take some comfort in that, when we are next faced with such decisions, the foundation for going forward will be more solid and justifiable.[1]

References

1   Albert J, Abrahamsson B, Nagy K, Aurelius E, Gaines H, Nystrom G, Fenyo EM: Rapid development of isolate-specific neutralizing antibodies after primary HIV-1 infection and consequent emergence of virus variants which resist neutralization by autologous sera. AIDS (Phila.) 1990; 4: 107 – 112.
2   Belshe RB, Bolognesi DP, Clements ML, Corey L, Dolin R, Mestecky J, Mulligan M, Stablein D, Wright P: HIV infection in vaccinated volunteers [letter]. JAMA 1994; 272: 431.
3   Bolognesi DP: Human immunodeficiency virus vaccines. Adv Virus Res 1993; 42: 103 – 148.
4   Carr CM, Kim PS: A spring-loaded mechanism for the conformational change of influenza hemagglutinin. Cell 1993; 73: 823 – 832.
5   Daniel MD, Mazzara GP, Simon MA, Sehgal PK, Kodama T, Panicali DL, Desrosiers RC: High-titer immune responses elicited by recombinant vaccinia virus priming and particle boosting are ineffective in preventing virulent SIV infection. AIDS Res Hum Retroviruses 1994; 10: 839 – 851.
6   Desrosiers RC: HIV with multiple gene deletions as a live attenuated vaccine for AIDS. AIDS Res Hum Retroviruses 1992; 8: 1457.
7   Francis DP, Fast P, Harkonen S, McElrath MJ, Belshe R, Berman P, Gregory T, the AIDS Vaccine Evaluation Group: MN rgp120 (Genentech) vaccine is safe and immunogenic—but will it protect humans ? [abstract]. In: Tenth Int Conf on AIDS; Yokohama Aug 7 – 12, 1994. Abstract Book Vol. 1, p90, abstr. 314A, 1994.
8   Francis DP, Hadler SC, Thompson SE, Maynard JE, Ostrow DG, Altman N, Braff EH, O'Malley P, Hawkins D, Judson FN, Penley K, Nylund T, Christie G, Meyers F, Moore JN, Jr, Gardner A, Doto IL, Miller JH, Reynolds GH, Murphy BL, Schable CA, Clark BT, Curran JW, Redeker AG: The prevention of hepatitis B with vaccine. Report of the Centers for Disease Control multi-center efficacy trial among homosexual men. Ann Intern Med 1982; 97: 362 – 366.
9   Girard M: 1994. Further studies on HIV-1 vaccine protection in chimpanzees. Presented at Tenth Int Conf on AIDS; Yokohama, Aug 7 – 12, 1994.
10   Hanson CV: Measuring vaccine-induced HIV neutralization: report of a workshop. AIDS Res Hum Retroviruses 1994; 10: 645 – 648.
11   Ho DD: Long-term non-progressors [abstract]. In: Tenth Int Conf on AIDS; Yokohama Aug 7 – 12, 1994. Abstract Book Vol. 1, p50, abstr PS10, 1994.
12   Hu SL, Abrams K, Barber GN, Moran P, Zarling JM, Langlois AJ, Kuller L, Morton WR, Benveniste RE: Protection of macaques against SIV infection by subunit vaccines of SIV envelope glycoprotein gp160.

Science 1992; 255: 456 – 459.
13 Koup RA, Safrit JT, Cao Y, Andrews CA, McLeod G. Borkowsky W, Farthing C, Ho DD: Temporal association of cellular immune responses with the initial control of viremia in primary human immunodeficiency virus type 1 syndrome. J Virol 1994, 68: 4650 – 1655.
14 Matthews TJ: Dilemma of neutralization resistance of HIV-1 field isolates and vaccine development. AIDS Res Hum Retroviruses 1994; 10: 631 – 632.
15 Matthews TJ, Wild C, Chen CH, Bolognesi DP, Greenberg ML: Structural rearrangements in the transmembrane glycoprotein after receptor binding. Immunol Rev 1994; 140: 93 – 104.
16 Natuk R, Robert-Guroff M, Lubeck M, Steimer K, Gallo R, Eichberg J: Adeno-HIV priming and subunit boost: 2nd generation AIDS Vaccines. [abstract]. In: Tenth Int Conf on AIDS, Yokohama Aug. 7 – 12, 1994. Abstract Book Vol. 1, p74, abstr. 248A, 1994.
17 Pauza D, Trivedi P, Johnson E, Meyer KK, Streblow DN, Malkovsky M, Emau P, Schultz KT, Salvato MS: Acquired resistance to mucosal SIV infection after low dose intrarectal inoculation: The roles of virus selection and CD8-mediated T cell immunity, p151 – 156. In: Girard M and Valette L (ed), Retroviruses of Human AIDS and Related Animal Diseases. 8e Colloque des Cent Gardes, Fondation Marcel Mérieux, Lyon, Oct 25 – 27, 1993.
18 Sattentau Q: 1994. Studies with monomeric and oligomeric forms of the HIV envelope from primary and cell line adapted viruses. Presented at Tenth Int Conf on AIDS; Yokohama, Aug. 7 – 12, 1994.
19 Schultz AM, Hu SL: Primate models for HIV vaccines. AIDS (Phila.) 1993 7: S161 – S170.
20 Steimer KS: Status of gp120 subunit vaccine development. Presented at Tenth Int Conf AIDS; Yokohama, Aug. 7 – 12, 1994.
21 Sullivan N, Wyatt R, Olshevsky U, Moore J, Sodroski J: Neutralizing antibodies directed against the HIV-1 envelope glycoproteins. AIDS Res Hum. Retroviruses 1994; 10 Suppl 3: S110, abstr 188.
22 Szmuness W, Stevens CE, Zang EA, Harley EJ, Kellner A: A controlled clinical trial of the efficacy of hepatitis B vaccine (Heptavax B): A final report. Hepatology 1981; 1: 377 – 385.
23 Tartaglia J, Franchini G, Robert-Guroff M, Abimuku A, Benson J, Limbach K, Wills M, Gallo RC, Paoletti E: Highly attenuated poxvirus vetor strains, NYVAC and ALVAC, in retrovirus vaccine depeloment 1993; p. 293 – 298. In: Girard M, Valette L (ed), Retroviruses of Human AIDS and Related Animal Diseases. 8e Colloque des Cent Gardes, Fondation Marcel Mérieux, Lyon. Oct 25 – 27, 1993.
24 Walker MC, Fast PE: Human trials of experimental AIDS vaccines. AIDS (Phila.) 1993; 7: S147 – S159.
25 Willerford DM, Bwayo JJ, Hensel M, Emonyi W, Plummer FA, Ngugi, EN, Negalkerke N, Callatin WM, Kresis J: Human immunodeficiency virus infection among high-risk seronegative prostitutes in Nairobi. J Infect Dis 1993; 167: 1414 – 1417.

Update on Antiretroviral Therapy

Stefano Vella

Retrovirus Department, Laboratory of Virology, Istituto Superiore di Sanità, Rome, Italy

In the 1980 edition of the *Goodman and Gilman's Textbook of Therapeutics*, only about three pages were devoted to antiviral agents among the over eighteen hundred pages of the volume: indeed, at the beginning of the AIDS pandemic, only a few antivirals were available to combat viral diseases. At that time, the identification of substances able to inhibit the replication of one of the most complicated class of viruses, such as retroviruses, appeared to be an even more difficult objective. Indeed, a number of biological and pathogenetic characteristics of HIV infection hamper the development of effective therapies against this virus. In particular, the fact that the disease caused by HIV is chronic and evolutive, that this particular retrovirus has a multiplicity of cellular targets, that the virus-host relationship changes over time, and that, at least in the late stages, there is a concurrence of other serious infections which make the picture even more complicated from a therapeutic point of view. Finally, for a long time, we have been lacking reliable markers for drug activity and clinical efficacy, a fact that has complicated the clinical evaluation of the few antiretroviral drugs that have been developed in recent years.

Despite all these difficulties, considerable progress has been achieved in the last few years. A number of active compounds have been introduced in clinical practice, namely zidovudine, didanosine (ddI), zalcitabine (ddC) and stavudine (d4T), all belonging to the class of nucleoside analogues which target a precise enzyme of HIV, the reverse transcriptase. Other nucleoside analogues like 3TC and other compounds of a different class but targeting the same enzyme, the non-nucleoside reverse transcriptase inhibitors (NNRTI) are currently under development. Among the major achievements of antiretroviral therapy the effect of zidovudine in reducing the materno-fetal transmission of HIV must be cited [1]. After the successful outcome of the ACTG 076 trial, future studies will hopefully help to determine more precisely the exact timing of fetal HIV infection and the possibilities to further reduce this transmission modality. At that point it will be mandatory to work out the availability and accessibility of antiretroviral drugs to HIV-infected pregnant women in the developing countries. Finally, new compounds inhibiting HIV replication through the effect on other viral enzymes, i.e. the protease inhibitors, are entering clinical research and have shown, in preliminary studies, a good tolerability and a strong antiretroviral effect. Hopefully, in the next few years, they will enter clinical practice and be combined with the already available antiretroviral drugs.

As has been the case also with other diseases of man, doctors began treating HIV infection when the disease was already in an advanced stage. Indeed, in the short term, clear beneficial effects with the use of nucleoside analogues were detected. We have been able to prolong survival and delay the progression of the disease administering zidovudine, and more recently ddI, ddC and d4T, late in the course of the disease. A number of indirect markers of disease progression, such as the CD4$^+$ lymphocyte count, are also favourably modified by these drugs [2 - 5].

Unfortunately, it rapidly appeared that the benefits obtained with monotherapy were of short duration and that they did not significantly modify the natural history of the disease in terms of progression to AIDS and survival.

The idea of using antiretrovirals earlier in the course of the disease is now supported by a very strong pathogenetic background. Fauci clearly showed that, in HIV disease, clinical latency does not reflect virological latency, that HIV infection is active within the lymphoid organs from the early phases, and that the deterioration of the immune system is progressive [6, 7]. More recently, it has been demonstrated that there is an incredibly high turnover of HIV, and that AIDS is primarily a consequence of continous, high-rate HIV replication, leading to virus and immune-mediated killing of CD4$^+$ lymphocytes [8 - 9].

Indeed, a number of controlled trials have been completed to address the issue of early intervention with antiretroviral monotherapy. The results of the first trial on this matter were published in 1990 in *The New England Journal of Medicine*, by Volberding and co-workers [10]. The study showed that, in the short term, there was a clear benefit for asymptomatic patients with less than 500 CD4$^+$ in using zidovudine versus placebo. However, subsequent studies demonstrated that this benefit was of limited duration [11]. The EACG 020 study, published in 1993 by Cooper and co-workers, showed a limited although sound benefit with respect to progression to AIDS [12] but, finally, in 1994, the ANRS–MRC Concorde Study demonstrated that although there was a significant benefit in terms of CD4$^+$ cell increase, no benefit was detected in terms of progression to AIDS and of survival between patients who were allocated to immediate treatment versus deferred treatment [13].

How can we reconcile these controlled observations with the actual knowledge about the pathogenesis of HIV disease? A few historical lessons can be learned by the review of the development of drugs for tuberculosis. Shortly after the discovery of streptomycin in 1944 - 45, the hope that this drug could defeat tuberculosis was subsequently deceived by the observation that the long-term outcome of patients treated with streptomycin was in fact poor. In 1950, an editorial in *The New England Journal of Medicine* stated that doctors should have stopped the 'uncontrollable compulsion' to resort to the use of streptomycin because there was 35% relapse of pulmonary tuberculosis within twelve months (table 1). The reality was that streptomycin, while an effective drug, was not potent enough when used in monotherapy to overcome a complicated disease such as tuberculosis. Only with the appearance of new drugs and with the development of combination chemotherapy did the treatment of tuberculosis became more successful a few years later [14].

What happened with tuberculosis is happening for HIV disease: therapeutic research is now turning to combination therapy, because monotherapy, although performed with active drugs, is not effective enough in shutting down HIV replication.

Several studies have already shown that combination therapy is better than monotherapy, at least in terms of CD4$^+$ and viral load levels. We have a number of studies now demonstrating that a combination of two nucleosides (zidovudine + ddI,

Table 1.

The first matter that this report re-emphasizes is that *streptomycin can never (or hardly ever) be counted on to cure tuberculosis.* This concept must be hammered home to all physicians (and patients alike, for that matter), in whom the establishment, or even suspicion of a diagnosis of tuberculosis invariably stimulates an uncontrollable compulsion to resort to streptomycin therapy. The most convincing proof of this is the fact that 35 per cent of all streptomycin-treated cases of pulmonary tuberculosis have relapsed within twelve months of completion of this therapy.

(Editorial. New Engl. J. Med. 1950; 242; 843.)

zidovudine + ddC, Zidovudine + 3TC) is more effective in decreasing the plasma HIV levels or in increasing the $CD4^+$ peripheral counts [15]. In particular, the results of combination studies with zidovudine and 3TC show that this combination may reduce the amount of virus in the blood to a much greater degree than zidovudine alone. In other combination studies thus far conducted, virus levels tend to return to baseline after a few weeks, but the effect of this particular combination persisted for at least 48 weeks.

From these preliminary data it is easy to predict that, although toxicity and tolerability problems may arise, triple combination may even be better than double combination to treat HIV disease. Indeed, the results of the ACTG 229 trial support the hypothesis that, at least from a virological point of view, a combination of two nucleoside analogues with a drug acting at a different level of HIV replication (in this case a protease inhibitor) may be even more effective than double combinations.

At the present time, there is preliminary evidence, mainly based on observational although potent studies, that combination antiretroviral therapy may also add benefits in terms of survival, but if we need definitive answers in terms of disease progression and survival, we will have to wait for the results of controlled studies such as the DELTA or ACTG 175, which are based on clinical endpoints. Unfortunately, these studies, as with all long and complicated studies, inevitably face very high withdrawal rates, so that a final lack of evidence to show small differences between treatments is becoming a possibility. Also, if therapy is initiated late in the course of the disease, combination therapy may not appear better than monotherapy. As an example, in the ACTG 155 study, patients who were very advanced, heavily pre-treated and randomized to zidovudine + ddC did not survive longer than patients randomized to zidovudine or ddC monotherapies. Possible explanations for the lack of efficacy of combinations at very low $CD4^+$ counts may include toxicity, the fact that immune system is already destroyed and, possibly, the presence of high-degree pre-existing zidovudine resistance.

However, this study should not be interpreted to mean that combinations do not work better than monotherapy; on the contrary it underlines the fact that if combination turns out to be the more effective strategy, it should be initiated early in the course of the disease.

Together with the incomplete suppression of viral replication, the emergence of reduced sensitivity to antiretroviral drugs is another possible reason for the time-limited efficacy of monotherapy. Indeed, the two events are linked: the emergenece of resistance is an

Table 2.   Mutations in HIV reverse transcriptase which confer drug resistance (adopted from Larder)

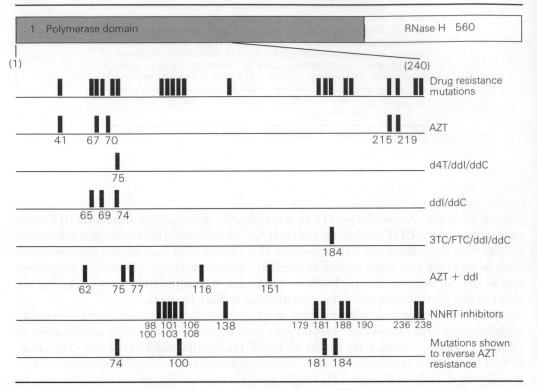

inevitable consequence of incomplete virus suppression. A number of mutations in the HIV reverse transcriptase gene have been described that confer resistance to the currently available nucleoside analogues and to NNRTI (table 2). Unfortunately, it has been also shown that HIV is able to generate new sets of mutations to escape from combinations of nucleoside analogues [16 – 20].

A few points need to be considered concerning the emergence of reduced sensitivity to antiretroviral drugs (table 3).

(A) Is drug-resistance clinically relevant? It seems today very clear that reduced sensitivity to antiretroviral drugs is indeed of clinical importance, even if other independent

Table 3.   Reduced sensitivity to antiretroviral drugs

- Clinical relevance
- Cross resistance
- Reversal of resistance
- Transmission of drug-resistant strains
- Delay of resistance
- Where to look for resistance ?
- Where does resistance arise ?

variables, such as the emergence of syncitium-inducing (SI) HIV strains, can also predict drug failure.

(B) Not all the nucleoside analogues select for the same mutations on the reverse transcriptase gene: the combination of drugs selecting for different mutations will be one of the driving rules for future therapy.

(C) An interesting phenomenon has been recently described, which is represented by the ability of particular RT mutations (i.e. mutation at codon 184 induced by 3TC) to counteract the resistance induced by other mutations (i.e. 215 mutation selected for by zidovudine).

(D) Where will resistance arise?   And where should one look for resistance?   These are two major questions that the ongoing studies on HIV pathogenesis are expected to answer.   Clearly, it has been shown that HIV has different replication compartments (PBMC; lymph nodes; monocytes; central nervous system) that may be not fully related to each other.

(E) Would it be possible to delay resistance to antiretroviral drugs?   Rapid turn-over of HIV results in increasing viral diversity with time.   Again, in tuberculosis therapy, the incidence of resistance strains to isoniazid was clearly decreased by the use of a combination of isoniazid and other anti-tubercular drugs.   Unfortunately, until now there is no evidence that a combination of nucleoside analogues is able to delay the emergence of resistant strains, so the benefits suggested by the results of the preliminary studies with combinations may be due only to the increased reduction of viral replication and not to the delay of the emergence of resistance.

Clearly, if we wish to achieve a dramatic impact on the natural history of HIV disease, we must look at new approaches and develop new drugs to be combined with the already available agents.

Indeed, a new class of drugs, the inhibitors of HIV protease, are currently under evaluation[21 – 22].   The HIV protease has the function of cutting itself and other structural and functional proteins out of the long polyprotein synthesized during virus replication.   In a double-blind randomized trial we evaluated the antiviral and immunological effects of one of these compounds, saquinavir, alone or in combination with zidovudine.   Antiretroviral-naive patients were randomized into five groups of different drug treatments.   Two groups received the protease inhibitor or zidovudine mono-therapies.   The remaining three groups received different doses of saquinavir in combination with zidovudine.   Saquinavir appeared to be very well tolerated, and the effects in terms of CD4$^+$ level and in terms of viral burden measured as a number of RNA copies in the plasma was much more pronounced in the high dose combination.   As with all effective drugs, resistant strains appeared during the course of the study, but we have been able to obtain a delay in the emergence of resistance with respect to the two drugs, in the combination arm.   Even though preliminary, these results tend to support the hypothesis that a strong reduction in viral load and in virus replication may also reduce the incidence of resistant strains over time.

At present, many protease-inhibitors are under clinical development, some of which appear to be very potent.   Even though resistance seems to occur quickly if these compounds are used in monotherapy, the hope is that by using them in multiple combinations, it may be possible to finally modify the natural history of this disease through a prolonged and sustained suppression of viral replication (which has been proven to be the

Table 4.   Criteria for selecting combination of antiretroviral drugs

- Antiviral synergy
- Differential phosphorilation of nucleosides
- Complementary activity in chronically or acutely infected cells
- Complementary activity in different body compartments
- Lack of cross-resistance
- Reversal of resistance
- Delay of the emergence of resistance (?)

major factor driving the pathogenesis of the disease).

The future of antiretroviral therapy will clearly be to switch from treating patients with advanced disease—when the immune system is already deteriorated—with a single drug, to the treatment of early disease—when the immune system is still functional—with a combination of drugs.   In this respect, the synergistic antiviral activity and the lack of cross-resistant mutations should not be the only driving issues: complementary activity in chronically versus acutely infected cells (i.e. in the monocyte-macrophage system) or in different body compartments (i.e. in the central nervous system) must also be considered (table 4).

The individualization of antiretroviral treatment will clearly be the next step: this should be based not only on clinical status and CD4+ counts, but also on immune function, HIV phenotype, drug susceptibility and the new quantitative markers of viral replication (table 5).   Recent data showing a close correlation between viral load measures and clinical

Table 5.   Individualization of antiretroviral treatment

- Clinical status
- CD4 (+ immune function)
- Viral load
- HIV phenotype
- Drug susceptibility

response are indeed very encouraging.   We will possibly have in our hands in the near future a number of virological and immunological markers that will perform as reliable indicators of drug activity and, possibly, of clinical efficacy (table 6).   They will surely help

Table 6.   Virological and immunological markers in HIV infection

	Natural history	Indicator of drug activity	Surrogate marker for clinical efficacy
CD4+	++	+	+/−
p24Ag/ICDp24Ag	+	+	+/−
PBMC viremia	+	+	?
Plasma viremia	+	++	?
HIV-RNA quantitation	+	++	?

Table 7.   HIV virology implication for controlled studies

- Entry criteria
- Stratification
- End-point
---

the fast and effective clinical evaluation of the new combinations of antiretroviral drugs (table 7).   Moreover, once validated in controlled trials, we will possibly be able to incorporate them into clinical practice, and to tailor antiretroviral therapy according to the stage and to the response of individual patients [23, 24].

As with tuberculosis, we can also obtain new ideas from the treatment of acute leukemia.   In this neoplastic disease, treatment protocols often include a remission induction polychemotherapy, followed by a maintenance treatment and by the follow up of the patients to detect leukemic relapses.   The concept of 'total cell kill' could possibly by applied also to HIV treatment.   Clearly, HIV disease is quite different from leukemia, but an 'oncological' approach should still be tested: with the new drugs and combinations that are becoming available, we should try to induce a very sharp and significant reduction of HIV viral load through a 'virological remission' polychemotherapy, switching thereafter the patient to a 'maintenance regimen,' and monitoring viral load for virological relapse.   If we can achieve this goal early in the course of the disease, we could possibly help the immune system do the rest of the job.

Finally, figure 1 shows the petrified footprints of two of our ancestors, an adult and a boy, walking together, some million years ago, near a volcano in an African region called Laetoli.   Man has come a long way since then, and the fight against AIDS probably will also have a long way to go.   Hopefully, one day in a future not too far, through the work and committment of dedicated scientists and of the people living with HIV, if we continue to reinforce the close relationship between basic research and therapeutic research, this infection will be controlled and defeated.

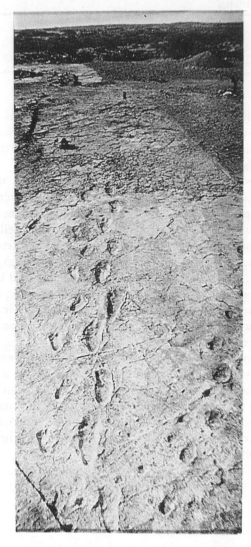

Fig. 1. Footprints of *Australopithecus afarensis* (Lucy) left on volcanic ash near Laetoli, in what is now Tanzania, 3 to 4 million years ago. (Courtesy of John Reader, National Geographic Society)

References

1   Zidovudine for the prevention of HIV transmission from mother to infant. MNWR 1994; 43: 285.
2   Fischl MA, Richman DD, Grieco MH, et al: New Engl J Med 1987; 317: 185.
3   Fischl MA, Richman DD, Hansen N, Collier AC, Carey JT, Para MF, et al: Ann Int Med 1990; 112: 727.
4   Kahn JO, Lagakos SW, Richman DD, et al: N. Engl. J. Med 1992; 327: 581.
5   Antiretroviral therapy for adult HIV-infected patients: Recommendations from a state of the art Conference. JAMA 1993; 270(21): 2583.
6   Pantaleo G, Graziosi C, Demarest JF, et al: Nature 1993; 362: 355.
7   Fauci AS; Science, 1993; 262: 1011.
8   Ho DD, Neumann AU, Perelson AS, Chen W, Leonard MJ, Markowitz M: Nature, 1995; 373: 123.
9   Wei X, Ghosh SK, Taylor ME, Johoson VA, Emini EA, Deutsch P, Lifson JD, Bonhoeffer S, Nowak MA, Hahn BH, Saag MS, Shaw GM: Nature 1995; 373: 117.
10   Volberding PA, Lagakos SW, Koch MA, et al:, N Engl J Med 1990; 322: 941.
11   Hamilton JD, Hartigan PM, Simberkoff MS, et al: N. Engl. J. Med 1992; 326: 437.
12   Cooper DA, Gatell JM, Kroon S, et al:, N Engl J Med 1993; 329: 297.
13   Concorde Coordinating Committe, Concorde, Lancet, 1994; 343: 871.
14   Crofton J, Br Med J 1960; 2: 679.
15   Collier AC, Coombs RW, Fischl MA, et al: Ann Int Med 1993; 119: 786.
16   Larder BA, Darby G, Richman DD, Science 1989; 243: 1731.
17   Richman DD, Guatelli JC, Grimes J, et al: J Inf Dis 1991; 164: 1075.
18   St Clair MH, Martin JL, Tudor-Williams G, et al: Science 1991; 253: 1557.
19   Richman DD, Antimicrob Agents Chemoter 1991; 37: 1207.
20   Larder B, J Gen Vir 1994; 75: 951.
21   Robins T, Plattner J, J Acquir Immune Defic Syndr 1993; 6: 162.
22   Vella S, AIDS 1994; 8 (suppl 3): S25 – S29.
23   Mulder J, McKinney N, Christopeherson C, Sninsky J, Greenfield L, Kwok S: J Clin Microbiol 1994; 32(2): 292.
24   Dewar RL, Highbarger HC, Sarmiento MD, Todd JA, Vasudevachari MB, Davey RT Jr., Kovacs JA, Salzman NP, Clifford Lane H, Urdea MS: J Inf Dis 1994; 170: 1172.

Gene Therapy for HIV Infection

Flossie Wong-Staal

UCSD, Clinical Science, La Jolla, CA, USA

I feel both optimistic and necessarily cautious to address a topic as forward looking as gene therapy. Originally, the concept of gene therapy was a replacement strategy for defective functions in genetic disorders. In its current expanded repertoire, gene therapy may provide long-term therapy for chronic infectious diseases, such as HIV infection. But we are still faced with many hurdles, both technical and conceptual, that relate to gene therapy in general and HIV infection in particular. The coming year or two will be critical as the feasibility of a number of gene therapy protocols will be evaluated in the clinic.

It is generally agreed that the virus, HIV, and host immunity are the two opposing forces that determine disease progression. Accordingly, the two arms of gene therapy are directed at boosting host immunity, either by immunization with genes encoding viral proteins or by adoptive transfer of T-cell clones that are genetically altered for greater safety or potency, and suppressing viral replication. In this presentation, I will focus on the antiviral approach, giving a brief overview of where things stand, and using work from my own laboratory to illustrate the kind of thinking and processes involved in the development of this potentially exciting therapeutic modality.

Antiviral gene therapy is sometimes referred to as intracellular immunization. The ultimate goal is to genetically alter most, if not all, potential target cells so that they would become resistant to virus replication. There are three steps to this process: design an inhibitory gene or gene combination, use or develop a high efficiency delivery system, and introduce the antiviral genes into either the mature target cells for virus infection, or their progenitor cells.

Table 1 summarize some of the potential antiviral genes under development. Many of these approaches take advantage of our understanding of the biology of the virus, a few are more general strategies for gene inhibition. The therapeutic agent may be a protein or a small RNA molecule. The transdominant proteins are defective viral proteins that interfere with wild-type function by competing for binding that their target sequences and effector molecules, or by oligomerizing with wild-type proteins to form inactive complexes. Soluble CD4 acts as a decoy for virus receptor binding, but a modification of the same molecule converts it into an intracellular trap for the virus envelope. The idea of trapping viral proteins intracellularly also underlies the design of single chain antibodies directed at various viral proteins. Interferon inhibits virus assembly and release. The use of inducible toxin genes does not really fit the concept of intracellular immunization but rather

169

Table 1.   Current approaches of anti-HIV gene therapy

RNA	Proteins
TAR and RRE Decoys	Transdominant Viral Proteins
	Rev[1], Tat
Antisense	Gag, Env
	Modified Cellular Proteins
Ribozymes[1]	sCD4
	sCD4·KDEL
	single chain Ab>Rev, Tat, Env, RT
	interferon
	Inducible Toxins
	(Suicide genes)

[1] Approved by the NIH RAC Committee for Phase 1 clinical trial.

aims at destroying the infected cells before active virus production.   The RNA therapeutics include decoy molecules for the RNA binding, regulatory proteins, Tat and Rev, and antisense and ribozyme molecules that be directed against many potential target sites of the HIV genome.   Currently, two of these approaches have obtained approval from the NIH RAC committee to proceed to a Phase I clinical trial: namely the transdominant Rev protocol that Gary Nabel developed at the University of Michigan, and the use of the hairpin ribozyme that my group has put forward.   It is anticipated that many more will make the transition from bench to bedside in the next two years.

No single approach is perfect, and it may well be that ultimately a combinatorial approach will confer the greatest efficacy.   Transdominant viral proteins suffer from the fact that they are likely to be immunogenic, and therefore the host immune response may eliminate the very cell population that one wants to protect.   Single chain antibodies as well as ribozymes and antisense RNA are susceptible to virus mutation and escape.   TAR and RRE decoys are known to also bind cellular factors and can therefore sequester these proteins and induce toxicity.   Interferon is a double-edged sword as it also down modulates immune function.

We were attracted to the idea of a ribozyme approach because unlike most of other strategies, which target a single step in the replication cycle, ribozyme can potentially act at many steps.   In fact, most other strategies only prevent virus expression from infected cells, but do not prevent infection of a new cells, while the ribozyme, by recognizing and cleaving viral RNA, can do so upon virus entry, after viral RNA transcription and at the time of viral RNA packaging.   It has often been advocated to inhibit both preintegration and post-integration events for greater synergy, and indeed the ribozyme can achieve synergy in a single molecule.

The ribozyme we have utilized is called a hairpin ribozyme, because of its structure, originally derived from the negative strand satellite RNA of the tobacco ring spot virus.   It has a minimal core sequence of 50 nt, recognizing a minimal target sequence of 14 nt.   It has a substrate recognition sequence, which forms two helices with the target, and can be engineered to match a target sequence.   In this regard, it resembles an antisense RNA.   However, it goes a step further: It also cleaves the substrate RNA catalytically, which means that one ribozyme can potentially inactivate many substrate molecules.   The substrate must contain a *GUC at this site for efficient cleavage, and this selectivity should also confer greater specificity and a lesser chance of cellular toxicity relative to antisense RNA.   The first ribozyme we designed was directed a highly conserved sequence in the U5 region of the HIV-1 LTR.   This ribozyme was shown to efficiently cleave the appropriate target sequence in vitro at a high substrate to enzyme ratio.

In previous studies for efficacy in cell lines, we showed that a functional ribozyme specifically inhibited HIV-1 expression in transiently transfected cells.   Interestingly, a disabled ribozyme with an intact substrate binding site did not have significant inhibitory activity, suggesting that the major antiviral effect was due to the RNA cleaving property of the ribozyme in vivo, rather than an antisense effect.   Transduced Jurkat and Molt 4 cells stably expressed the ribozyme gene long term, and these cells were now resistant to both infection and cytopathic effect by geographically diverse HIV-1 strains and clinical isolates. In the best situation, we observed a greater than four logs reduction of viral titer.   We demonstrated that the ribozyme indeed inhibited both pre-integration and post-integration events, possibly resulting in a synergistic antiviral effect.   And contrary to initial fears, we did not observe the rapid emergence of resistant mutants, i.e., the virus that did breakthrough was as sensitive to the ribozyme in a re challenge experiment as in the primary infection.

Once we validated the potential efficacy of an antiviral gene, the next step is to choose a gene delivery system.   There are many potential means of gene transfer, including direct physical methods, which are safe and simple.   However, they are limited by their still relatively low efficiency, and more problematically, the lack of integration and persistence. However, one arm of the transdominant Rev protocol calls for the delivery of the gene by ballistic gold particles into T-lymphocytes, and it will be interesting to follow the results from this clinical trial.

There are also a number of viral vectors that can transduce cells efficiently.   I have limited the consideration to three that would allow integration and may be appropriate for HIV infection.   Murine retrovirus vectors have so far been the workhorses of gene therapy because of their efficiency, persistence and broad host range.   As a result, there is also extensive safety data, not only in animals but also in man with these vectors.   One potential limitation is that they would not transduce non-dividing cells, while one of the major target cells for HIV is the terminally differentiated macrophage.   AAV can supposedly infect non-dividing cells, but it is still questionable whether integration occurs in these cells.   It has a small cloning capacity, but this should not be a problem with expression of the small RNA molecules: decoys, ribozymes or antisense.   An HIV vector is of course attractive for delivering therapeutic genes to the very target cells one wants to protect, and furthermore, the vector is reusable and can be disseminated to new target cells even when protection is not complete.

We inserted the U5 ribozyme gene into the LNL6 MLV vector under the expression of an internal tRNA promoter (fig. 1).   We have tried a number of promoters to test for optimal gene expression and antiviral potency, and found that the intragenic tRNA promoter worked the best, probably due to a combination of high level and ubiquitous expression as well as greater stability of the ribozyme RNA since it is fused to the tRNA sequence.   We generated amphotropic viral vectors in the PA317 packaging line.

Now the challenge is to introduce the therapeutic gene into the relevant target cells for

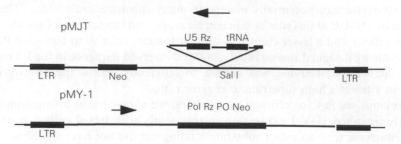

Fig. 1. Ribozyme and control vector constructs.

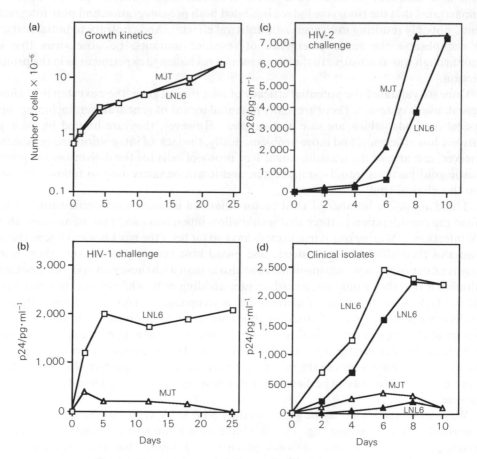

Fig. 2. Transduction and challenge of primary lymphocytes.

HIV infection: namely, primary T lymphocytes and macrophages.   However, since MLV vectors cannot transduce macrophages, we tried to transfer the gene into hematopoietic progenitor cells.   Of course, ideally, targeting the true stem cell may allow for permanent immune reconstitution.   Short of that, gene transfer into committed progenitors should still provide more sustained protection as well as accessing cells of the monocyte/macrophage lineage.

We obtained peripheral blood lymphocytes from normal donors, transduce with the retroviral vectors with or without the ribozyme gene and selected for stably transduced cells. Figure 2 summarizes the results.   First, we wanted to be sure that ribozyme expression did not have any deleterious effects on cell proliferation or function.   Here we showed that cells transduced by the control vector or the ribozyme vector had identical proliferation kinetics.   The lymphocytes were still IL-2 dependent and responsive to T cell activation. We then challenged with both a laboratory HIV strain, HXB-2, as well as different clinical isolates.   As you can see, virus expression was significantly suppressed in the ribozyme protected cells.   To rule out the possibility that the apparent inhibition was due to an incidental selection of non-infectable cells, we used HIV-2, which has the same biology as HIV-1 but is sufficiently divergent that it should not be recongized by the ribozyme, and indeed infection by HIV-2 was not inhibited.

To obtain the progenitor cells, we took advantage of the fact that both the primitive and committed progenitor cells express the CD34 antigen.   This allows for enrichment of this cell population by immunoselection.   Initially, we used several sources of progenitor cells: adult bone marrow, umbilical cord blood and mobilized peripheral blood.   More recently, we focused on the umbilical cord blood as a source for reasons I will discuss later.   CD34$^+$ cells were enriched using the immunomagnetic beads developed by Baxter.   The cells were then transduced in the presence of different combinations of growth factors, SCF, IL-3, IL-

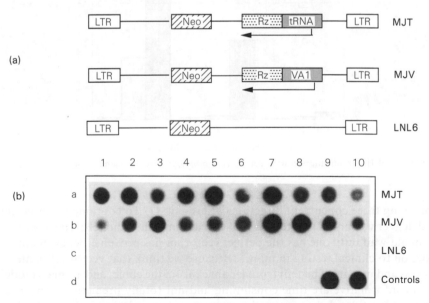

Fig. 3.   *a.* Schematic representation of the retroviral vector constructs.   *b.* Ribozyme expression assay by RNA PCR.

6, and then allowed to proliferate and form colonies, which can then be assayed for transduction efficiency or for expression of the transgene.

We found that these CD34$^+$ cells obtained from cord blood, in particular, were transduced at quite high efficiency.   Figure 3 shows that of ten randomly selected clones transduced by two ribozyme vectors, the MJT vector and MJV, which has the ribozyme driven by another Pol III promoter, the Adeno virus VA1 promoter, all were expressing detectable levels of the ribozyme gene.   The variability may be in part due to the different sizes of the colonies, which usually comprise 100 – 500 cells.   As a point of reference, these spots represent 1000 transduced Jurkat cells that are known to be resistant to HIV-1 infection.   Cells transduced by the control vector or omitting the RT step were negative, suggesting that these signals represent specifically expression of ribozyme RNA.

While the CD34$^+$ cells themselves are not infectable, or at least not efficiently infected by HIV-1, one can induce them to differentiate along the monocyte/macrophage lineage by supplying GM–CSF and selecting for adherent cells in vitro.   After 10 – 14 days, one can end up with a relatively pure population of terminally differentiated macrophages, which one can then challenge with a monocyte-tropic HIV-1.   Indeed, the ribozyme transduced cells showed significantly reduced virus expression (fig. 4).   And this inhibition could be accounted for the persistent expression of the ribozyme gene throughout differentiation. It has been observed previously that many promoters, including the MLV LTR, are turned off in progenitor cells.   Here, we observed that expression from the MLV LTR was indeed much lower than that from the Pol III promoters (data not shown).

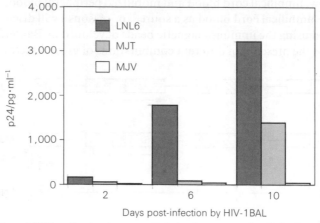

Fig. 4.   Inhibition of HIV replication in stem cell derived monocytes by the leader sequence ribozyme.

We are pursuing three concurrent directions at present: (1) To continue to refine gene constructs and deliver vectors; (2) To test in vivo efficacy in animal models; The question is whether one should wait until one has the perfect vector, or has proven efficacy in animals before one goes on to clinical testing in man.   Because we think that vector refinement is an endless process and may itself benefit from feedback from the clinic, and animals models, although may be informative are time consuming and not totally predictive of what can happen in man, we have decided to proceed simultaneously to a Phase 1 clinical trial.

A major concern in the development of anti-HIV therapy, whether it is drug therapy or gene therapy, is the ability of the virus to mutate and become resistant.   There are several strategies to minimize this possibility: choice of highly conserved sites, which one can do since there are many potential sites on the HIV genome for ribozyme cleavage; as emphasized by others for antiviral drugs, it is important to treat early in infection, when the viral burden is relatively low, and early intervention is very appropriate for a gene therapy approach; finally, it is expected that a combinatorial approach that targets multiple sites of the HIV genome will be more effective.   We have designed a double ribozyme vector that expresses in addition to the U5 ribozyme another ribozyme that recognizes a sequence in the Pol gene.   As shown in figure 5, the double ribozyme works better than either of the parental ribozyme vector.   Although we cannot address the issue of resistance since we have not seen resistant mutants generated in culture even with single ribozymes, we hope that for in vivo long-term therapy, this greater antiviral potency also correlates with greater difficulty for the virus to escape.

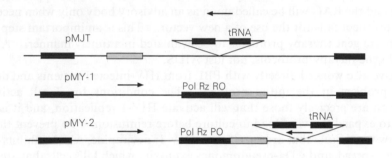

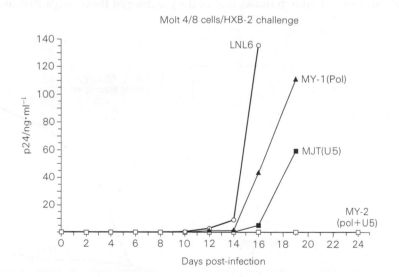

Fig. 5.   Inhibition of HIV replication by single and double ribozyme vectors.

The first Phase 1 clinical protocol we developed involved ex vivo T cell therapy. It is essentially a test for the safety and feasibility of this approach: Is there any acute or chronic toxicity, is the ribozyme expressed in vivo and if yes for how long? Efficacy will be measured only at a cellular level. We would take PBL from infected patients and infect them with either the control vector or the ribozyme vector, mix the two populations of cells and reinfuse them back to the same patient. Efficacy of the ribozyme will be measured by the relative survival of the ribozyme transduced cells and their resistance to virus infection.

At present, all gene therapy protocols have to go through four levels of regulatory approval in the U.S., institutional human subjects and recombinant DNA committees and additionally by the NIH Recombinant DNA Committee and the Federal Food and Drug Administration. This lengthy process of approval makes it difficult to have rapid feedback between bench and bedside, which is exactly what one needs in a novel area of development such as gene therapy. At a recent meeting of the National Task Force for AIDS Drug Development, the NIH Director and the FDA Commissioner have agreed to work together to streamline this process. The proposal on the table is that a single application will go to the FDA, and the RAC will be called upon as an advisory body only when necessary, e.g., when the protocol calls for the use of a new vector. This is an important step forward in allowing more gene therapy protocols to be evaluated in a timely manner. And this will benefit all gene therapy protocols, not just AIDS.

We have also worked directly with PBL from HIV-infected patients and detected one potential problem in the initial protocol. The conditions for T-cell activation and transduction are precisely those that will activate HIV-1 replication, and it is cleary not desirable to expand the viral load in culture before reinfusion. To prevent this, we have included two antivirals that are specific for HIV-1: nevirapine, which inhibits its RT and blocks virus spread, and CD4-pseudomonas exotoxin, which kills cells that are expressing the viral env protein. Figure 6 shows that in the presence of these two antivirals, no HIV

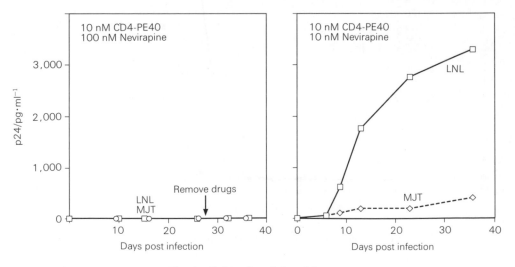

Fig. 6. Culture from infected donors.

expression was detected over 30 or more days.   Even when the drugs were removed at day 25, no virus breakthrough was observed, suggesting that we had effectively eliminated the infected cell population.   Interestingly, when the concentration of one of the antivirals was lowered, virus expression was detected in the cells transduced by the control vector, but cells transduced by the ribozyme vector still held.   This result indicates that the ribozyme is also effective against HIV acquired in vivo.

Although the first ex vivo T cell therapy protocols will be very informative for the feasibility of the general approach, there are a number of issues that may be problematic for the concept of ex vivo T-cell therapy.   First is the question whether one can forestall disease progression or whether an irreversible program of immune damage sets in once infection has occurred.   I think our clinical experience with antiviral compounds, as well as a vast body of studies in animals showed that a reduction in viral burden can confer clinical benerfits.   The second issue is whether one can access enough of the CD4$^+$ cells to make an impact on the viral burden.   It has been estimated that less than 10% of the total T-cells in the body can be replaced at a single infusion, and with repeated infusions at regular intervals, this may not be sufficient for immune reconstitution.   The answer again is not known, since we really do not know what the threshold of virus load is for disease progression, and at what point the immune system can kick in and take care of the bulk of the infected cells.   Infection of the brain is another confounding factor, and one only hopes that an intact immune system can again keep infection here at bay.   Future efforts may be directed at using vectors that target the CNS.   We have stressed time and again the importance of early intervention, but early intervention also raises the problem of how one can determine the clinical endpoints of a gene therapy trial in a patient population that usually takes 10 to 20 years to progress to the full blown disease.

Some of these concerns can be addressed by targeting the stem or progenitor cells, which would allow for more thorough and sustained immune reconstitution.   My colleagues and I have developed a second protocol, which has been approved by the UCSD Human Subjects Committee, and now awaits RAC and FDA approval.   This protocol calls for the autologous reinfusion of CD34$^+$ cells derived from placental/umbilical cord blood into infants infected in utero with HIV-1.

There seem to be several advantages in using placental/umbilical cord blood as source of hematopoietic stem cells for transplantation.   First, procurement of the CD34$^+$ cells is non-invasive to the donor.   Second, it has been shown that PUBC is more enriched in the more primitive progenitor cells and that stem cells from this source are better able to engraft and less prone to allorecognition in an allogenic transplantation setting.   So although the initial trial is for autologous reinfusion, the prospect of allogenic stem cell therapy is also feasible in the long term.

There are several features of CD34$^+$ cell trial in the pediatric population that should be mentioned.   First, we will only proceed with the trial after the HIV infection status of the infant is verified.   Second, this represents an early intervention strategy, as it will be carried out within days to weeks after birth.   Since disease progression is usually a very rapid in this patient population, the mean age of progression to AIDS being 2, this trial should also provide an earlier assessment of clinical efficacy.   Of course, the initial parameter to determine would be whether the transduced CD34 cells will engraft and depopulate long term after reinfusion.

A frequent criticism of gene therapy and a valid one is that the requirement for ex vivo manipulations makes it impractical even irrelevant for the developing world so our long term good would be to develop an injectable vector that can home into the right target cells a high titer HIV vector for example.   If that happens then one can argue that gene therapy makes even greater sense for the developing world in conferring a simple, effective and sustained therapeutic modality.   It is hoped that the urgency of the AIDS epidemic will provide impetus to further accelerate the development of this powerful technology.

References

Ojwang J, Hampel A, Looney, D, Wong-Staal, F, Rappaport, J: Inhibition of human immunodeficiency virus type-1 (HIV-1) expression by a hairpin ribozyme.   Proc Natl Acad Sci USA 1992; 89: 10802 – 10806.

Yu M, Ojwang J, Yamada O, Hampel A, Rappaport J, Looney D, Wong-Staal F: A hairpin ribozyme inhibits expression of diverse strains of human immunodeficiency virus type 1.   Proc Natl Acad Sci USA 1993; 90: 6340 – 6344.

Yu M, Poeschla E Wong-Staal F: Progress toward gene therapy for HIV-1 infection.   Gene Therapy, 1994; 1: 13 – 26.

Yamada O, Yu M, Yee J-K, Kraus G, Looney DJ, Wong-Stall F: Intracellular immunization of human T-cells with a hairpin ribozyme against human immunodeficiency virus type 1.   Gene Therapy 1994; 1: 39 – 45.

Leavitt M, Yu M, Yamada O, Kraus G, Looney D, Poeschla E, Wong-Staal F: Transfer of an anti-HIV-1 ribozyme into primary human lymphocytes. 1994.   Human Gene Therapy 1994; 5: 1151 - 1120.

Yu M, Leavitt M, Maruyama M, Yamada O, Young D, Ho A, Wong-Staal F: Intracellular immunization of human hematopoietic stem/progenitor cells with a ribozyme against HIV-1.   Proc Nat Acad Sci USA 1995 92: 699 – 703.

HIV Drug Resistance: Molecular Basis and Clinical Significance

Mark A. Wainberg[1], Marilyn Smith[1], Julio S.G. Montaner[2], Kazushige Nagai[1], Avrum Spira[1], Horacio Salomon[1] and Zhengxian Gu[1]

[1] McGill University AIDS Centre, Jewish General Hospital, Montreal, Quebec, Canada and
[2] St. Paul's Hospital, University of British Columbia, Vancouver, B.C., Canada

The development of HIV-1 resistance to drugs was predictable on the basis of similar experience with other viruses including influenza [1], herpes simplex viruses (HSV) [2] and cytomegalovirus (HCMV) [3,4]. In each instance, continuous selective pressure exerted by anti-viral chemotherapy enables the amplification of mutated viral strains that possess a drug-resistance phenotype.

HIV Reverse Transcriptase (RT) as a Target

Most of the drugs that antagonize viral RT activity are DNA chain terminators that prevent the synthesis of viral (proviral) DNA from a genomic RNA template. By being incorporated into newly-made viral DNA in the place of the usual nucleotide, e.g. thymidine triphosphate, compounds such as the triphosphates of zidovudine (ZDV) and dideoxyinosine (ddI) act as competitive inhibitors and chain terminators, causing an arrest in the formation of proviral DNA. At higher concentrations, certain of these drugs can also competitively inhibit the function of certain cellular DNA polymerases, helping to explain some of the toxicities associated with these compounds. This problem has now diminished as lower doses of viral chemotherapeutic agents are being prescribed [5,6].

CD4 Count and Drug Resistance

Between 60 – 75% of patients with advanced disease including AIDS may possess drug-resistant variants after one year of therapy with ZDV [7 – 10]. When CD4 counts fall below $100/mm^3$, this figure may exceed 90% [9,11,12], while asymptomatic individuals may display ZDV resistance only 20% of the time after 1 year of treatment [7,12]. IC_{50} comparisons of paired isolates from the same patients, obtained prior to and following treatment, demonstrated that degree of resistance increased with time [13], with over 100-fold resistance reported in some patients on ZDV monotherapy after 18 months [13 – 16].

Figure 1 presents data from a cohort of 72 initially asymptomatic patients with CD4 counts over 300 cells/mm^3, who received 500 mg/day of ZDV. Viruses were considered resistant if they possessed post-treatment IC_{50} values for ZDV at least 30 times over those

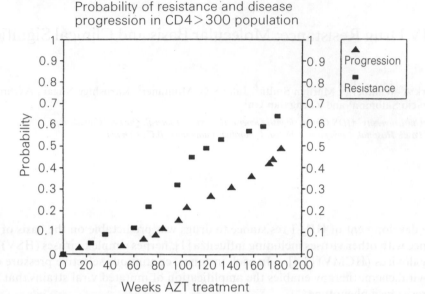

Fig. 1. Probability of disease progression, as assessed by occurrence of an opportunistic infection, and of zidovudine resistance in initially asymptomatic patients. Resistance defined as presence of isolate with IC_{50}>30-fold higher than pre-therapy isolate. Data are replotted from reference [15].

of pre-treatment isolates. The probability of developing drug resistance increased in relation to that of becoming symptomatic and both trends were observed in concert with drops in CD4 count [15]. The occurrence of resistance was found to be an independent marker of disease progression, even after adjustment for baseline CD4-to-CD8 ratio.

Early in treatment, relatively few viruses isolated from patients may be drug-resistant. The selective pressure of therapy will augment the percentage of viruses that possess such a phenotype.

To assess drug resistance, most laboratories first isolate HIV in the absence of drug by co-cultivation of patient peripheral blood mononuclear cells (PBMC) with donor PBMC or cord blood mononuclear cells (CBMC) that serve as targets for amplification of viral stock over several replication cycles. The ability of these viruses to replicate in the same targets at a variety of drug concentrations is then assessed, permitting a IC_{50} value to be calculated, on the basis of levels of viral p24 antigen and/or RT acivity in culture media [14 – 20].

Patients in whom drug-resistant isolates of HIV-1 were demonstrated yielded such viruses for as long as the same type of monotherapy was continued [7] and for periods up to 15 months after ZDV was discontinued [7,13]. Some viral isolates became more sensitive to ZDV while developing resistance to ddI in individuals whose therapy was switched from one to the other [21]. Resistance to both ddc and ZDV has been detected in some patients on alternating therapy [22].

The Genotypic Basis for HIV Drung Resistance

Comparisons of paired isolates, obtained before or after ZDV treatment, revealed five mutations at codons 41, 67, 70, 215 and 219, whose presence could be correlated with ZDV resistance.   Site-directed mutagenesis studies, performed with the infectious molecular clone pHXB2, confirmed the biological relevance of these mutations, since recombinant viruses that contained these mutations possessed high level resistance to ZDV [23].   The acquisition of these mutations was also demonstrated in viruses from patients receiving ZDV.   Both the site 41 and site 215 changes seem to be more important than the others in predicting declines in CD4 counts and clinical failure [19,24,25].

Cell-free RT assays in which the active form of ZDV, i.e. ZDV-triphosphate, is utilized to block the synthesis of DNA oligonucleotides have so far failed to distinguish between the RTs of drug-resistant and -sensitive strains of HIV-1.   More recent work with recombinant RTs mutated at either codon 74 or 65, conferring resistance against ddI and ddC, respectively, suggest that these enzymes may discriminate against the triphosphate forms of these drugs [26,27].   In addition, the RTs of resistant variants usually have increased K_i and K_i/K_m values, suggesting that changes in binding efficiency to nucleotide substrate may have occurred [11,27,28].   Additional research that uses viral RNA instead of synthetic RNA as a primer should be performed with ZDV-triphosphate and other drugs.

The polymerase chain reaction (PCR), together with appropriate primer pairs, specific for wild-type and mutated sequences, can be used to directly identify resistance-conferring viral genotypes.   The 215 mutation is present in the co-culture DNA or viral RNA of asymptomatic patients on chronic ZDV chemotherapy [19,23,26].   We can identify the presence of resistance-conferring mutations by gene amplification prior to isolation of viruses that possess a drug-resistance phenotype [18,25,26].

Work with uncultured patient PBMCs, patient plasma virus RNA [29], plasma culture DNA [30], and tissue culture-propagated viruses have documented mutations at positions 41, 67, 70, 215 and 219.   Usually, mutations at positions 41, 70 and 215 preceded the occurrence of mutations at the other sites [25].   The use of step-wise increases in drug concentrations and in vitro selection protocols have yielded similar findings; namely, ZDV-resistant variants have been grown out from initially wild-type isolates through such manipulations [31,32].   PCR studies have also shown that mixtures of genotypes may frequently be present, reflecting the large number of quasi-species seen after infection by HIV.

Several groups have documented mixtures at each of several codons during the transition from largely wild-type to mutated sequences in individual patients [20,25]. Mutational analysis of viral genomes derived from either PBMC or plasma culture showed that significant variations at each position can occur within individual patients [33].

Drug-resistant viruses can maintain a resistance phenotype, even when passaged over long periods in the absence of drug [7,12,14,26,34,35].   Although shifts in individual genotypic patterns have been reported in the absence of drug pressure [20,26] the 215 mutation was shown to persist in all 81 clones analyzed of viral RT obtained from four patients whose therapy was changed from ZDV to ddI for up to 15 months [33].   Most of these sequences were derived from plasma-derived viruses, implying the continuous replication of drug-resistant viruses in these subjects.   The persistence of the 215 mutation was noted in 7 of 8 clones derived from co-cultured DNA of a single patient 26 months after a change in therapy from ZDV to ddI [36].   Others showed a slow reversion of mutations starting 9 – 18 months after discontinuation of ZDV treatment [29], and resistant isolates were obtained 6 months after treatment from each of 10 patients who had received ZDV for 12 – 35 months [37].   Thus, the 215 mutation appears to be stable and viruses that possess it can replicate at rates similar to those of parental wild-type variants [23,26].

Resistance-conferring mutations have been detected from various sources, including uncultured PBMC DNA [38], co-culture DNA [11,31], plasma culture DNA [30], and plasma viral RNA [29].   Furthermore, individual mutations may be detected in plasma samples prior to their appearance in PBMC [39].   This is consistent with data suggesting that the greatest burden of HIV in infected individuals is not in PBMC but rather in lymphoid organs such as lymph nodes and spleen [40].   Viruses that become mutated in these organs may find their way to the blood before the migration of PBMCs that harbor these same mutated forms.   Such mutations may also be more frequent in serum than in PBMCs [39].

PCR methodology may be used to quantitate levels of HIV RNA in patient serum or plasma [41].   Virus which is present in such fluids is first ultracentrifuged, following which viral RNA in the pellet is reverse transcribed to yield DNA.   The latter can then be amplified through the use of quantitative PCR reactions, controlled for the numbers of copies generated, to provide a sensitive indication of viral burden and to quantitate the amount of virus possessing resistance-conferring mutations, relative to wild-type strains in the plasma of HIV-infected individuals [41].   Viral burden has been shown to increase concurrently or prior to CD4 decrease [42].   High viral burden does not appear to be necessary for the 215 mutation to occur; the 215 mutation and high viral burden may independently predict CD4 decline [39].

Cross-Resistance to Other Drugs

ZDV-resistant strains of HIV may simultaneously possess altered sensitivity to other nucleosides.   Extensive cross-resistance has been seen with compounds that possess a 3′-azido moiety, e.g. 3′-azido-2′,3′-dideoxyuridine (AZdU), 3′-azido-2′,3′-dideoxyinosine (AZA), and 3′-azido-2′,3′-dideoxyguanosine (AZG) [9].   Similar results have been found with some ZDV-resistant isolates and 2′,3′-dideoxy-3′-didehydrothymidine (d4T) [14]. These variable patterns of susceptibility and cross-resistance are probably due to variations in the genotypes that account for diminished sensitivity to ZDV.

Although no significant cross-resistance has been found between ZDV and either ddI or ddC among laboratory strains of HIV-1 [7,9,11,14,22], isolates from patients on prolonged ZDV therapy may display resistance to ddI [10].   A controlled trial of continued ZDV or ddI in adults (asymptomatic or ARC), with previous ZDV treatment history, reported fewer new AIDS-defining events and deaths in those assigned to 500 mg per day ddI than those who continued to receive ZDV (600 mg per day), although the efficacy of ddI was unrelated to the duration of previous ZDV therapy [44].

Table 1.   Isolation of HIV variants resistant to ddI or ZDV

Number of patients	Drug	Number of patients studied	Percentage of patients with resistant virus[†]	Average IC_{50} prior to treatment	Average IC_{50} after treatment	Ratio of IC_{50} values post: pretreatment
140	ZDV	104	74	0.05	3.9	78
48	ddI	23	27	1.6	14.8	9.2

† Determinations for resistance were carried out after 12 months of treatment.

Resistance to Other Drugs

Resistance to ddI has been observed in patients undergoing prolonged therapy with this drug [21,45].   Resistance to ddI has also been selected for through the use of step-wise increases in drug concentrations in tissue culture, and generally ranges between five- and twenty-fold, i.e. lower than for ZDV [19,32,46].   Neither is the percentage of patients who develop resistance to ddI as high as for ZDV (table 1) [32], as shown with 48 patients with CD4 counts below 300 who received ddI for at least one year after having been treated with ZDV for at least 6 months.   Resistance to ddI was seen in only 27% of subjects compared to 74% of patients manifesting resistance to ZDV.   Furthermore, the extent of resistance was generally less than that for ZDV.   In another study, some patients receiving ddI for up to 29 months showed no increase in ddI resistance in their isolates [36].

A mutation at *pol* site 74 confers resistance to ddI [19], as demonstrated in a patient who had initially been treated with ZDV and who was switched to ddI.   Viruses possessing the mutation were not only resistant to ddI (up to 26-fold change in IC_{50}) but also demonstrated increased sensitivity to ZDV [36].   Interestingly, the addition of a mutation at site 74, into a background containing the 215 mutation, increased sensitivity to ZDV (IC_{50} of 2.3 µM vs 32 µM), while resulting in a small reduction in sensitivity to ddI (IC_{50} of 22 µM vs 17 µM) [19].

Our lab first identified a mutation at position 184 (Met⟶Val) that confers 500 – 1000 fold resistance in tissue culture against 2′,3′-deoxythiacytidine (3TC) [32,47,52] and 5 – 10-fold resistance to each of ddC and ddI [49 – 52].   Cross-resistance against ZDV was not demonstrated, consistent with previous observations on ddI resistance [13,14,32].   Mutations at codon 184 (from Met to Val or isoleucine) after passage in the presence of 3TC or (−)-FTC also occurs [50].   The 184 valine mutation has also been detected in the virus *pol* sequence of patients who have received 3TC therapy for several months [50].   In a scenario reminiscent of mutation 74, introduction of the 184 Val mutation into a virus that was resistant to ZDV (due to mutations at sites 41 and 215) caused resistance to 3TC alongside a restoration of ZDV sensitivity [51].

A change at codon 69, in close proximity to some of the ZDV resistance mutations, has been identified as conferring an approximately 5-fold level of resistance to ddC [53].   A mutation at position 65 (Lys⟶Arg) has also been shown to encode resistance to ddC and is likely to be more important clinically than the site 69 alteration; these results have been confirmed by site-directed mutagenesis using infectious HIV DNA [54].   Mutagenesis and in vitro selection procedures have also pointed to a mutation at codon 89, that confers

Table 2. List of mutations associated with HIV drug resistance

Mutation site	Drug	Wild-type amino acid	Replacement amino acid
41	ZDV	methionine	leucine
65	ddC, ddI, 3TC	lysine	arginine
67	ZDV	aspartic acid	aspargine
69	ddC	threonine	aspartic acid
70	ZDV	lysine	arginine
74	ddI	leucine	valine
75	d4T	valine	threonine
89	ddG	glutamic acid	glycine
181	Nevirapine	tyrosine	cysteine
184	ddI, ddC, 3TC	methionine	valine or isoleucine
215	ZDV	threonine	tyrosine or phenylalanine
219	ZDV	lysine	glutamine or glutamic acid

resistance of HIV-1 RT to ddG triphosphate [55].   A codon change at position 75 is associated with resistance to d4T [56].

HIV resistance has also been reported in vitro against a family of non-nucleoside compounds that antagonise RT by acting as non-competitive inhibitors of DNA chain elongation [57 – 60].   These drugs can inhibit HIV replication at low concentrations and are non-toxic, but can repidly give rise to up to 1000-fold resistance following in vitro passage in their presence [61,62].   Resistance has also developed rapidly against these drugs in clinical trials [63,64].   Sequencing and mutagenesis have revealed that mutations at codons 103, 181 and 188, among others, are involved in conferring such resistance [61,62]. The mutations at positions 181 and 188 may simultaneously increase sensitivity to ZDV [65].

High level resistance and the appearance of the site 181 mutation have been indentified after as little as seven days of replication in tissue culture in the presence of these drugs. HIV-resistant variants that are generated against one member of this family commonly show cross-resistance against other drugs in the family as well, e.g. pyridinone inhibitors and Nevirapine [61,62].   Amino acids 101 – 106 of RT may interact with residues 155 – 217, and each category of compound may display subtle differences with regard to binding interactions at amino acids 176 – 190 [66].   Table 2 presents a partial summary of mutation sites and corresponding amino acid changes identified to date as accounting for HIV drug resistance, as confirmed by site-directed mutagenesis.

Combination Therapy

Combinations which utilize ZDV plus either ddC, 3TC or ddI have strong rationale, since studies have shown that ZDV plus any of ddC, ddI, 3TC and/or interferon-2α (IFNα) are synergistic for inhibition of both wild-type and drug-resistant variants.   Nor do drug combinations permit the outgrowth of resistant strains using the in vitro scheme of viral replication in increasing concentrations of anti-viral agents [32,67]. However, several groups have successfully generated viruses that are simultaneously resistant to ZDV, Nevirapine, and ddI on the basis of sequential selection procedures and/or site-directed mutagenesis [68,69].

Combinations may need to be carefully chosen for therapeutic purposes. One of four patients who received alternating weekly regimens of ZDV and ddC developed resistance to both drugs; a far lesser incidence of resistance was seen in subjects who received the same two drugs simultaneously [36]. Drug combinations including ZDV/ddI and ZDV/IFNα can act synergistically against both wild-type and ZDV-resistant variants of HIV-1 [70 – 75]. The interactions among various resistance-conferring mutation sites are complex. In the case of ZDV, high-level resistance is evident only when combinations of mutations at sites 41, 67, 70, 215 and 219 are present. In contrast, for other mutations, it is apparent that introduction of codon changes that confer resistance to 3TC or ddI may actually increase sensitivity to ZDV.

Clinical Significance

PCR or other nucleic acid amplification techniques may eventually be used to identify patients in whom drug resistance occurs. Genetic screening might identify relevant viral sequences before resistance is demonstrable biologically and prior to possible clinical deterioration.

PCR technology will not be limited to the detection of mutations that confer resistance to antagonists of viral RT. Compounds directed against other targets within the HIV replication cycle will probably suffer from problems of drug resistance as well. Indeed, resistance to both peptide and cyclic urea-based inhibitors of the HIV protease has been detected and responsible mutations have been characterized [76 – 80].

The sensitivity of PCR and other nucleic acid amplification techniques may not necessarily be translated into useful diagnostic advances. First, implementation of genotypic resistance screening on a widespread basis may be impractical, since the number of mutations known to confer drug resistance is large and doubtless incomplete. The numbers of primer pairs potentially needed for screening might be inordinately high, although direct sequencing of PCR amplified products may serve to detect some mutations preferentially [29,81]. In addition, these assays are costly, although less expensive than the phenotype-based tests. Potential problems also exist in interpretation of results, due to the multitude of viral quasi-species, many of which may possess different drug resistance-conferring mutations. Treatment with other drugs may also contribute to the presence of mutations, whose significance may not be clear once changes to therapeutic regimens have been made.

The occurrence of HIV drug resistance commonly precedes clinical deterioration and is likely to be at least partially responsible for treatment failure. Various confounders, however, make the precise relationship between clinical progression and HIV resistance difficult to interpret. As stated, patients with low CD4 counts, who have progressed to more serious disease, while on ZDV, are most likely to harbor ZDV-resistant viruses. Some subjects who were clinically stable while on ZDV had a preponderance of resistant viruses, although HIV-1 titers in plasma and mononuclear cells were generally not elevated

[82].   Both high viremia and drug resistance have been reported in patients who progressed to more serious illness [82].   Progressions and deaths occurred most commonly in children from whom drug-resistant variants of HIV-1 had been obtained [16].

Whether the use of antivirals in asymptomatic patients with high CD4 counts will induce drug resistance at relatively early time points is unknown.   Nor is it understood whether concerns about drug resistance should cause clinicians and patients to delay the use of anti-retrovirals until CD4 counts have fallen significantly.

The error-prone nature of the RT enzyme underlies all mutations in the viral genome, including those that confer drug resistance in the RT gene itself [86 – 89].   For example, mutations in *env* that cause extensive variability in antigenicity of viral gp120 are due to errors by RT [86 – 89].   While the V3 loop has been most prominent in analyses of envelope variability, other gp120 domains may also vary.   Naturally, responsibility for conferring resistance against both nucleoside and non-nucleoside inhibitors of RT lies with mutations in RT.

Such mutations occur each time the virus goes through a replication cycle at an estimated frequency of 10^{-4}.   Since many of the changes which take place may be lethal, these mutations may not always be detectable in patient material.   Non-lethal mutations that confer either drug resistance or changes in antigenicity may also go undetected, unless they can be amplified against a wild-type viral background.   In regard to *env* gene mutations, the selection pressure which permits such amplification is provided by the immune system, e.g. specific anti-HIV immune responsiveness in the form of cytotoxic T lymphocytes and neutralizing antibodies.   In the case of drug resistance, selective pressure is exerted by anti-viral drugs against viruses that cannot efficiently replicate in the presence of these compounds.

Drug resistance mutations will occur as a function of both the rate of viral replication and total viral burden.   Distinct viruses may replicate at different rates and possess RT enzymes that differ with regard to their infidelity [90].   Subjects with high viral burden will usually possess higher numbers of viral quasi-species with potential heterogeneity in degree of fidelity of their RT's and rates of replication.   Increased numbers of replication events will occur in such individuals, making it more likely that relevant resistance-conferring mutations will be found. However, facile interpretation of the relationship between disease progression and drug resistance is not possible, because viral replication is thought to be controlled by specific anti-HIV immune responsiveness as well as chemotherapy.

Thus, reductions in CD4 counts and loss of operational anti-HIV immune responsiveness may lead to increased viral burden, driving the development of drug resistance.   Hence, HIV drug resistance could result from, rather than cause, disease progression and treatment failure.   Nor can the possibility that HIV drug resistance and CD4 reduction might proceed in tandem be ruled out, since the occurrence of drug-resistant variants might give rise to increased viral burden in the face of chemotherapy, contributing, in turn, to loss of $CD4^+$ lymphocytes.

Properly designed prospective clinical trials may provide answers to some of these issues. Heightened anti-HIV immune responsiveness, through the use of immunomodulators, may impact on development of HIV drug resistance.   In this context, viral resistance to ganciclovir and acyclovir occur most often in patients whose immune systems are already compromised.   Notwithstanding, problems of HSV and CMV drug resistance are still important clinically, regardless whether pre-existing immunosuppression

Table 3. Confounding variables in HIV drug resistance

1. Rate of replication of distinct viruses.
2. Total viral burden.
3. Error-prone nature of viral reverse transcriptase (RT); individual viruses may have enzymes that are more error-prone than others; mutated forms of HIV, responsible for drug resistance, may possess RT enzymes that are more or less error-prone than those found under conditions of non-treatment.
4. Drug selection pressure.
5. Drug dosing and pharmacokinetics.
6. Anti-HIV immune response and CD4 count.
7. Co-development of other genotypic and phenotypic changes, e.g. SI vs NSI phenotype.

was involved. The occurrence of HIV drug resistance may be similarly responsible for treatment failure and compromise in clinical status, even if immune deterioration was initially responsible for the emergence of HIV drug resistance.

Resistance to ZDV occurs slowly and not abruptly; this also contributes to difficulties of interpretation. Various levels of ZDV resistance could have variable significance at different times following initiation of treatment. The use of non-nucleosides provides the best evidence that drug resistance can result in treatment failure. Treatment led to an early increase in CD4 counts and decline in viral burden that was quickly reversed in concert with appearance of viral drug resistance [91]. A list of confounding factors in assigning clinical significance to HIV drug resistance is found in table 3.

Unresolved Issues

It is of concern whether drug-resistant variants of HIV-1 are transmitted to significant extent by horizontal or vertical means. Ethical considerations have precluded addressing sexual transmission in a straightforward way. Since we are not yet certain of the clinical significance of HIV drug resistance, it may not be ethical to inform patients that they harbor drug-resistant variants. Proper counselling of HIV-infected individuals to practice safe sex may, of course, impede our ability to detect such transmission. Although drug-resistant variants of HIV-1 have been demonstrated in human vaginal fluid and ejaculate, this does not prove sexual transmission [92], although primary infection with ZDV-resistant HIV-1 has been reported [93]. Drug-resistant HIV-1 has also been transmitted vertically from a mother on prolonged ZDV therapy to her infant [94]. The recent findings that AZT usage during the third trimester of pregnancy may prevent maternal transmission of HIV are encouraging [95]. However, there is concern that this may be a short-term benefit if AZT-resistant viruses become increasingly prevalent in the population.

The virulence and pathogenicity of drug-resistant variants of HIV-1 are also important. Although such strains may be predominant in individuals suffering from disease progression, this does not mean that such viruses will necessarily mediate infection or cause disease in people to whom they are spread. Culture studies have not indicated any loss in virulence or replication ability on the part of ZDV-resistant variants [7]. A recent study suggests, however, that drug-resistant variants which are propagated over many cycles may contain more cytopathogenic viruses yet fewer replication-competent [35], while other data show similar particle-to-plaque-forming unit (PFU) ratios for mutant and wild-type particles.   The fact that ZDV-resistant viruses can continue to replicate in the body, 15 months after a switch from ZDV treatment, may be indicative of the fitness of these particles [33].

Many patients who progressed from an asymptomatic carrier state to AIDS yielded isolates that possessed enhanced syncytium-inducing (SI) capacity for cultured lymphocytes in comparison with those of matched non-progressing controls [21,96–98]. A change from non-syncytium-inducing (NSI) to SI phenotype may correlate better with disease progression than drug resistance, although cause and effect relationships are difficult to establish.   Reductions in CD4 counts and/or immune effector capacity may be causally related to the appearance of SI variants.   Recombination may be postulated to occur between SI mutants and drug-resistant mutants, producing viruses with both characteristics and with the ability to enhance disease progression in individuals with high levels of viremia.

Drug-resistant HIV-1 may be found in tissues other than blood.   The presence of resistant variants of HIV-1 in ejaculate may have public health implications.   Similarly, resistant viruses may be present in the central nervous system (CNS) of patients with HIV neurological manifestations.   Such viruses may originate independently within the CNS under conditions of drug pressure or be transported to the CNS from the blood.   Work on both freshly biopsied material as well as cerebrospinal fluid (CSF) of infected donors may prove fruitful.   Such tissues may also yield fewer ZDV-resistant particles than found in blood, due to reduced blood-brain barrier penetration and less opportunity for replication. Clinical significance has ultimately been assigned to all previously documented cases of drug resistance in infectious disease.

Acknowledgments

Our research has been supported by the Medical Research Council of Canada, Health and Welfare Canada, and the Fonds de la Recherche en Santé du Québec.

References

1   Belshe RB, Burk B, Newman F, Cerruti RL, Sim SI: J Infect Dis 1989; 159: 430.
2   Derse D, Bastow KF, Cheng Y-C: J Biol Chem 1992; 257: 10251.
3   Biron KK, Fyfe JA, Stanat SC, Leslie LK, Sorrell JB, Lambe CU, Coen DM: Proc Natl Acad Sci USA 1986; 83: 8769.
4   Collins P, Larder BA, Oliver NM, Kemp S, Smith IW, Darby G: J Gen Virol 1989; 70: 375.
5   Fischl MA, Richman DD, Grieco MH: N Engl J Med 1987; 317: 185.
6   Richman DD, Fischl MA, Grieco MN: N Engl J Med 1987; 317: 192.
7   Rooke R, Tremblay M, Soudeyns H, DeStefano L, Yao X-J, Fanning M, Montaner JSG, O'Shaughnessy M, Gelmon K, Tsoukas C, Gill J, Ruedy J, Wainberg MA: AIDS 1989; 3: 411.
8   Land S, Treloar G, McPhee D, Birch C, Doherty R, Cooper D, Gust ID: J Infect Dis 1990; 161: 326.
9   Larder BA, Chesebro B, Richman DD: Antimicrob Agents Chemother 1990; 34: 436.
10   Japour AJ, Chatis PA, Eigenrauch HA, Crumpacker CS: Proc Nat Acad Sci USA 1991; 88: 3092.
11   Larder BA, Darby G, Richman DD: Science 1989; 243: 1731.
12   Richman DD, Guatelli JC, Grimes J, Tsiatis A, Gingeras TR: J Infect Dis 1991; 164: 1075.

13 Richman DD, Grimes JM, Lagakos SW: J Acquir Immune Defic Syndr 1990; 3: 743.
14 Rooke R, Parniak MA, Tremblay M, Soudeyns H, Li X, Gao Q, Yao X-J, Wainberg MA: Antimicrob Agents Chemother 1991; 35: 988.
15 Montaner JSG, Singer J, Schechter MT, Raboud JM, Tsoukas C, O'Shaughnessy M, Ruedy J, Nagai K, Salomon H, Spira B, Wainberg MA: AIDS 1993; 7: 189.
16 Tudor-Williams G, St Clair MH, McKinney RE: Lancet 1992; 339: 15.
17 Japour AJ, Mayers DL, Johnson VA: Antimicrob Agents Chemother 1993; 37: 1095.
18 Boucher CAB, Termette M, Lange JMA: Lancet 1990; 336: 585.
19 Larder BA, Kellam P, Kemp SD: AIDS 1991; 5: 137.
20 Lopez-Galindez C, Rojas JM, Najera R, Richman DD, Perucho M: Proc Natl Acad Sci USA 1991; 88: 4280.
21 St Clair MH, Martin JL, Tudor-Williams G: Science 1991; 253: 1557.
22 Dimitorv DH, Hollinger FB, Baker CJ: J Infect Dis 1993; 167: 818.
23 Larder BA, Kemp SD: Science 1989; 246: 1155.
24 Kellam P, Boucher CAB, Larder BA: Proc Natl Acad Sci USA 1992; 89: 1934.
25 Boucher CAB, O'Sullivan E, Mulder JW: J Infect Dis 1992; 165: 105.
26 Gu Z, Fletcher RS, Arts EJ, Wainberg MA, Parniak MA: J Biol Chem (accepted for publication).
27 Wainberg MA, Tremblay M, Rooke R, Blain N, Soudeyns H, Parniak MA, Yao X-J, Li X-G, Fanning M, Montaner JSG, O'Shaughnessy M, Tsoukas C, Falutz J, Stern M, Belleau B, Ruedy J: Ann N Y Acad Sci 1990; 616: 346.
28 Martin JL, Wilson JE, Haynes RL, Furman PA: Proc Natl Acad Sci USA 1993; 90: 6139.
29 Albert J, Wahlberg J, Lundeberg J, Cox S, Sandström E, Wahren B, Uhlén M: J Virol 1992; 66: 5627.
30 Smith MS, Koerber KL, Pagano JS: J Infect Dis 1993; 167: 445.
31 Larder BA, Coates KE, Kemp SD: J Virol 1991; 65: 5232.
32 Gao Q, Gu Z, Parniak MA, Li X, Wainberg MA: J Virol 1992; 66: 12.
33 Smith M, Koerber KL, Pagano JS: J Infect Dis 1994; 169: 184.
34 Nielson C, Gotzsche PC, Nielsen CM, Gerstoft J, Vestergaard BF: Antiviral Res 1992; 18: 303.
35 Tremblay M, Rooke R, Wainberg MA: AIDS 1992; 6: 1445.
36 Shirasaka T, Yarchoan R, O'Brien MC: Proc Natl Acad Sci USA 1993; 90: 562.
37 Land S, McGavin C, Lucas R, Birch C: J Infect Dis 1992; 166: 1139.
38 Meyerhans A, Cheynier R, Albert J: Cell 1989; 58: 901.
39 Kozal MJ, Shafer RW, Winters MA, Katzenstein DA, Merigan TC: J Infect Dis 1993; 167: 526.
40 Pantaleo G, Graziosi C, Demarest JF, Butini L, Montroni M, Fox CH, Orenstein JM, Kotler DP, Fauci AS: Nature 1993; 362: 725.
41 Kaye S, Loveday C, Tedder RS: J Med Virol 1992; 37: 241.
42 Connor RI, Mohri H, Cao Y, Ho DD: J Virol 1993; 67: 1772.
43 Mayers DL, McCutcheon FE, Sanders-Buell EE: J Acquir Immune Defic Syndr 1992; 5: 749.
44 Kahn JO, Lagakos SW, Richman DD: N Engl J Med 1992; 327: 581.
45 McLeod GX, McGrath JM, Ladd EA, Hammer SM: Antimicrob Agents Chemother 1992; 36: 920.
46 Reichman RC, Tejani N, Lambert JL: Antiviral Res 1993; 20: 267.
47 Gu Z, Gao Q, Li X, Parniak MA, Wainberg MA: J Virol 1992; 66: 7128.
48 Wakefield JK, Joblonski SA, Morrow CD: J Virol 1992; 66: 6806.
49 Gao Q, Gu Z, Hiscott J, Dionne G, Wainberg MA: Antimicrob Agents Chemother 1993; 37: 130.
50 Schinazi RF, Lloyd RF Jr, Nguyen M-H: Antimicrob Agents Chemother 1993; 37: 875.
51 Tisdale M, Kemp SD, Parry NR, Larder BA: Proc Natl Acad Sci USA 1993; 90: 5653.
52 Gao Q, Gu Z, Parniak MA, Cameron J, Cammack N, Boucher C, Wainberg MA: Antimicrob Agents Chemother 1993; 37: 1390.
53 Fitzgibbon JE, Howell RM, Haberzettl CA, Sperber SJ, Gocke DJ, Dubin DT: Antimicrob Agents Chemother 1992; 36: 153.
54 Gu Z, Gao Q, Fang H, Salomon H, Parniak MA, Golberg E, Cameron J, Wainberg MA: Antimicrob Agents Chemother 1994; 38: 275.
55 Prasad VR, Lowry I, Deloaantos T, Chiang L, Goff SP: Proc Natl Acad Sci USA 1991; 88: 11363.
56 Lacey SF, Larder BA: Antimicrob Agents Chemother 1994; 38: 1428.
57 Babba M, DeClercq E, Tanaka H: Proc Natl Acad Sci USA 1991; 88: 2356.
58 Merluzzi VJ, Hargrave KD, Labadia M: Science 1990; 250: 1411.
59 Pauwels R, Andires K, Desmyter J: Nature 1990; 343: 470.
60 Boyer PL, Currens MJ, McMahon JB, Boyd MR, Hughes SH: J Virol 1993; 67: 2412.
61 Nunberg JH, Schleif WA, Boots EJ: J Virol 1991; 65: 4887.
62 Richman DD, Shin C-K, Lowry I, Rose J, Prodanovich P, Goff S, Griffin J: Proc Natl Sci USA 1991; 88: 11241.
63 Kappes JC, Chopra P, Campbell-Hill S: Eight Int Conf on AIDS, Amsterdam, 19–24 July 1992, Abstract PoB 3021.

64   Richman DD: VIII Int. Conf. on AIDS, Amsterdam, 19–24 July 1992, Abstract PoB 3576.
65   Larder BA: Antimicrob Agents Chemother 1992; 36: 2664.
66   Condra JH, Emini EA, Gotlib L: Antimicrob Agents Chemother 1992; 36: 1441.
67   Gao Q, Parniak M, Gu Z, Wainberg MA: Leukemia 1992; 6: 1926.
68   Larder BA, Kellam P, Kemp SD: Nature 1993; 365: 451.
69   Gao Q, Gu Z, Salomon H, Nagai K, Parniak MA, Waingerg MA: Arch Virol 1994; 136: 111.
70   Hartschorn KL, Vogt MW, Chou TC, Blumberg RS, Byington R, Schooley RT, Hirsch MS: Antimicrob
     Agents Chemother 1987; 31: 168.
71   Dubreuil M, Sportza L, D'Addario M, Lacoste J, Rooke R, Wainberg MA, Hiscott J: J Virol 1990; 179: 388.
72   Johnson VA, Merrill DP, Videler JA: J Infect Dis 1991; 164: 646.
73   Eron JJ Jr, Johnson VA, Merrill DP, Chou T-C, Hirsch MS: Antimicrob Agents Chemother 1992; 36: 1559.
74   Johnson VA, Merrill DP, Chou T-C, Hirsch MS: J Infect Dis 1992; 166: 1143.
75   Smith MS, Kessler JA, Rankin CD, Pagano JS, Kurtzburg J, Carter SG: Antimicrob Agents Chemother
     1993; 37: 144.
76   Kaplan AH, Michael SF, Webbie RS, Knigge MF, Paul DA, Everitt L, Kempf DJ, Norbeck DW, Erickson
     JW, Swanstrom R: Proc Natl Acad Sci USA 1994; 91: 5597.
77   Ho DD: Second International Workshop, Noordwijk, 3–5 June 1993, p18.
78   Michael S, Kaplan A, Kempf D: Second International Workshop, Noordwijk, 3–5 June 1993, p19.
79   Webbie R, Petit S, Michael S, Kaplan A, Swanstrom R: Second International Workshop, Noordwijk, 3–5
     June 1993, p20.
80   Otto MJ, Garber S, Stack S, Winslow D: Second International Workshop, Noordwijk, 3–5 June 1993, p21.
81   Jung M, Augut H, Candotti D, Ingrand D, Katlama C, Hutraux J-M: J Acquir Immune Defic Syndr 1992;
     5: 359.
82   Mohri H, Singh MK, Ching WTW, Ho DD: Proc Natl Acad Sci USA 1993; 90: 25.
83   Preston BD, Poiesz BJ, Loeb LA: Science 1988; 242: 1168.
84   Roberts JD, Bebenek K, Kunkel TA: Science 1988; 242: 1171.
85   Takeuchi Y, Nagumo T, Hoshino H: J Virol 1988; 62: 3900.
86   Desai SM, Kalyanasman VS, Casey JM, Srivivasan A, Andersen PR, Deurne SG: Proc Natl Acad Sci USA
     1986; 83: 8380.
87   Javaherian K, Langlois AJ, LaRosa GJ: Science 1990; 250: 1590.
88   LaRosa GJ, Davide JP, Weinhold K: Science 1990; 249: 932.
89   Laman JD, Schellekens MM, Abacioglu YH: J Virol 1992; 66: 1823.
90   Lacey SF, Reardon JE, Furfine ES: J Biol Chem 1992; 267: 15789.
91   Richman DD: Antimicrob Agents Chemother 1993; 37: 1207.
92   Wainberg MA, Beaulieu R, Tsoukas C, Thomas R: AIDS 1993; 7: 433.
93   Erice A, Mayers DL, Strike DG: N Engl J Med 1993; 328: 1163.
94   Frenkel LM, Demeter LM, Wagner L: Keystone Symposia: HIV Pathogenesis in infants and children,
     March 29–April 2, 1993. Albuquerque, NM, QZ 102, p96.
95   Morbidity and Mortality Weekly Report, Aug 5, 1994.
96   St. Clair MH, Hartigan PM, Andrews JC, Vavro CL, Simberkoff MS, Hamilton JD: J AIDS 1993; 6: 891.
97   Koot M, Keet IPM, Vos HV: Ann Intern Med 1993; 118: 681.
98   Termette M, De Goede REY, Ap BJM: J Virol 1988; 62: 2026.

Care and Preventive Activities

Interface between HIV/AIDS and Prostitutes: Micro Level Analysis in the Red-Light Context

Priti Patkar

Prerana Municipal School, Bombay, India

Prerana, an NGO, works for the Welfare and Development of Red-Light Area (women) Prostitutes (RLAP) and their children since June 1986. Its programs for the above children include Night Care Center, Formal Education Support Project, Placement in Institutions of Residential Care (away from the red-light area), personality development, etc. Programs for the prostitutes include Health Awareness, General Social Awareness/ Education, Environmental Development, Liaison with Civic Authorities, Establishing Human and Civic Rights of the RLAP, e.g. right over public distribution system, etc., participating in policy making affecting RLAP and prostitution in general, educating the general public over RLAP, representing the RLAP at governmental and international policy-making bodies such as the UNICEF, ESCAP, WHO, IAF, UNDP, etc.

Red-light area prostitutes (RLAP) in India are essentially a deprived lot, stripped of scioeconomic and psychological well-being.

Personal health status is generally a strong and direct indicator of an individual's economic and environmental situation in developing countries like India. The red-light areas are environmentally worse than the typical slums of the metropolises in India. The status of physical infrastructure, basic amenities, primary health care services, demographic situation and private sector medical care, etc., are hostile to a prostitute's health.

Prerana holds strongly that every possible step must be taken to wipe out the institution of prostitution from the earth. Prerana is obviously therefore against the legalization of prostitution in principle. Prerana opposes legalization of prostitution even as a short-term practical measure because not only it is non-practical but it will lead to corruption and many other undesirable practices besides reinforcing the institution. It believes that prostitutes have been wrongly held individually responsible for their professional practice and considered as deviants. The fact that a prostitute as a victim of the exploitative patriarchal social structure and prostitution constitutes the worst form of sexual slavery is conveniently neglected. In a variety of ways the evil practice is perpetuated by attributing to it the functional role of a safety valve. Even today, one finds a number of NGO's and policy makers favoring legalization of prostitution. It would not be wrong to state they are not concerned with the safety and welfare of the prostitutes, but to combat the spread of STD/ HIV and protect largely the male clients.

Certain Facts about RLAP

(1)   The lives of the RLAPs are entirely controlled by the underworld through the brothel keepers and their henchmen/women.   The client is the King.   In almost all cases the prostitutes earnings go to the brothel keeper.   At a much later stage when the woman is not of much use to the brothel keeper and if she is not indebted to the brothel keeper and mony lender, then fifty percent of a prostitutes income goes to the brothel keeper, ten percent to the pimp, ten percent for housekeeping and the the remaining thirty percent is left for herself.

(2)   A prostitute in the RLA above 30 years of age earns about Rs. 15 to 20 per client and on average entertains 6 – 7 clients per day.

(3)   Demand for virgin prostitutes has gone high, allegedly after the influx of Arab visitors.   Moreover, there is the belief that a man can cure himself of venereal disease and sterility by having sex with minors.   Demand for child prostitutes has become more widespread because of the global HIV/AIDS scare.   Many clients think they are not likely to get the deadly disease if they have sex with young prostitutes, especially virgins.   A minor RLAP easily earns anything between Rs. 100 to 500 per client.

(4)   With the onset of HIV/AIDS there has been yet another change in the status of the prostitutes.   They are now called 'Commercial Sex Workers.'   The change in terminology is an attempt to normalize the sexual exploitation and marketing of women's bodies as a given and normal component of the labor market.   This 'economic' change has made no improvement in their existing condition.   With the onset of AIDS, and its popular association with prostitution, the income of the RLAPs has gone down significantly.

(5)   It has always been impossible for the RLAP to discuss the use of condoms even as a form of contraception to their clients.

(6)   Prostitutes prefer abortion over other methods of contraception, as none of the contraceptives are compatible with their day-to-day living and profession.

(7)   Most prostitutes visit private practitioners in case of ill health, because in public hospitals, in their opinion, they are humiliated with many 'offending' questions.   Doctors, health educators and many social workers express surprise as to why a prostitute of all people should feel insulted or hurt by their intimate questions.   Why should the prostitutes feel shy to hold a condom or participate in condom demonstration, they ask.

(8)   Injection of whatever kind is a sure form cure.   A belief cultivated and perpetuated by a cluster of licensed and unlicensed medical practitioners in and around the RLA.

(9)   It is a popular feeling that as clients don't like publicizing their visit to the RLAP, involving their sex partners the prostitutes is the right way to communicate with the client and prevent HIV/AIDS.

(10)   The socio-economic, cultural, political status of most Indian women leaves them entirely at the receiving end even in sexual relations.   They are thus more vulnerable to HIV infection and are grossly disadvantaged in terms of protecting themselves from HIV infection.   Prostitutes are the lowest in rank among these women.

It is erroneous to think that without intevening into the overall context of the existence of the RLAP they can be made to use condoms and make clients use condoms merely by teaching them high tech communication skills.   This is a non-social, non-political and unscientific diagnosis of their existence.

(11)   There are several clients who still don't use condoms and a prostitute will invite the wrath of the brothel keeper by pressing the clients to use condoms.

(12)   Findings from the women and AIDS Research Programme suggest that initiating condom use is not practical for many women around the globe.   The studies have found that domestic violence and non-concensual sex are most common realities in the lives of many women.

(13)   In Bombay, HIV prevalence among prostitutes has increased from one percent in 1986 to at least 38 percent currently.

(14)   Most prostitutes are fatalistic.   They find their current life more agonizing than the possibility of death through AIDS.

(15)   Even today besides the lay public, the media, the public health sector and policy makers, all regard the prostitutes as the 'reservoirs' and 'major carriers' of infection.   They are not considered either as victims, or as those most exposed to risk and in dire need of help.

(16)   Long before HIV/AIDS came into the lives of the prostitute she had still has several other problems, like lack of sufficient water, poor and inadequate sanitation facilities, a hostile public health sector, insufficient space to live in, an environment which breeds numerous kinds of infection, total lack of cleanliness, etc.   As a result she has always remained unperturbed with HIV especially because she knows she can't do anything to prevent infection, and she is at the mercy of other, i.e. her clients.

Prerana started its work on HIV/AIDS prevention and control in the year 1989, when it was discovered that the prostitutes from the R.L.A. of Kamathipura, Bombay seeking treatment were being forced or deceived into giving blood samples to public health service centers. We intervened at both ends, the health department and the patient.   We informed the prostitutes that they had every right to seek explanation from the public health functionary the purpose of collecting blood samples, and to refuse to give blood for testing if a proper explanation was not forth coming.

We believe that the RLAP (with reference to HIV) are involved in 'high risk behavior,' not of their own free will but out of situational compulsion and helplessness. Their clients are definitely involved in 'high risk behavior' of their own free will.

HIV/AIDS has created near mass hysteria in the world, giving sudden and forceful boost to a series of international events and actions.   In the eyes of the international planners, advisors and organizations the RLAP became very important as they were called the group involved in 'high risk bahavior.'   Practically the turmoil was guided by one dominant equation: prostitutes are the fastest and most powerful carriers of HIV/AIDS. The prostitutes were least perturbed with the menace of AIDS but certainly much irritated with the new status they had been given.

Prerana incorporated HIV/AIDS awareness activity into the health and social awareness sessions for the RLAP.   In 1992, Prerana carried out a 'Pilot Project on Peer Group Education' training for 100 RLAPs on behalf of the AIDS/STD Control and Prevention Cell of the Municipal Corporation of Greater Bombay.   All the 100 women were known to Prerana for more than 4 – 5 years and their brothel keepers allowed them to attent these meetings because the issues were health-related.   Taking into consideration Prerana's past experience of a total health awareness programme, HIV/AIDS awareness was incorporated into a health awareness programme along with communication skills.   It was also an attempt to understand women's empowerment possibility vis-a-vis HIV/AIDS control and prevention.

Some of the important responses of the RLAP expressed in these sessions are:

(1)   Information on different health problems was very helpful and well understood.

(2)   The women showed a lot of apprehension about speaking to their peers and also mentioned that it would upset their brothel keepers if they spent their time educating their peers instead of resting or attending customers.

With Reference to HIV, the Reaction was as Follows:

(1)   Who are the interventionists primarily concerned about — the prostitutes or the clients ?   It is the conviction of the RLAP that these are two different worlds connected by a one-way exploitative relationship.

(2)   HIV/AIDS education package for the red-light area stinks of a limited and opportunistic intervention of the outside world.   Overall health education and intervention is urgently required.

(3)   Who decides the use of a condom ?   In the red-light area power structure the prostitute is stripped of her basic dignity and human right.   How can she decide the use of a condom against the wishes of the clients, particularly when the latter are supported by the brothel keepers ?   A Women's Empowerment Program is meaningless unless handled in the totality of their existence although it is crucial for the success of HIV/AIDS prevention and control.

(4)   Their historical fatalism makes them so resigned that they feel there is little to be additionally lost by contracting HIV/AIDS.   The way the packets of condoms are being dumped on their doorsteps in the red-light areas the RLAP feel that they are singularly being held responsible for the spread as well as control of HIV/AIDS.

(5)   During the pilot project we discovered that there exist several myths among RLAP regarding sexual behavior, which get better clarified in a setting characterized by an integrated approach.

In a nutshell, continuation of the PGE & WEP restricted to the 'limited' sphere of HIV/AIDS and RLAP will continue to suffer from serious inherent shortcomings in their effectiveness.   Merely dumping condoms at the doorstep will only make the RLAPs hostile and alienate them further from the work of HIV/AIDS prevention and control.

In the field of HIV/AIDS prevention and control the WEP expects the prostitutes to negotiate with the clients over the use of condoms.   In an isolationist approach such empowerment is impossible and meaningless and hence makes HIV/AIDS prevention and control work ineffective.

Integrated intervention in the life of the RLAP achieved by Prerana has given certain positive results.   Previously, the RLAP considered themselves merely as objects of sexual attraction by the managers of the flesh trade and the clients.   Their perception of their own children was very peculiar.   The girl child was to grow into a prostitute, a boy child was to be a recruiter for the flesh market and the underworld.   The retired and exhausted prostitute was to become a begger, die a premature death.   Their self-perception was that of a condemned soul and body.   Their self-perception had become so distorted that they unmistakably joined the bandwagon of the other elements of the flesh trade in celebrating the birth of a girl child to a prostitute because it was a free and frictionless recruit to the flesh trade.

Empowerment first and foremost means change of self-perception, acquisiton of vision, setting of short- and long-term goals. building faith in transformation.   Prerana's continuity and totality of approach provided the first point of reference for the prostitutes to start charting the graph of their future.   The shocking rate of non-enrollment in primary school, adsenteeism, dropout, waste and stagnation of the children of RLAP started improving significantly.   The enrollment at the Night Care Center, which was opposed and perceived as a threat by most of the constitutents of the flesh trade, improved and attendance became regular.   The mothers started asserting themselves against the reluctance of the brothel keepers.   Today there is a long waiting list at the NCC.

Another important step in protecting the children of RLAP and also assuring some future security to the RLAP was to shift the children away from the RLA and place them into institutions for residential care.   This was an open declaration that the child was lost to the flesh trade.   Prerana has placed over 100 children, primarily girls and many boys, at different and at times quite far-off institutions of residential care.   The only individual keen on this was the mother.   The rest of the flesh trade community was in strong opposition to any such loss to their trade.   Obviously the prostitute mothers asserted themselves and chose a different path for their children.

Most of their daily food would come from the open market with no discipline about who should eat what when and how.   A large number of petty food vendors thrived on the indiscreet eating habits of the prostitutes and their children.   Prerana's efforts made a definite difference.   The prostitute mothers have become nutrition conscious.   They prepare the tiffin for their children and regularly attend social/health education classes.   Their new eating habits, routine, and practice is in conflict with their general previous style.   The RLAP mothers of children covered by Prerana asserted themselves and started cooking decent food for their children and taking responsibility to personally deliver the same to the school.

Their perception vis-a-vis the state sought to be corrected.   Previously the state was representaed by petty policemen and unwilling health personnel from public clinics and hospitals.   Today the police station refers to the lawbook before summoning an RLAP mother under Prerana to the police station once eveing stes.   The RLAP mothers refuse to comply to the unreasonable demands of the medical and paramedical personnel who strive to extract blood samples from them for their ulterior goals.   The most significant step in this journey was to deal with the public distribution bureaucracy and assert and get ration cards, thereby establishing their identity as a citizen and also getting legitimate access to the subsidized commodities sold at the authorized ration shops.   These are just a few indicators of the results of Prerana's intervention.   The RLAP mothers have become assertive.

The EWP, an isolated intervention in the life of the RLAP with a view to protect the client, is bound to fail.   It is illogical to expect that the prostitutes will become assertive vis-a-vis the clients and/or use their limited communication skills to persuade the client to use a condom.

A gradual development of self-confidence, self-image and vision among the RLAP will someday reach a level where they will be able to successfully assert themselves against the other dominant element of the flesh trade to ensure protection for themselves.   This, however, requires integrated and continuous intervention in the life of the RLAP.

Prerana's work in the Field of HIV/AIDS Prevention and Control

(1)   As mentioned earlier Prerana has incorporated the HIV/AIDS awareness activity into its general health awareness program, which is given to them through periodical sessions, individual counseling.   These sessions go a long way in breaking the myths about HIV/AIDS.   Many of them still think that penetration sex is safe, while oral or anal is unsafe sex.   Condom demonstration forms a part of these sessions, so that they can use their knowledge of the proper use of condoms with a willing client.   We used to make condoms available for women, but now with the social marketing of condoms, there is almost "door-to-door" sales of condoms, and therefore we have withdrawn ourselves from the supply.

(2)   Carrying out HIV/AIDS Awareness Programmes with the help of posters, street play and songs, outside railway stations, in slum communities, among street children and industrial workers.

(3)   Organizing training programmes for students, community workers and child-care workers helping them understand the problem and helping them incorporate HIV awareness programmes within their existing activities for their communities.

(4)   Incorporating HIV awareness into sex life education and social awareness sessions for the adolescent girls and boys of the RLA.

(5)   Working for a broader and better network and functioning of STD clinics. Calling it an STD clinc itself keeps many prostitutes away.   We are submitting to the public health authorities to convert the existing STD clinics into multipurpose clinics, with facilities to attend to the common health problems of the RLAP and their children.

Prerana has been continuously working with the public hospitals to make them admit and treat the HIV/AIDS patients much against the reluctance of these authorities.   Another important area of intervention with the public hospitals and clinics is prohibiting forced testing of the RLAP for HIV infection.   It is an undesirable and unethical medical practice gaining popularity at these public places of health care.   It is hated by the RLAPs.

Unfortunately, the mass media have portrayed the red-light areas as the centers and origins of the HIV/AIDS infection, thereby adding to their previous notoriety.   This is most unfortunate.   The mass media must be made more responsible and sensitive since, as vanguards of social renaissance, they are expected to adopt a positive role in alleviating the pain and plight of the red-light areas.   Prerana is working on this front also.

At different fora of public policy making Prerana has been advocating against legalization of prostitution.   Besides the several demerits of such a step legalization is sure to open up a new ground for corruption in the police, bureaucracy and medical profession and will force the HIV/AIDS-affected prostitutes go underground thereby negatively affecting the HIV/AIDS prevention and control mission.

Eighteen Months After the Pilot Project, Focus Group Interviews were Conducted with 50 Prostitutes

Womens reactions:

(1)   Many prostitutes still like to believe that condoms are for having sex with 'the

other/irregular clients' and not with the regular or stable clients.

(2) If both men and women involved in unprotected sex have the danger of contracting HIV, then why are only the prostitutes being singled out especially when the preventive measure has to be used only by men.

(3) Women now state there is an increase in the number of men using condoms, but not because they (i.e. the prostitutes) have convinced the clients to do so, but because it is their own decision.

(4) As of 1989 – 90 there is a definite increase in their knowledge of HIV transmission and prevention, but even then they continue to be helpless before the clients and cannot make the clinet use a condom.   They have always that there is no question of objecting to their clients not using condoms, as they are never allowed to object to anything related to their profession.

(5) Prostitutes fear that if their blood is found to be HIV-positive, the government will force them to leave the profession, if their brothel keeper doesn't do so first.

It is neither enough for the brothel keepers to say that 'all the clients visting my girls use condoms,' nor for the NGO's and health educator to say that the situation has improved. It is important that the prostitutes agree that all their client have started using condoms. That is not the case today and the vulnerability of the prostitutes remains.

Higher incidence of condom use, it can be safely assumed, provides a higher protection to the client but not necessarily to the prostitutes in the same degree.   A single infected non yielding client can expose the prostitutes to the serious danger of contracting the HIV/ AIDS infection.

Heavy concentration on attempting to get prostitutes to work towards HIV/AIDS prevention is not out of concern or compassion to protect them, but out of concern for male health.

Conclusions and Suggestions:

(1) Prostitutes have always been regarded to be the 'reservoir and carriers' of disease and never as victims, potential or otherwise.   There is an urgent need to change the perception, emphasis, and posture vis-a-vis prostitutes, particularly the RLAPs in all intervention programmes and AIDS prevention and control is no exception.

(2) Merely giving them the knowledge about HIV/AIDS and imparting communication skills of negotiating with their clients is not going to protect them, especially when enforcing such measures is difficult in a relationship outrightly based on inequality and exploitation.

(3) Prostitutes require a protective technology which they can use without having to negotiate or persuaded the clients at the same time without getting disqualified in their current market.

(4) All the above-mentioned suggestions should go hand-in-hand with efforts to improve the prostitutes' environmental conditions, health services, socioeconomic status, structural imbalances, rather than as a strategy 'fix' that precludes the need for broader structural change.

(5) Men who have unprotected sex with their primary and other partners should be the focus of intervention and not the prostitutes.   With their existing socioeconomic

handicaps the RLAPs are placed in jeopardy by the behavior of the clients.   Men must be involved in discussions that will help them understand how a multiplicity of sex partners increases not only their own chances of getting HIV, but also that of their partners.

Evaluation of Harm Reduction Methods among Injecting Drug Users

Palaniappan Narayanan

Ikhlas/Pink Triangle, Kuala Lumpur, Malaysia

When we started IKHLAS/Pink Triangle we didn't know anything about evaluation. In fact we didn't even think about it. We were just hard working people with good intentions wanting to do something about the situation. We just adapted a logical model of intervention and worked on it.

Evaluation was alien to us. We believed it was not a part of our work. It was something social scientists should do and not social workers on the streets.

So we carried on doing what we do. And now we ask ourselves;

(1)   Is this method working?
(2)   Why are we facing all these problems?
(3)   Why are we getting tired?
(4)   How can we move forward?

We then realized that we needed to evaluate our programs. To check if the method was effective, if it is working or should we alter or change it. Evaluate to identify the areas which we should concentrate on and the directions we should move.

So we started to do something we don't do very often — read books on evaluations. And we realized why we have never read them before. All these books had words like design, models, structures and quantitative. Forcing ourselves to read them, we realized:

'Hey! we don't have to be afraid of it. We do it all the time.' In fact we are the EXPERTS because:

(1)   We are with our clients
(2)   We are working with the community
(3)   And we know what is happening.

Therefore we need to do our own evaluation. And evaluation to us means 'To check on the harm reduction methods being utilized, to see if it is working effectively given the resources available and the social conditions present.'

Allow me to explain further using IKHLAS Center as a point of reference.

IKHLAS Drop-in Center (a project under Pink Triangle Malaysia) is a non-governmental organization dealing with the prevention of HIV/AIDS among injecting drug users and sex workers. We are a user friendly center which creates a safe space for drug users to gather and receive information. Counseling, food and medical treatment and other support services. Street outreach is also conducted on a regular basis.

The harm reduction method that we use is cleaning of needles with bleach. Bleach is distributed through street outreach and at the center.

To evaluate the effectiveness of this method, we must have proper documentation. And to have an effective evaluation documentation is vital. In IKHLAS we have outreach forms for outreach workers. This simple, time saving, volunteer friendly when completed gives information on the number, age, race of clients met, number of bleach bottles and other materials distributed. And it supports other aspects of the program. Outreach workers note what they have seen, heard of felt and how they reacted to it. This encourages the worker as he feels that his/her views are important. It also keeps everyone in the organization informed about the community.

This form of documentation also helps us understand the daily happening at the site and prepare us to face unexpected situations in the future. Training module for CHOWs can also be prepared by taking into account this documentation.

In the center, we do form filling as well. We have the drop-in form and the medical report form. The drop-in form, when the data are collected, will show us if we are reaching out to one particular group or more than one group, it also gives us the breakdown of who we are meeting and who we want to meet, should there be an expansion. Medical report form on the other hand shows us if our message of safe injecting practices are getting through to the community. It also allows us to justify and validate the medical program.

Next we produce stories out of the observation and the experience that we have made and had. We write the ordinary and out-of-the-ordinary stories about the issues in the community. This is important for three reasons:

(1)   It encourages staff to listen to clients.
(2)   We receive valuable information.
(3)   It is so much more fun to do a story than a report.
(4)   People prefer to read stories than books on evaluation.

The stories written about the women makes us understand the situation of women clients better and from there on work to provide support for these women.

We must always remember that the most important people in any program are the clients. So talk to your clients and they can guide you and inform you on what their problems are, what their needs are and what we can do. They can also tell us if our methods are working.   How do we do it ? Have interviews in a structured or unstructured manner.   However, interviewing clients requires training, a topic I will touch on later.

In evaluating our programs we need to check on the objectives.   And with meeting and workshops we must always ask,

(1)   Have we reached the objectives ?
(2)   Have we been over-ambitious or must we change our objectives ?
(3)   Can we bandle what we have set out to do ?
(4)   And what is the next step we must take ?

These are important questions of evaluation because being community based, street type programs where there has been no previous successful models, we are in the process of creating change.

And therefore, it is important for us not to be discouraged when the objectives are not met but instead to understand why and to be practical and creative in developing objectives and goals that are challenging but not impossible.   Through evaluation we at IKHLAS have realized that while providing support for harm minimization, the elements of care and support cannot be ignored.

Resources are an important factor in evaluation.

Firstly, human resources.   Do you have it and does it have what it takes.   The right attitude is important especially working with IVDUs where we often find that lack of understanding in the issues prevents service providers from being effective.   If the program fails because of lack of skills then we know there is nothing wrong with the method; it is the machines we have to change and alter.

Next, money, Do you have enough of it?   If not, how can we be efficient in using what we have.

Proper materials.   Are they available?   Where can we obtain them?   Should we beg, buy or steal?

All these resources depend on social conditions and we must study the social conditions of that particular community.   And evaluation enables us to see this.

The harm reduction that we use must have a perspective that is understanding and sensitive to the community and its needs.

For example, in Kuala Lumpur we have been dealing with prevention of HIV/AIDS among injecting drug users when a large portion of the community are already HIV$^+$.   If it was not for evaluation we would not have realized this.   And evaluation of harm reduction method has enabled us to shift some resources from prevention to providing care and support.

The harm reduction method needs to consider other factors such as class, financial resources, gender and society's perception and how these issues affect self-esteem of clients. Self-esteem is a major contributor to the success of any harm reduction program among injecting drug users.   In Malaysia, due to society's perception and constant harassment, the users have very low self-esteem and IKHLAS believes that any form of harm reduction method will not be effective if the self-esteem of users is not elevated.   It is therefore of utmost importance that care givers and service providers maintain a friendly and non-judgmental attitude towards their clients.   For a drug user who has lost all hopes of rehabilitation and return to society a friend who is willing to listen and treats him as a respectable human being is like a light shining at the end of the tunnel.   Only when he is able to see this distant light will he be able to accept and support for behavioral change.

Harm reduction method needs to have a proper understanding of the community. Therefore we also need to evaluate attitude and perception of the wider community in terms of values, beliefs and laws.

For IKHLAS, we are using bleach as the harm reduction method not because needle exchange is not effective but because of the laws and polities that surround us.   And we need to understand the elements of failure due to social constraints.   If we need to think of needle exchange, evaluation will force us to consider whether resources are available and can be shifted into advocacy for needle exchange.   If your organization is involved in front-line service provision and you feel a need to do evaluation but unsure about it, these are the things you can do:

(1)   Network with other similar organizations who have done similar programs or made it part of their programs.

(2)   Speak to HIV/AIDS agencies and funders asking for evaluation support and training.

After 12 years of AIDS existence, there are many resources in terms of human skills, finance and technology.   Make these evaluation resources available to you.

Conclusion

Implementation of harm reduction methods surely varies according to culture, laws and other factors.   Therefore a successful model must take these factors into consideration and work to make the best possible Possible effective ways of harm minimization.   Harm reduction method among drug users is still very new in developing countries.   Minimal work is being done for IVDUs.   However, we see programs being carried out, have energy, creativity and sheer guts.   Let us not lose the momentum.   Evaluating will help us learn from each other and ensure effective and efficient IDU programs.

Promoting Health among Out-of-School Youth: Recognizing Individual and Common Needs for HIV Prevention

Ana Filgueiras

Brazilian Center for the Defense of the Rights of Children and Adolescents, Ipanema, Rio de Janeiro, Brazil

Just like adults, young people are not a homogenous group. This is often said, but practice shows that many adults still tend to view all young people as inherently irresponsible, rebellious, and risk-taking, always in a permanent search for immediate pleasure. With this attitude, the responsibility of an eventual HIV infection is ultimately placed on young people themselves. In many cultures and within specific constraints, young people might be exposed or protected because of adult pressure, an over-protective family, or religious beliefs.

Although not homogeneous, young people have some factors in common. They are growing and developing in specific cognitive stages that correspond to particular patterns of behavior. An understanding of the different abilities and difficulties within the distinct stages of development is crucial in order to help any child or young person develop and adopt skills to cope with daily life. This includes the ability to adapt behavior in order to avoid the risk of HIV infection.

Despite a diversity of cultures and socio-economic situations, all adolescents experience the passage into adulthood. They must all learn to cope with physical changes, get used to emergent sexual desire, and deal with the changes associated with puberty. Adolescence is always a period of life where the exploration of feelings, desires, possibilities, limits, and social and gender role expectations occur.

Sex Education and Condoms

As young people experience life, including sex, adults ask themselves if adolescents should know about or ignore sex. Instead of assessing what their practices are and what kind of knowledge they might need, adults often deny them access to adequate information. The World Health Organization recently compared 19 studies from Australia, Europe, Thailand, and the United States to look at the impact of sex education on the sexual behavior of young people. The conclusions showed that sex education does not promote or increase sexual activity, but in some cases may in fact incourage young prople to delay penetrative sex, to reduce the number of sexual partners, or to have safer sex. By refusing to provide accurate information and skills, adults leave young people exposed to abuse, unwanted sex, or sex early in life. Rather than question when they should or should not be sexually active, it is more effective to focus efforts on learning what young people want to discuss and to be informed about so that they themselves can adopt safer practices.

The same occurs when people question whether condoms should be available for young people. Instead, this question should be directed at young people themselves. Young prople will not cease to be sexually active because of a lack of condoms. They will continue to exercise their sexuality, but possibly in an unsafe manner and without the use of condoms. Merely distributing condoms is not sufficient, and we must also speak openly about other forms of safer sex, including the possibility of abstinence, masturbation, and nonpenetrative sex.

Distinct Vulnerabilities

What makes out-of-school or socially apart youth[1] distinct from other young people, and what factors add to their vulnerability? These are often young people living in poverty with little or no access to the most basic social and health sevices. They are overwhelmed early in life by hard word and other responsibilities in order to help support the family. Homelessness is common and can be due to civil conflicts and unrest, famine, or because families fall apart. Domestic abuse, the loss of parents, migration, violence, use of drugs to cope with physical and emotional pain, stress caused by fatigue, fear, a lack of self-esteem, ill health including untreated sexually transmitted diseases—the list is very long.

Whatever the reason, vulnerability is often increased because these youth must rely on contacts with the adult community, increasing their exposure to potential adult exploitation, including that of the sex trade.

Two specific groups of young people with particular needs are often ignored and deserve particular attention.

Young Women

One third of people living with HIV are women, and more than half are under the age of 25. Up to 60% of all infections in females occur by the age of 20.[2] In sub-Saharan Africa, there are studies showing that 60% of new infections are among people between the ages of 15 and 24, and of these more women than men are seropositive. Young women between the ages of 15 and 19 are four times more likely to be HIV infected than their male counterparts.

There are several reasons for this increased vulnerability. Gender inequality results in

---

[1] Expressions such as street kids, children in difficult circumstances, marginalized youth, and several others have been invented to try and describe the vulnerable situations facing many of the world's young people. With the addition of HIV/AIDS, these labels fail to emphasize the common and primary factor exposing these distinct groups to HIV infection, which is that they are all outside the social system and lacking access to services and information. A new term, 'socially apart youth', may illustrate this point more clearly, whether referring to a refugee, an abused child, a kid on the streets or an adolescent in institutional care.

[2] From the speech of Dr. Michael Merson, Director of the Global Programme on AIDS, World Health Organization, presented at the 10th International Conference on AIDS in Yokohama, Japan, August 1994.

less opportunities and less power for women to avoid unsafe sex or negotiate for safer sex. There is evidence that women are pushed to become sexually active at earlier than men, adding to their risk of exposure to HIV infection at a younger age.   Older men in many countries are now seeking out young women for sex in the belief that these girls are less likely to be infected with HIV.   Young women's vulnerability to HIV infection is also higher because of the physical trauma caused by sex at an early age.   This is happening all over, but especially where AIDS is having a visible impact.

The rates of pregnancy and sexually transmitted diseases among young women are high and reflect the potential exposure to HIV through unprotected sexual intercourse.   In Africa, one third of all teenage girls become pregnant before the age of 17.   Every year 5 million abortions occur among women between the ages of 15 and 19, with many illegal, a factor which for most women results in unsafe and life-threatening conditions.   One in 20 teenagers worldwide is estimated to have a sexually transmitted disease, although the actual figures are probably much higher but difficult to calculate because young women have difficulty recognizing symptoms, or else they do not seek treatment because in many settings treatment is equated with the stigmatization of being sexually active.

Female genital mutilation, part of traditional rites in many African and Arab countries, is another practice increasing physiological risks of infection.   It is estimated that between 85 and 114 million women have suffered genital mutilation worldwide, usually performed when they were between 4 and 8 years old.   Women who have suffered genital mutilation are often forced to engage in anal sex while vaginal intercourse is not possible, thus adding to their vulnerability to HIV infection.   Also, in an attempt to avoid pregnancy, or also for reasons of pleasure, and intercourse is commonly practiced but rarely acknowledged.

Pregnancy and childbearing is a major factor forcing young women to drop out of school, depriving them of education and skills needed to gain employment and often leaving little choice but to sell sex for survival.   Young women are deprived of the same educational opportunities as boys often because parents lack of the economic means to pay school fees or because their attendance at school is not seen as important compared to men due to social norms.   The traditional status and tole of women means that they are expected to carry the burden of domestic tasks and care for the family.

Poverty and miserable living conditions deprive young girls of even minimal privacy, exposing them to the risk of sexual assault and rape—often by family members where incest is one of the most accepted or silent abuses.   Girls who suffer from rape are usually socially outcast and rejected by the family and community.   In many cases these young women leave home to escape this abuse or to avoid depriving the family of the breadwinner or mother's companion.   Homeless and without any means of social support, these young women become subjected to the risks of constant abuse and potential HIV infection while living on the street.

Gay and Lesbian Youth

The second group rarely discussed is gay and lesbian youth.   Too often young people in developing or developed countries are pushed out of their homes, their communities, or even their countries because of their sexual preference or because they are searching for their sexual identity.   They are discriminated against and abused in schools with the silent complicity of teachers until they drop out of school.   They are humiliated and ignored in programs traditionally devoted to working with young people by the constant denial or lack of understanding by youth workers.   They are sexually abused by adults working in penal institutions, refugee camps, or in war areas.   The lack of awareness, understanding, and support of gay youth forces many to be socially apart and at increased exposure to HIV infection.

Innovative programs, particularly in developing countries, must be implemented which seek to understand and take into account areas which until now have been constantly denied or ignored by those working with young people.   This includes programs that are sensitive and non-judgmental, and which are rooted in the needs of gay and lesbian youth.   This requires that we bravely stand against the widespread but false notion that people make a choice about their sexuality, and that in the case of young people they can be influenced or manipulated to adopt a homosexual identity.   In fact, anyone who has ever really listened to a young gay person will be convinced that sexual preferences are not about choice. Instead, it will be apparent that our role is not about trying to convince them what is right or wrong, but to respect their rights to live and be as they are.   Only when we learn to accept and respect diversity can we hope to make progress against the spread of HIV, and this includes the acceptance of gay and lesbian youth.

Empowering Youth

The concept of empowerment is often used without a full appreciation of its meaning and importance.   Empowerment means supporting a person's ability to cope with constraints, such as discrimination on any basis such as race, gender, religious affiliation or sexual identity.   It is the support one must have in order to manipulate social mechanisms for the defense of individual and social rights.   In the case of young people, this notion must be specifically redfined, especially when, like socially apart youth, they are deprived of any family, adult or community support.   For these children and adolescents to fully develop their potential, empowerment must be viewed as a concept to create a supportive environment whcih allows them to express their needs, desires, pleasures or pains and the other full range of emotions leading to the growth of their self-esteem.

Sometimes HIV positive youth are encouraged to be open about their status, despite the possibility that they may be living in a discriminatory and abusive environment.   In another instance, a young sexually abused girl may be told that it is good to speak out against her abuser, even though protective measures to ensure her safety and well-being can not be guaranteed.   Street children have been shot at by the police because, with the backing of outreach workers, they dared to point out police corruption and torture to the press.

In each of these cases, it is clear that young people must never be encouraged to confront their oppression and abuse when there are insufficient measures to ensure their safety and survival.   Without these guarantees, the concept of empowerment becomes nothing more than a cruel and empty promise, and is sometimes an abuse itself.

What Measures Can Help to Reduce Vulnerability ?

• Any educational strategy addressing socially apart youth must be designed, planned, and implemented with the active participation of the young people themselves.   However, youth must not be used to merely legitimize the ideas and agendas of adults.   The tokenistic involvement of youth in programs and services is offensive and counterproductive. Instead, we must support young people by developing their skills in communication and negotiation so that they can participate fully and as equals

• HIV positive young people need to be involved in programs and services to guarantee quality and relevance.   Avoid creating situations where young people are made to feel responsible or guilty for their serostatus, and acknowledging their specific needs

• work to change attitudes towards young people's sexuality, including lesbian and gay youth

• provide legal advocacy, especially in developing countries where huge numbers of young people are denied their primary human rights such as access to existing health services.   Such advocacy initially designated to support the defense of individual and social rights can be most effective in opening pathways to clinical, educational, and welfare services when available but blocked by the bureaucratic and discriminatory net

• reinforce joint programs between NGOs, governments, bilateral and international agencies.   Education, prevention, and care must be planned and provided in an integrated way.   Programs should be expanded to mobilize society as a whole as well as individuals

• researchers must be mobilized and key data used to advocate for concrete responses to the needs of young people

• define a common agneda on human rights to abolish abusive practices and behaviors.

Children and adolescents, like other human beings, are unique individuals.   Each child and each adolescent establishes and develops different relationships either with their peers, their family, their community, and their environment.   That is why our biggest challenge is to be able to design programs and services in such a way that they will have a positive impact on the promotion of health of that youth community, while at the same time being meaningful to each unique child, adolescent, and young adult within that same community.

Out-of-school youth, children in difficult circumstances, street kids, children who are refugees, or the expression socially apart youth, whatever label we place on them, the common denominator is that they are young people.   They have needs, desires, and dreams as children in any culture and in any part of the world.   Like all children they need to be loved and listened to.   They need for us to leave behind our preconceived ideas and prejudices about them, and to approach them and their problems on their level as individuals.   They need our trust, without moral judgment that will inhibit them and lock their fears inside.   To ensure this, we must provide a safer, supportive, and sustained environment.

To incorporate:

• social prejudice, together with institutional barriers, makes access to public services difficult

• flexible outreach programs using face-to-face approaches promoting bahavior change/safer practices

• address basic survival needs and wants, from education to care, which are rooted in the current experience of the youth

• conclude with listen to youth (again).

Future Strategies Regarding Children Affected by HIV/AIDS

Mazuwa A. Banda

Churches Medical Association of Zambia, Lusaka, Zambia

Introduction

The purpose of this paper is to discuss HIV/AIDS as it affects children and identify ways in which the impact of HIV/AIDS on children could be minimized, especially in the African context where the problem is greatest at the moment. The paper starts off by discussing some of the ways in which HIV/AIDS affects children, then identifies some measures being undertaken to address the problem of HIV/AIDS among children and gives some suggestions on further development in prevention, care and support to children affected by HIV/AIDS.

For the purpose of this discussion, children affected by HIV/AIDS include:

• children who are infected with HIV or ill with IIIV related disease,

• children who have parents, siblings or some other close relative, infected with HIV or ill with HIV related disease,

• children who have lost one or both parents, sibling(s), or some other close relative to HIV/AIDS and

• children living in communities where HIV/AIDS is evident.

It was estimated that by December 1993 there were about 1 million children infected by HIV and 500,000 cases of pediatric AIDS cases worldwide. The number of infections in children is expected to rise to 5 – 10 million by the year 2000. It was also estimated that there were 2 million uninfected children who are or will become orphans and this figure may rise to 20 million at the end of this century.

Sero-prevalence data and case reporting on HIV/AIDS do not in themselves provide a complete picture of the impact of HIV/AIDS on children. It may have been due to reliance on such data that in the early stages of the HIV/AIDS pandemic that the problem among children was underrated.

Impact of HIV/AIDS on Children

HIV disease in children generally takes a more aggressive course and is much more difficult to treat than in adults. Children experience immense psychological and emotional trauma to see a loved one, who may be a mother, father, brother, sister or some other close relation suffer a debilitating illness and die, and to witness the collapse of their family unit.

Children often lose the right to land and other assets which belonged to their parents. The drop out of school because there is no one to meet the costs, thereby missing an opportunity that would have enabled them earn a decent living in future and so sealing their fate to a life of poverty and misery.

Children who have lost parents due to HIV/AIDS are much likely to being abused than children with parents.   They may be exploited as cheap labor.   Many of these youngsters find themselves in a situation where they would easily exchange sex for money.   Sexual abuse of children places them at risk of children getting infected with HIV, other sexually transmitted diseases and unwanted pregnancies.

The total effect of HIV/AIDS on children is therefore very severe, it attacks their bodies, their personality, their potentials and their future.   HIV/AIDS kills many children while they are still living.   HIV/AIDS can transform young lives from a fairly tale to a reality of never-ending horror.

Current Efforts

A number of effort are being made by non-governmental organizations, community groups, government agencies, and donor agencies to address the problems of children affected by HIV/AIDS.   Some of these measures are described here, they are divided into two groups as institutional and non-institutional forms of support to affected children.

Institutional Forms of Care and Support

Institutional forms of child care and support involve classical child care institutions such as orphanages or children homes.   These institutions recruit orphans or other disadvantaged children from the community to live in the institution.   The institution tries to meet all the needs of the children until they reach an age where they are let out of the institutions to go and live on their own or referred to other types of institutions.

Institutions of child care are a relatively new phenomenon in most developing countries and are of limited value in providing support to disadvantaged children.   In the Kagera region of Tanzania about 4.1% of orphans were found to be under institutional care while in Lusaka about 2.9% of orphans were under institutional care.   The apparent limited role that institutions have is due to the fact that other forms of care and support already exist.

Child care institutions in Africa are considered inappropriate because they detach children from the community, and develop artificial lifestyles whcih make it difficult for the children to fit back into society.   Institutions may also be very expensive to develop and run.   However, there are some instances where institutions may be the more appropriate options.   Such situations may include care of very young children, children who are completely destitute (or have no home at all), in cases of specific problem situations such as medical care, drug addiction, sexual abuse or violence.

Non-Institutional Forms of Child Care and Support

Various forms of non-institutional child care exist some of which have existed for ages and others being new inventions.   Non-institutional care aims at providing care and support to disadvantaged children while keeping them within their respective communities. Forms of non-institutional support include the extended family systems, foster parenting, older sibling support, day care centers, skills training centers, peer support.

(A) *Extended family/kinship support systems:* In most traditional African societies no real orphans or destitute existed. This is because family and kinship systems were such that each person was considered to be a member not only of a basic biological family unit but a larger one involving near and distant relatives. This concept of family sometimes extends to cover a whole clan or village. It was the responsibility of the other members of this family to take care of any disadvantaged members in their midst as they would be a close relative. Orphans therefore would be taken up by members of this extended family and would continue to lead a life close to what they had when their parents were alive. The extended family system is still taking care of disadvantaged children today. The system works well in predominantly farming or subsistence communities where almost every member has a role to play in contributing to the livelihood of the whole family.

However the extended family system has come under increasing stress in recent times that it is not always able to cope with the problem of children affected by HIV/AIDS. As more and more adults die from HIV/AIDS, the family effectively breaks down. This is compounded by the adverse economic conditions obtaining in most developing countries which greatly undermine the capacity of the family to care for itself.

Efforts are being made to support the extended family. These include providing additional resources to families that are looking after other children. These resources may be in the form of cash, food, clothes, blankets, school expenses, other material requirements or counselling.

(B) *Foster parenting/adoption:* Some children are being looked after by foster parents. The children may live in the home of foster parents, in their original home or in a different place. There are efforts also being made to encourage families who have the means to adequately care for children to adopt children that are in need. However, fostering and adoption are still not very commonly practiced in African settings. One of the reasons being that most families always have other extended family relatives who they need to support before they can care for someone not at all related to them.

(C) *Support through older siblings:* Older siblings, who are in their teens, may be identified as head of the family. Material and emotional support is given to such siblings so that in turn they support the younger siblings. The older siblings are also assisted to retain and maintain the estates of their parents.

(D) *Day Care Centers:* Are often established as places where children can go to some time during the day and receive therapy, food, encouragement and probably schooling. Day care centers would exist not very far from where the children live so that they are easily accessible. Day care centers may also be expensive to run, though not as much institutions such as orphanages and children homes.

(E) *Skills training centers:* These are developed specifically to impart some skills on the affected children so that they are able to make a living. Children may be attending a skills training center daily from their homes or they may reside at the center for some length of time. Sometimes skills training centers impart skills which, in practice, the children are not able to make a living out of.

(F) *Peer support:* Groups of children are encouraged and provided opportunities to discuss their individual situations and how they can help themselves and each other. This may be done at day care centers or through special projects.   The children may form support groups or cooperatives to generate income.

Non-institutional strategies often require strong community support and involvement in order to be successful and sustainable.   However, communities often need to be assisted in their efforts because they usually face a host of other challenges to their survival and resources to effectively dealt with the challenges are often very limited.

Suggestion for Future Strategies

The major challenge for the present and future in providing care and support to children affected by HIV/AIDS is to expand existing initiatives to match the scale of the problem.   I do not wish to recommend specific strategies as these may be numerous and vary with local conditions.   I, however, wish to suggest some general principles that need to be considered when developing strategies for children affected by HIV at present and in the future.

Identify and Concentrating on Priority Needs of Affected Children in a Particular Setting

It is obvious that the needs of children affected by HIV/AIDS are numerous and complex.   However, in order to have meaningful effect it is important to identify what the priority needs of the children are.   Priority needs are those which if adequately met will cause the most significant positive change in the lives of the children and may also minimize the negative effect of the other unmet needs.

The priority needs of children may vary with age and local social conditions.   For instance babies or small children may have as the most crucial needs, food and warmth, without which they may not live.   For other children the most crucial needs in one setting may be continuing in school or skills training, while in another setting the priorty may be to deal with drug abuse.   In other situations (such as in rich countries) the priority may be emotional or psychological support.

Identifying and concentrating on priority needs enables program implementors and communities to place the most energies and resources where it matters most.   This is especially important in a situation of greatly limited resources in which most of us find ourselves.   Identifying and concentrating on priority needs also may enable greater improvement skills or approaches in addressing those needs.

Begin with Existing Resources and Structures

It is important that strategies employed in supporting children affected by HIV/AIDS consider existing resources and structures at the beginning.   This may be necessary for some initiatives to get started at all and to be sustained.

Strategies that primarily depend on resources from outside tend to alienated and disempower the people they intend to assist.   They appear foreign to the local people and so the local people do not feel confident to play active roles in the scheme.   The local often passively wait to be instructed on what to do by the people who know best.   This in turn leads to creation of a dependency situation where the local people or the affected children see themselves merely as recipients of the benefits without much responsibility in the venture.

Strategies which begin with existing resources, on the other hand, will appear familiar to those they intend to assist. The communities or affected children will often be able to see how they fit in and what contributions they could make. They are more likely to actively participant and positively influence the development of the initiative. The role of external support must be to increase the capacity of local systems to deal with the problems at hand.

However, it may sometimes be necessary that existing systems be completely changed or totally new ones introduced in order to best meet prevailing challenges. This may occur in crisis situations where very quick action may be necessary or where traditional systems have completely broken down.

Need to Invest more in Children in HIV/AIDS Efforts

In the past significant effort and resources have been placed in addressing the consequences of HIV/AIDS in adults. There have been comparatively fewer resources devoted to meeting the needs of children. There is need for local communities and the international community to invest in children because doing that is investing in the real sense of the word. This does not in any way imply that efforts dealing with HIV/AIDS in adults need to relent, but that a lot more resources should be mobilized to more for children as well. There are some good reasons why it is important to invest in children:

(A)   *It may be easier to reduce or prevent transmission of HIV/AIDS in children than in adults.* It is well known that children learn new things much more readily than do adults. Children also have not developed particular rigid lifestyles so that they are more easily amenable to change. It may therefore be more expedient to put much effort into trying to prevent HIV/AIDS in children.

(B)   *Children are a vulnerable group.* Children are not able to adequately take care of themselves, they are not able to provide for all their needs or protect themselves. They are also not able to adequately speak for themselves or effectively lobby for the safeguarding of their interests, especially children who are not in proper homes. Left to themselves children will soon meet disaster of one form of another. Someone else needs make deliberate effort to safeguard the welfare of these children. That someone else is all of us. In the middle of a serious crisis such as the HIV/AIDS pandemic it is necessary that while measures are being taken to support the affected adult populations, extra efforts are devoted to protecting children as children are also affected in a big way.

(C)   *Children are the future generation.* A whole generation of society may be lost if children are not adequately prepared for adulthood. The consequences of that may pass on for many generations.

Investing in children can be done in many ways. One way is by providing more support to existing effort to care and support children so that the measures cover a large number of the children in need and increase in effectiveness. It is obvious that the large majority of initiatives currently in place to support children are carried out by NGOs and community groups. Current international support for HIV/AIDS activities has been largely ineffective because it is mainly targeted at or channelled through governing authorities. Even where there has been the best of intentions, assistance through governing authorities has not adequately reached those in need.

There is need for complete realignment of the international support system if there is any seriousness in the intention to assist communities and individuals affected by HIV/

AIDS.   A system needs to be devised where the international community could channel assistance more directly to NGOs and community groups that are working on the ground.

A second way of investing in children is to build and expand infrastructure which enhance the growth and development of children.   Such infrastructure include schools, skills training, children recreation centers or children homes.   Boarding schools, in particular, may require special consideration.   In an HIV/AIDS situation, boarding schools may provide a suitable environment where affected children could best concentrate on their schooling.   Affected children often experience numerous stresses in the home which may prevent them from giving adequate attention to school work.   Though boarding schools remove children from the daily stresses of life yet they do not completely cut off children from community life.   This is because children always mix back into society and so still maintain their family ties and contacts.   Boarding schools also have the advantage that they make it easy for others to provide support to children.   I would therefore argue for development of more boarding schools, at least in developing countries.

Control of the HIV/AIDS Pandemic

The fourth major principle in supporting children affect by HIV/AIDS is by controlling the HIV/AIDS pandemic.   This has proved very difficult to achieve especially in developing countries.   I want to suggest that efforts to control HIV/AIDS have not appeared very effective because there are a number of phases the campaign needs to go through before maximum effect can be realized.

The first phase is the creation of awareness about HIV/AIDS among specific population groups and the total population.   This phase is what has been largely achieved in the past decade of AIDS control efforts.   The second phase involves enlisting actual participation of population groups and communities in the HIV/AIDS campaign.   This is beginning to be achieved in the present time with groups such as commercial sex workers, people living with HIV/AIDS, women groups and others beginning to take active role in the campaign against HIV/AIDS.   Involvement of communities in the campaign leads to the third phase which that of changing underlying socioeconomic factors which facilitate the propagation of HIV/AIDS.   The underlying factors include poverty, discrimination, stigmatization, certain cultural, religious, political beliefs and practices.   Positively altering the underlying factors would create a conducive environment for appropriate behavior change which would result in reduction in the transmission of HIV/AIDS and strengthening of support efforts.

Each preceding phase consolidate the succeeding one and each phase may take a duration about 2 to 5 years.   It is possible that more than one phase can be achieved simultaneously.   Sometimes one particular phase may have sufficient impact on the whole course of the epidemic.

Conclusion

In conclusion, HIV/AIDS affects children in a much more profound way than is often apparent at the surface.   Children are a vulnerable group, they are completely helpless in the face of the HIV/AIDS pandemic.   The impact of HIV/AIDS on children today is likely to have consequences for many generations to come.   It is therefore necessary that appropriate and adequate measures be put in place now and more resources be devoted to protecting the children.   Investing in children is investment in the true sense of the word. There are many things that are lovely and heart warming to look at, one of them is the smile of a child.   Please let us not allow that to disappear.

References

Children and AIDS: An Impending Calamity. UNICEF 1991, UN Plaza, New York, USA.

Chiodo F, et al: Vertical transmission of HTLV-III. Lancet 1986; 1: 739.

European Collaborative Study. Mother to child transmission of HIV infection. Lancet 1988; 2: 1029-42.

Global Programme on AIDS, The HIV/AIDS Pandemic: 1993 Overview. WHO/GPA/CNP/EVA/1993; 93, 1.

Gutman LT, et al: Human immunodeficiency virus transmission by child sexual abuse. Am J Dis Child Feb 1991; 145: 137-41.

Hunter SS: Orphans as a window on the AIDS epidemic in Sub-Saharan Africa: Initial results and implication of a study in Uganda. Soc Sci Med 1990; 31(6): 681 – 690.

Iranganyama BM: Socio-economic factors as a function of HIV/AIDS transmission among street children. Int Conf AIDS in Africa, Dec 1994 (abstract no. M.O.P 25).

Lusaka Workshop Report, Support to Children and Families affected by HIV/AIDS. Centre International de l'Enfance 1994, Chateau de Longchamp, 75 016 Paris, France.

Mataka E: Assessment of the needs of children in distress. 2nd SANASO Conf Report 1993. SANASO, Harare, Zimbabwe.

Mann J. Tarantola DJ, Netter T: AIDS in the World, Global Report. Harvard University Press, Cambridge, Massachusetts, USA, 1992.

Mukoyongo MC, Williams G: AIDS orphans. Strategies for hope No. 5. Action Aid, AMREF, World in Need. 1991.

Mutembei IB: AIDS Orphans: The case study of orphans caring in Kagere, Tanzania. Int Conf AIDS 8(2) 1992, PG D414 (abstract no. P.o.D5162)

Preble EA: Impact of HIV/AIDS on African children. Soc. Sci. Med 1990; 31(6): 671 – 680.

Preble EA: The African Family and AIDS: a current look at the epidemic. AIDS 1991; 5 (suppl 2): S263 – S267.

Rwechungura C: Assistance to AIDS orphans. Int Conf AIDS 8(2) 1992, PG D414 (abstract no. P.o.D5163).

Scott BA, et al: Survival in children with peri-nataly acquired human immunodeficiency virus type-1 infection. N Engl J Med 1989; 321: 1791-6.

Tovo PA, et al: Prognostic factors and survival in children with peri-natal HIV-1 infection. Lancet May 1992; 339: 1249-53.

Methods of Protection against Sexual Acquisition of HIV: Options Available for Women

Zena A. Stein, M. A., Helga V. Saez

HIV Center for Clinical and Behavioral Studies, New York State Psychiatric Institute and the School of Public Health, Columbia University, New York, USA

At its most general, methods of protection that women may use are also those that both women and men may use together. Lifetime mutual monogamy is such a method and it is often the method of choice. The key word here, however, is 'mutual.' A woman on her own is powerless to achieve mutuality. From her standpoint, protection requires not only that she is faithful but that he also is.

Therefore for many women, lifetime mutual monogamy is an unattainable strategy and not one on which to rely, to halt the transmission of HIV.

Another strategy is for the woman to urge her partner to use a condom. But men in many cultures have the right to dominance in sexual relationships and this right includes the privilege of using or not using a condom [1].

Some societies are changing, albeit slowly in respect of reciprocal rights between women and men, but not fast enough to stem the epidemic. So women need something more, and we summarize below the current status of barrier methods, which would be within the control of women, and hence reduce their vulnerability. With these methods, women explicitly take responsibility for their own protection.

First we describe physical barriers (the vaginal diaphragm, the cervical cap) and in particular, the newly-introduced woman's condom, with preliminary reports of its acceptability and method effectiveness. Next we discuss the available chemical barriers that might be protective, also in terms of acceptability and effectiveness. Critical biological, social and psychological questions still need resolution before the potential of these highly desirable methods of protection can be fully realized.

Physical Barriers

The vaginal diaphragm and the cervical cap, usually lubricated with a spermicide, were widely used as contraceptives before the advent of oral contraceptives. Although they have to be individually fitted, once prescribed, a device may be reused for years. The failure rate in contraception has been comparable to that of the other barriers, higher than with the oral contraceptives. They may be used without negotiation with the partner. Control trials and considerable observational experience has established the protective role of the diaphragm against gonorrhoea, chlamydia and perhaps also against other sexually transmitted diseases [2].   However, there are no observations that clearly separate the protective role of the device alone from that of the spermicide-microbicide lubricant that is usually used together with it.   Nor are there data on their potential for protection against HIV.

More thorough protection could in theory be afforded by the woman's condom, very recently on the market in the U.S., Reality and a year before in Europe (Femidom).   The woman's condom, available in one size only, is sold over the counter; no prescription, clinic visit or fitting is needed.   It consists of a 6 inch polyurethane sheath, with flexible rings located at either end.   In laboratory tests, it protects against HIV, chlamydia, cytomegalovirus and other sexually transmitted diseases, in much the same way as does the male condom; human tests for contraception also show results similar to the male condom (Trussel, et al; 1994) [3].   However, protection afforded by the woman's condom as with the condom for men, depends on correct and consistent use.

This device cannot be comfortably used without male co-operation.   Carefully explained, in clinic and family planning settings, it should fill a niche.   It permits women to take the initiative which, if carried out with tact and care, does not need to flout the rights of the man.   Volunteers have been willing to try it out (Liskin, 1993) [4].   In the U.S., small groups have participated in short-term trials (Shervington; Gollub, Stein, El-Sadr) [5, 6].   Much more experience in counselling is now needed, to see if use is maintained.   Also, since the purchase price remains too high for many women, we await tests of re-usability of this device.

Chemical Barriers

Because chemical barriers do not require the consent, active or passive, of the man, they are potentially 'clandestine' strategies.   Still, a woman would feel more secure if she disclosed her use of a barrier, less afraid of repercussions if the man should accidentally discover it.   Disclosure would depend on the circumstances, which is for the woman to judge.

There are various available chemical barriers or microbicides, of different strengths and composition.   Desiderata for such barriers have been formulated [8] in conversations with a wide range of women.

First, covert use must be possible, since this is necessary in some cases.   Hence the substance should preferably be tasteless, odorless, and not too messy.   It should be simple to apply, easy to store, disposable.

It should be effective against a wide range of sexually transmitted diseases.

It should be affordable.

There should be little if any irritation or harmful effects associated with its use.

It should be appropriate for use with anal, vaginal or oral sex.

Finally, barriers should not necessarily be contraceptive.   Many women who need protection against infection, may wish to become pregnant.   This issue is discussed again below.

No currently available or tested product meets all these desiderata.   Among those available are: Nonoxynol-9, Butylurea, Octoxynol-9, Polyanionic Polysaccharides, Benzalkonium Chloride, Myeloperoxidase, Menfegol, Gossypol, Protectaid Sponge, Gramicidin.

The chemical most widely used in the U.S., Nonoxynol-9 or N-9 was developed as a contraceptive or spermicide, and is sold over the counter as a suppository, a sponge, a foam, a film, a tablet, a gel.   In the laboratory, even at low doses, N-9 destroys the HIV (and also several other organisms involved in sexually transmitted diseases) [9, 10].   Field trials of its effectiveness against gonorrhoea and chlamydia have been published and are convincing [11, 12].

For some time N-9 is likely to remain as the only available preparation, certainly in the U.S., and questions have been raised as to its safety and effectiveness.   Regarding N-9, there are three interlocking themes to consider: one is that, given the proven protective role of N-9 in preventing other sexually transmitted diseases (gonorrhoea, chlamydia, genital ulcers), may we assume that N-9 will automatically, if indirectly, protect against HIV transmission?   Two what is the evidence for unintended consequences of N-9? Specifically, in respect of local effects such as reported irritation, or disruption of the vaginal epithelium, both the circumstances that cause these and the role they may play in interfering with expected benefits of N-9.   Three, what is the evidence for reduction in HIV incidence, with N-9?

First, We Deal with N-9 and Other Sexually Transmitted Diseases:
Following on a number of placebo controlled trials of N-9, in the US, in Thailand and Kenya, it may be inferred (as noted above) that the incidence of gonorrhoea, and probably chlamydia too, and several other sexually transmitted diseases seems to be reduced, with regular use and dosage of N-9 preparations.   Similar findings were recently reported from a prospective observational study in the Cameroons [13].

New episodes of ulcerative and non-ulcerative sexually transmitted diseases are so frequently associated, in women and in men, with seroconversion from HIV⁻ to HIV⁺, as to make a causal connection convincing [14].   Recently Laga and colleagues [15] published their 3-year prospective study of women sex-workers in Kinshasa, Zaire: embedded in this article is confirmation of their previous report that sexually transmitted diseases facilitate transmission of HIV-1, as confirmed by the time relationships in the incident cases of other sexually transmitted diseases and HIV.   So, if N-9 reduces infections with other sexually transmitted diseases we would expect it to reduce HIV infection.

Second: We Must Consider the Unintended Consequences:
Controlled trials that used N-9 to protect against other sexually transmitted diseases, mentioned above, made little mention of adverse symptoms (irritation, itchiness and burning) or of observed findings (disruption of the epithelial lining of the cervix or genital ulcers).

The first and only controlled trial of N-9 and HIV, used the 'Today Sponge' (1000 mgm N-9 applied up to several hours before use, and left in, certainly for 24 hours, probaly longer).   The intervention was carried out among 138 Nairobi sex-workers [16] beginning in 1987, who were randomized so that 74 used the N-9 sponge, 64 a suppository or cream without N-9.   At the time, 85% of the population were already HIV⁺.   Women were to report to the clinic every month, and if sexually transmitted diseases were discovered, they would be treated.   Altogether, 116 women saw the trial through, visiting the clinic an average of 9 times.   The rate of gonorrhoea declined significantly among N-9 users: but nearly half complained of irritation and an excess of ulcers on the vulva were noted.   The trial was stopped when it became clear that HIV infection would not decline: it was in fact, slightly higher among sponge-users, although the increase was not significant.

This important study is still understood imperfectly.   Why, if gonorrhoea was significantly reduced, was HIV infection not reduced?   Could it be that the irritation caused by the sponge was the explanation?   That the irritation provided a point of entry for this virus, despite the absence of gonorrhoea (and to some extent, chlamydia)?

And if that is true, then why was there irritation and ulcers, with the sponge?   The literature on the sponge is quite extensive and surprisingly bland.   Very little in the way of local irritation and no ulcers, were reported.   In post-marketing trials, women used a lower dose schedule than did the Nairobi sex-workers; if they followed instructions, they could have used twice the recommended dose.   These and other explanations were advanced by investigators.

Third: What Other Evidence do We have about N-9 and HIV Infection?

A prospective observational study of 303 sex workers in the Cameroons [18, 19] is the most recent evidence.   Women in the Cameroons were counselled on the use of the male condom, and were invited to return monthly for examination, further counselling and supplies.   All women were given in addition, suppositories of 100 mgm N-9 and carefully instructed in their use.   Use of condom and spermicide were monitored on coital logs. Protection against gonorrhoea was clearcut [13].   Also, little in the way of irritation was reported by these women, and no excess ulcers.

In figure 1 the results are shown.   On the horizontal, women are grouped according to whether condoms were used 'mostly' (>75% of times), 'sometimes' (50 – 74% of times) or 'seldom' (less than half the time).   The black bars are 'mostly' users of spermicide, the white bars 'sometimes' users, the gray bars 'seldom' users.   When the condom was seldom used, as on the extreme right hand, the contrast for spermicide use is most evident; very few new cases occurred among the 'mostly' users of suppository, moderate numbers among the 'sometimes' used, and many cases among the 'seldom' users.

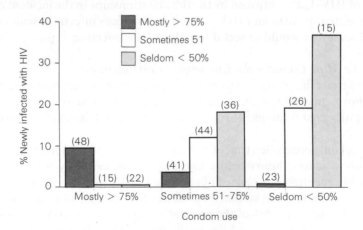

*273 Sex workers in the Cameroons, observed monthly for 1 year, and counselled to use condoms and spermicides

Adapted from Feldblum, Weir: AJPH, 1994, p.1032.

The worst strategy may be for women to use nothing at all.   But we need more trials of safety and efficacy.

There are products probably better than N9: gramicidin, long in use as a contraceptive gel in Russia and found recently to inactivate HIV-1, at doses apparently much lower than N-9 [20].   Polyanionic polysaccharides seem particularly promising, and the gel is colorless, odorless, and in vitro, non-disruptive to cervical or vaginal epithelium [21].

Some critical biological questions still await resolution.

One, mentioned briefly above, is that a microbicide should not necessarily be a contraceptive.   Related to this need, is the important, still unresolved question [22, 23]: Is the sperm involved in transmission and how often?

A second question is whether and to what degree, infection of the female genital tract takes place in the absence of pre-existing ulceration, or breach of the mucosa [21, 24]?

Third, which structures of the genital tract must be protected?   With young women, the mucosal epithelium of the endocervix, which is columnar, is more exposed than at older ages, at which time the stratified squamous epithelium of the vagina is more exposed.   Is increased exposure of the columnar epithelium, known as 'ectopy', a factor in susceptiblity?

Fourth, is there variation in susceptibility and transmission at different stages of the menstrual cycle?

Fifth, what is the role of the pH and the flora of the vagina in protection?   What ill-effects may the microbicide have on the vaginal flora [28]?

Besides knowledge of these biological phenomena, behavioral and socioeconomic variables of potential women and men users must be studied.   We need communication between behavioral scientists, laboratory scientists and public health professionals to establish an integrated program of research and development into methods that women may use.

Acknowledgment

This research was supported in part by grant 5-P50-MH43520 and in part by 5-T32-MH19139.

References

1   Abdool Karim Q, Zuma N, Preston-Whyte E, Stein Z, Morar N: Women and AIDS in Natal/Kwazulu: Determinants to the adoption of HIV protective behavior.   Network of AIDS Researchers of Eastern and Southern Africa (NARESA) Newsletter 1994, 12.
2   Rosenberg MJ, Davidson AJ, Chen JH, Judson FN, Douglas JM: Barrier contraceptives and sexually transmitted diseases in women: A comparison of female-dependent methods and condoms.   Amer J Pub Hlth 1992; 82: 669 – 674.
3   Trussel J, Sturgen K, Strickler J, Dominik R: Comparative contraceptive efficacy of the female condom and other barrier methods.   Fam Plann Persp 1994; 26: 66 – 72.
4   Liskin L: Using female condom for AIDS prevention: Promises and problems.   TOP 28, 14 Dec 1993. VIIIth Int Conf on AIDS in Africa. 12-16 Dec, Marrakesh, Morocco.
5   Shervington D: The acceptablilty of the female condom among low-income African-American women.   J Nat Med Asso 1993; 85: 341 – 347.
6   Gollub EL, Stein Z, El-Sadr W: Acceptability of the Reality female condom among women living or working

in Harlem, New York City.   (in press).

7   Stein Z: HIV prevention: The need for methods women can use.   Amer J Pub Hlth 1990; 80: 460 – 462.

8   Elias CJ, Heise LL: Challenges for the development of female-controlled vaginal microbicides.   AIDS 1994; 8: 1 – 9.

9   Hicks DR, Martin LS, Getchell JP, Heath JL, Francis DP, McDougal JS, et al: Inactivation of HTLV III/LAV-infected cultures of normal human lymphocytes by nonoxynol-9 in vitro.   Lancet 1985, 2: 1422 – 1423.

10 Malkowsky M, Newell A, Dalgleish AG: Inactivation of HIV by nonoxynol-9.   Lancet 1988; 1: 645.

11 Louv WC, Austin H, Alexander WJ, Stagno S, Cheeks J: A clinical trial of Nonoxynol-9 for preventing gonococcal and chlamydial infections.   J Inf Dis 1988; 158: 518 – 523.

12 Rosenberg MJ, Rojanpithayakorn W, Feldblum PJ, Higgins JE: Effect of the contraceptive sponge on chlamydial infection, gonorrhea and candidiasis: A comparative clinical trial.   JAMA 1987; 257: 2308 – 2312.

13 Weir SS, Feldblum PJ, Zekeng L, Roddy RE: The use of Nonoxynol-9 for protection against cervical gonorrhoea.   Amer J Pub Hlth 1994; 84: 910 – 914.

14 Wasserheit JN: Epidemiological synergy: Interrelationships between human immunodeficiency virus infection and other sexually transmitted diseases.   Sex Transm Dis 1992; 19: 61 – 77.

15 Laga M, Alary M, Nzila N, Manoka AT, Tuliza M, Behets F, Goeman J, St. Louis M, Piot P: Condom promotion, sexually transmitted diseases treatment, and declining incidence of HIV-1 infection in female Zairian sex workers.   Lancet 1994; 344: 246 – 248.

16 Kreiss J, Ngugi E, Holmes KK, et al: Efficacy of Nonoxynol-9 contraceptive sponge use in preventing heterosexual acquisition of HIV in Nairobi prostitutes.   JAMA 1992; 268: 477 – 482.

17 North B, Edelman DA, Vorhauer BW: Longterm use of the Today contraceptive sponge.   Adv Contracep 1986; 2: 355 – 361.

18 Zekeng L, Feldblum PJ, Oliver RM, Kaptue L: Barrier contraceptive use and HIV infection among high-risk women in Cameroon.   AIDS 1993; 7: 725 – 731.

19 Feldblum PJ, Weir SS: The protective effect of Nonoxynol-9 against HIV-infection.   Amer J Pub Hlth 1994; 84: 1032 – 1034.

20 Bourinbaiar AS, Lee-Huang S: Comparative in vitro study of contraceptive agents with anti-HIV activity: Gramicidin, Nonoxynol-9 and Gossypol.   Contraceptive 1994; 49: 131 – 132.

21 Pearce-Pratt R, Phillips DM: Studies of adhesion of lymphocytic cells: Implication for sexual transmission of the human immunodeficiency virus.   Biol Reprod 1993; 48: 431 – 445.

22 Anderson DJ: Mechanisms of HIV-1 transmission via semen.   J NIH Res 1992; 4: 104 – 108.

23 Scofield VL: Sperm as vector and cofactors for HIV-1 transmission.   J NIH Res 1992; 4: 105 – 111.

24 Phillips DM, Bourinbaiar BS: Mechanisms of HIV spread from lymphocytes to epithelia.   Virologie 1992; 186: 271 – 273.

25 Clemetson DBA, Moss GB, Willeford M, Hensel M, Emonyi W, Holmes KK, et al: Detection of HIV DNA in cervical and vaginal secretions.   Prevalence and correlates among women in Nairobi, Kenya.   JAMA 1993; 269: 2860 – 2864.

26 Hooton TM, Fennel CL, Clark AM, Stamm WE: Nonoxynol-9: Differential antibacterial activity and enhancement of bacterial adherence to vaginal epithelial cells.   J Inf Dis 1991; 164: 1216 – 1219.

27 Klebanoff SJ: Effects of the spermicidal agent Nonoxynol-9 on vaginal microbial flora.   J Inf Dis 1992; 165: 19 – 25.

28 Voeller B, Anderson DJ: Heterosexual transmission of HIV.   JAMA 1992; 267: 1917 – 1918.

Controlling the Emergence of Tuberculosis (TB) in HIV-Infected Patients

José M. Gatell

Infectious Disease Unit, Hospital Clinic, Barcelona, Spain

The existence of tuberculosis (TB) was established in mummies dating from 2000 to 4000 years BC [1,2]. Since then it has probably been, and still is, the leading cause of death attributable to a single infectious agent [1,2]. It was recognized as a transmissible infection by the end of the last century. Its incidence (number of new cases of active disease per year and per 100,000 population) has been steadily declining since the beginning of this century due mainly to the improvement of socio-economic conditions [1]. The first active anituberculosis agents (namely streptomycin, isoniazid and *p*-aminosalicylic acid) were introduced 'recently' (in the late 40's or early 50's) and dramatically improved the mortality directly attributable to TB. The most active and useful agents (namely isoniazid, rifampin and pyrazinamide) were not introduced, or widely used for combination therapy, until the late 60's or early 70's.

According to World Health Organization (WHO) estimations [1–3], in 1990 tuberculosis still remains the largest cause of death attributed to a single infectious agent. Roughly 30% to 50% of the total world population has been infected (almost always silently) by *Mycobacterium tuberculosis* and remains with a latent infection (TB infection) capable of reactivation. In 1990 nearly 8 million people developed a new active infection (TB disease) accounting for an incidence ranging from 5 to more than 200 new cases per 100,000 people [1,4]. The prevalence (total number of cases in a given moment) of TB disease may be as high as 20 million people [1,4]. The fatality rate of the disease ranges from 0–10% (5–8) in adequately diagnosed and treated people, to 50–100% in immunocompetent untreated hosts and to almost 100% in immunosuppressed untreated hosts [5,9]. This means a total number of about 2.5 million deaths per year attributable to TB [1–4]. More than 95% of the problem is concentrated in the developing world, mainly in Africa and Southeast Asia. By the year 2000 an increase of about 30% in the incidence of TB, and of mortality attributable to TB, has also been estimated by the WHO [4].

In the United States (US) as well as in most of the Western European countries the incidence of TB has been steadily declining during the last few decades leading to the hope of near eradication of the disease whithin the first quarter of the next century [10–13]. By 1989 it became evident, however, that the incidence of tuberculosis was not only no longer declining but in fact increasing with a cumulative excess of about 50,000 unexpected cases only in the US by 1992 [10]. In Barcelona (Spain) the incidence rose from approximately 40 cases per 100,000 people in 1985 to about 60 cases in 1992 [13]. The perception of this sharp and apparently unexpected increase in the incidence of TB in the developed world together with some preliminary data confirming an increase in the initial and secondary resistance rates [14 – 18] to major antituberculosis agents was felt as a defeat in the battle against TB.   In fact, in several parts of the developing world the struggle has made little headway.

Depending on the geographical area, from 10% to as many as 67% of the reported incident cases of TB develop in patients infected with the Human Immunodeficiency Virus type 1 (HIV-1) [13,19,20].   Five to 50% of HIV-1 infected patients will develop TB before AIDS (CDC criteria of 1987) as an AIDS indicator event or present TB later on during the evolution of the HIV-infection [19,21].   Consequently, an epidemiological linkage between the raising incidence of TB and the HIV-1 epidemic can easily be accepted.

In fact, before the AIDS era it was already known that the risk of developing TB is much higher in several types of immunosuppressed hosts as compared with the general population [22,23].   The overall risk in HIV-1-infected patients in general, and in AIDS patients in particular, might be more than 100 times higher.   We now have compelling evidence that the natural history of TB can be dramatically modified by the profound, progressive and irreversible immunodepression due to HIV-1 infection.   A samller inoculum or a shorter exposure period may be enough to infect HIV-1-positive patients.   A rapid progression of a newly (first time) acquired infection is frequent (less than 5% in immunocompetent hosts) [24 – 27].   The risk of reactivating an old latent infection is much higher (at least 30 times higher when compared with the general population) [28 – 30].   Reinfections are possible and may be frequent [14,31].   Isoniazid-resistant strains and multidrug-resistant strains do not seem to be less virulent at least in the HIV-1-infected population.   This means that the whole HIV-1-infected population [at least 10 – 20 million worldwide] and particularly those coinfected with both *M. tuberculosis* and HIV-1 (at least 4 million worldwide) represent an important reservoir for future cases of TB [4,32].   To make things even worse, less than 1/3 of dually infected people (with HIV-1 and *M. tuberculosis*) have a positive PPD skin test (due to skin anergy) as compared with almost 90% to 100% in the general population [28 – 30,33].

When TB disease develops in HIV-1-infected people about 2/3 are extrapulmonary or disseminated forms [7,34] and may be treated using the standard regimens for the developed world (isoniazid + rifampin 6 to 9 months plus pyrazinamide during the first 2 months) [6,35].   Adding a fourth drug (namely ethambutol or streptomycin) during the first two months does not provide additional benefit in terms of efficacy [7] and should only be used when the initial resistance to isoniazid is above a given arbitrarily chosen threshold (about 4%) [35,36].   Relapse rate, although reported to be relatively low [6] in several studies, is at least 3 – 5 times higher than expected in the immunocompetent hosts able to complete the treatment [5].   If future antiretroviral treatments [37] or other treatments [38,39] are aable to prolong life in HIV-infected people, the TB relapse rate may be high enough to consider maintenance therapy (secondary prophylaxis) for life as we are currently doing with several other opportunistic infections in HIV-1-infected patients [40,41].

The most cost-effective step in the prevention of TB (and the best marker of an efficient prevention program) is the early identification of active pulmonary cases (sputum smear positive), and adequate treatment [1 – 3].   In the Western world emphasis has also been put in trying to avoid the reactivation of latent TB infection (with a risk of about 10% during normal lifespan in immunocompetent hosts).   In this setting isoniazid given from 6 to 12 months is able to prevent 90% of the reactivations in compliant patients, and is considered indicated in at least those subgroups of PPD-positive patients with the highest risk of reactivation [42]. Finally the BCG vaccination early after birth is able to prevent disseminated and severe forms of tuberculosis and to decrease the mortality. It may be considered indicated in the developing world and is still administered in several developed countries with a relatively low incidence of TB (43 – 47). All these preventive steps can be applied to HIV-infected patients with the following additional considerations. Since at least 1/3 of TB incident cases may be rapid progressions of newly acquired infections [25 – 27] (first time or even reinfections) major emphasis should be put on early diagnosis, isolation measures (while the sputum smear is positive), adequate treatment (supervising treatment directly if necessary [48 – 51] and considering the possibility of resistant strains thus making sensibility testing mandatory) as well as surveillance of contacts. In coinfected people with a positive PPD test, isoniazid (9 – 12 months) should be administered and has proven effective at least while being administered and shortly therafter [28,29,52 – 54]. The duration of its protective effect remains to be determined [29] and the possibility of using shorter (to achieve a better compliance) regimens with a single more effective drug or combining 2 or 3 drugs are currently being tested in ongoing studies [55,56]. Some subgroups of coinfected people with a PPD-negative test and skin anergy may have a risk of developing an active TB high enough (above 5 – 10 cases per 100 patient-years) to also be considered for chemoprophylaxis [28,33]. Special care should be taken to avoid TB transmission in health care facilities and those procedures able to generate aerosols (e.g. sputum induction, administration of aerosolized pentamidine) may be particularly dangerous [57].

On the other hand, since 1989 at least 16 outbreaks of multidrug-(two or more drugs including in general isoniazid and rifampin) resistant tuberculosis (MDRT) have been reported in the US (mainly in New York, New Jersey and Miami) [9,58] and one in France [59]. Most have occurred in hospitals or other health facilities and have been traced to an index case. 241 patients (most of them with HIV-1 infection) and 17 health care personnel (most of them also with HIV-1 infection or immunosuppressed for other reasons) developed an active TB with a mortality rate of over 70% [9,58]. The PPD conversion rate in non-HIV-infected health care workers involved in the care of these patients or working in the areas frequented by them ranged from 22% to 50% [9,35].

The level of initial resistance has been steadily increasing in several areas of the US [14,16,17] and the level of secondary resistance may be very high even in places like Barcelona where the level of initial resistance still remains below the 'safety boundaries' [15,18]. Thus, the potential for multidrug-resistant tuberculosis to spread exists almost everywhere. When a multidrug-resistant strain is suspected it may be advisable to add two additional drugs (one should be a quinolone) to the standard four-drug regimen [35,36]. In this setting, chemoprophylaxis if considered indicated (on the basis of evaluating the risk of a newly acquired infection with a multidrug-resistant strain and the risk of developing active disease) should include at least two drugs (e.g. a quinolone plus pyrazinamide or ethambutol)[35,36].

Finally, I believe we should emphasize that prevention and treatment of tuberculosis is probably the most cost-effective health intervention in the developing world and that some of the classical antituberculosis programs in the developed world need to be rescheduled and refunded. In addition, we should also recognize that HIV-1 infection is only responsible for part of the unexpected new cases of TB [4]. The rest may be attributed the demographic changes including immigration and social and health care system disruption including poverty and unemployment as well as lack of availability of expensive drugs [4]. More rapid and accurate diagnostic methods and new antituberculosis agents should be targeted as research priorities.

References

1   Bloom BR, Murray CJ: Tuberculosis: commentary on a reemergent killer. Science 1992; 257: 1055-64.
2   Lee Tynes L: Tuberculosis: the continuing story. JAMA 1993; 270: 2616 – 7.
3   Snider DE, La Montagne JR: The neglected global tuberculosis problem. A report of the 1992 World Congress on Tuberculosis. J Infect Dis 1994; 169: 1189 – 1196.
4   Dolin JP, Raviglione MC, Kochi A: A review of current epidemiological data and estimation of future tuberculosis incidence and mortality. (WHO, TB unit; in press).
5   Chan SL: Chemotherapy of tuberculosis. In: PDO Davies, (ed: Clinical tuberculosis. 1 ed. London: Chapman and Hall Medical, 1994, pp141 – 156.
6   Small PM, Schecter GF, Goodman PC, Sande MA, Chaisson RE, Hopewell PC: Treatment of tuberculosis in patients with advanced human immunodeficiency virus infection. N Engl J Med 1991; 324: 289 – 294.
7   Gatell JM, Gonzalez J, De Witt S, Clumeck N, ENTA 05 Tuberculosis Study Group: Tuberculosis in HIV-infected patients in Europe. Clinical characteristics and efficacy of three vs a four drug regimen. In press.
8   Styblo K: Recent advances in epidemioligical research in tuberculosis. Adv Tuberc Res 1980; 20: 1 – 63.
9   Dooley SW, Jarvis WR, Martone WJ, Snider DE: Multidrug-resistant tuberculosis. An Inter Med 1992; 117: 257 – 259.
10 CDC: Tuberculosis morbidity. United States 1992. MMWR 1993; 42: 696 – 704.
11 CDC: Expanded tuberculosis surveillance and tuberculosis morbidity. MMWR 1994; 43: 361 – 366.
12 CDC: Tuberculosis—Western Europe, 1974 – 1991. MMWR 1993; 42: 628 – 632.
13 Cayla JA, Galdos H, Jansa JM, Garcia P, Diez E, Plasencia A: La tuberculosi a Barcelona. Informe 1992. 1 ed. Barcelona: Area de Salut Publica. Ajuntament de Barcelona, 1994: 53.
14 Frieden TR, Sterling T, Pablos-Mendez A, Kiburn JO, Cauthen GM, Dooley SW: The emergence of drug-resistant tuberculosis in New York City [published erratum appears in N Engl J Med 1993 Jul 8; 329(2): 148] [see comments]. N Engl J Med 1993; 328: 521 – 6.
15 Ausina V, Riutort N, Viñado B, Manterola JM, Ruiz J, Rodrigo C ,et al: Prospective study of drug-resistant tuberculosis in a Spanish urban population including patients at risk for HIV infection. Europ J Clin Microb Infect Dis. In press.
16 Sepkowitz KA, Telzak EE, Recalde S, Armstrong D: Trends in the susceptibility of tuberculosis in New York city, 1987 – 1991. Clin infect Dis 1994; 18: 755 – 759.
17 Bloch AB, Cauthen GM, Onorato IM, Dansbury KG, Kelly GD, Driver CR, et al: Nationwide survey of drug-resistant tuberculosis in the United States. JAMA 1994; 271: 665 – 670.
18 Guelar A, Gonzalez J, Gatell JM, Jimenez Anta T, Soriano E: Patterns of resistance of mycobacterium tuberculosis in human immunodeficiency virus Spanish patients infected with HIV. In press.
19 Theuer CPE, Hopewell PC, Elias D, Schecter GF, Rutherford GW, Chaison RE: Human immunodeficiency virus infection in tuberculosis patients. J Infect Dis 1990; 162: 8 – 12.
20 Harris AD: Tuberculosis and human immunodeficiency virus infection in developing countries. Lancet 1990; 335: 387 – 390.
21 Buira E, Gatell JM, Zamora L, Mallolas J, Miro JM, Guelar A, et al: Caracteristicas y supervivencia de los 1000 primeros casos de SIDA. Med Clin (Barc) 1994. In press.
22 Kaplan MH, Armstrong D, Rosen P: Tuberculosis complicating neoplastic disease: A review of 201 cases. Cancer 1974; 33: 850 – 858.
23 Ortbals DW, Marr JJ: A comparative study of tuberculosis and other mycobacterial infections and their associations with malignancy. Am. Rev. Respir. Dis 1978; 117: 39 – 45.
24 Daley CL, Small PM, Scheter GF, Schoolnik GK, McAdam RA, Jacobs WR, et al: An outbreak of tuberculosis with accelerated progression among persons infected with the human immunodeficiency virus. N Eng J Med 1992; 326: 231 – 235.
25 Small PM, Hopewell PC, Singh SP, Paz A, Parsonnet J, Ruston DC, et al: The epidemiology of tuberculosis in San Francisco. N Eng J Med 1994; 330: 1703 – 1709.
26 Alland D, Kalkut GE, Moss AR, McAdam RA, Hahn JA, Bosworth W, et al. Transmission of tuberculosis in New York city. N Eng J Med 1994; 330: 1710 – 1716.

27 Hamburg MA, Frieden TR: Tuberculosis transmission in the 1990s. N Eng J Med 1994; 330: 1750 – 1751.
28 Moreno S, Baraia J, Bouza E, Parras F, Perez-Tascon M, Miralles P, et al: Risk for developing tuberculosis among anergic patients infected with HIV. Ann Inter Med 1993; 119: 194 – 198.
29 Guelar A, Gatell JM, Verdejo J, Podzamczer D, Lozano L, Aznar E, et al: A prospective study of the risk of tuberculosis among HIV-infected patients. AIDS 1993; 7: 1345 – 49.
30 Selwyn PA, Hartel D, Lewis VA, Schoenbaum EE. Vermund SH, Klein RS, et al: A prospective study of the risk of tuberculosis among intravenous drug users with human immunodeficiency virus infection. N Eng J Med 1989; 320: 545 – 554.
31 Small PM, Shafer RW, Hopewell PC, Singh SP, Murphy Desmond E, et al: Exogenous reinfection with multidrug-resistant mycobacterium tuberculosis in patients with advanced HIV infection. N Eng J Med 1993; 328: 1137 – 1144.
32 de March Ayuela, Garcia Gonzalez. [Clinical course of HIV infection/AIDS in developed countries. Impact on tuberculosis]. Med Clin (Barc) 1993; 100: 187 – 93.
33 CDC: The use of preventive therapy for tuberculosis infection in the United States. Recommendations of the Advisory Committee for Elimination of Tuberculosis. MMWR 1990; 39 (RR-8): 9 – 12.
34 Soriano E, Mallolas J, Gatell JM, Latorre X, Miro JM, Pecchiar M, et al: Characteristics of tuberculosis in HIV-infected partients: a case-control study. AIDS 1988; 2: 429 – 432.
35 CDC Initial therapy for tuberculosis in the era of multidrug resistance. MMWR 1993; 42: 1 – 8.
36 Wolinsky E: Statement of the Tuberculosis Committee of the Infectious Diseases Society of America. Clin Infect Dis 1993; 16: 627 – 628.
37 Fischl MA, Richman DD, Grieco MH, Gottlieb MS, Volberding BA, Laskin OL, et al: The efficacy of azidothynidine (AZT) in the treatment of patients with AIDS and AIDS-related complex: A double-blind, placebo-controlled trial. N Eng J Med 1987; 317: 185 – 191.
38 Cooper DA, Pehrson PO, Morini M, Pedersen C, Moroni M, Oksenhendler E, et al: The efficacy and safety of zidovudine alone or as cotherapy with aciclovir for the treatment of patients with AIDS and AIDS-related complex: a double-blind, randomized trial. AIDS 1993; 7: 197 – 207.
39 Studies of Ocular Complications of AIDS Research Group. Mortality in patients with the Acquired immunodeficiency syndrome treated with either Foscarnet or ganciclovir for cytomegalovirus retinitis. N Engl J Med 1992; 326: 213 – 220.
40 Fischl MA, Dickinson GM, La Voie L: Safety and efficacy of sulfamethoxazole and trimethoprim chemotherapy for Pneumocystis carinii in AIDS. JAMA 1988; 259: 1185-89.
41 Pedrol E, Gonzalez JM, Gatell JM, Miro JM, Mallolas J, Soriano E: Central nervous system toxoplasmosis in AIDS patients. Efficacy of an intermittent maintenance therapy. AIDS 1990; 4: 511 – 517.
42 Anonymous: Isoniazid prevention of tuberculosis. Lancet 1983; 1: 395 – 396.
43 Schwoebel V, Hubert B, Grosset J: Impact of BCG on tuberculous meningitis in France in 1990. Lancet 1992; 340: 611.
44 Koch-Weser D: BCG vaccination. Can it contribute to tuberculosis control? (editorial review). Chest 1993; 103: 1641 – 2.
45 Colditz GA, Brewer TF, Berkey CS, Wilson ME, Burdick E, Fineberg H.V., et al: Efficacy of BCG vaccine in the prevention of tuberculosis.   Meta-analysis of the published literature. JAMA 1994; 271: 698 – 702.
46 Fine PE, Rodrigues LC: Modern vaccines. Mycobacterial diseases. Lancet 1990; 335: 1016 – 1020.
47 Clemens JD, Chuong JJ, Feinstein AR: The BCG controversy. JAMA 1983; 249: 2362 – 2369.
48 Nardell EA: Public health policy and the treatment of the individual patient tuberculosis. Am Rev Respir Dis 1993; 148: 2 – 5.
49 Chaulk CP, Chaisson RE, Lewis JN, Rizzo RT. Treating multidrug-resistant tuberculosis: compliance and side effects. JAMA 1994; 271: 103-4; di.
50 Iseman MD, Cohn DL, Sbarbaro JA: Directly obseved treatment of tuberculosis. We can't afford not to try it. N Eng J Med 1993; 328: 576 – 578.
51 Alwood K, Keruly J, Moore-Rice K, Stanton DL, Chulk CP, Chaisson RE: Effectiveness of supervised, intermittent therapy for tuberculosis in HIV-infected patients. AIDS 1994; 8: 1103 – 1108.
52 Selwin PA, Sckell BM, Alcabes P, Friedland GH, Klein RS, Schoenbaum EE: High risk of active tuberculosis in HIV-infected intravenous drug users with cutaneous anergy. JAMA 1992; 268: 504 – 509.
53 Jordan TJ, Lewit EM, Montgomery RL, Reichman LB: Isoniazid as preventive therapy in HIV-infected intravenous drug abusers. JAMA 1991; 265: 2987 – 2991.
54 Pape JWPM, Jean SS, Ho JL, Hafner A, Johnson WD: Effect of isoniazid prophylaxis on incidence of active tuberculosis and progresssion of HIV infection. Lancet 1993; 342: 268 – 272.
55 Lecoeur HF, Truffot C, Grosset JH: Experimental short-course preventive therapy of tuberculosis with rifampin and pyrazinamide 1,2. Am Rev Respir Dis 1989; 140: 1189 – 1193.
56 de March Ayuela P: ¿ Puede acortarse la quimioprofilaxis de la tuberculosis? a la busqueda de una quimioprofilaxis corta de la tuberculosis. Arch Bronoconeumol 1991; 27: 210 – 213.
57 CDC. Guidelines for preventing the transmission of tuberculosis in health-care settings, with special focus

on HIV-related issues. MMWR 1990; 39: 1 – 29.

58   CDC. Nosocomial transmission of multidrug-resistant tuberculosis among HIV-infected persons—Floreida and New York, 1988 – 1991. MMWR 1991; 40: 585-90.

59   Bouvet E, Casalino E, Mendoza-Sassi G, Lariven S, Vallee E, Pernet M., et al: A nosocomial outbreak of multidrug-resistant *Mycobacterium bovis* among HIV-infected patients. A case-control study. AIDS 1993; 7: 1453-60.

Counseling/Social/Psychology/Support

Human Rights Violations as a Barrier to Effective Policies in Prevention and Care

Arnaud Marty-Lavauzelle

AIDS Fédération Nationale, Paris, France

Thank you—It is great honor for me to give a speech before you. Allow me to speak in my mother language. It is very difficult to speak for a very important person, also very difficult to speak for a patient. But this may be a challenge for us when we confront the epidemic.

I ask for your generosity if you find some errors in the slides and mistakes in my speech.

I also ask you to find in this speech the energy and the ardent participation of the volunteers and of the group I am working with.

We have the right to have common thoughts and emotions proper to each culture and to each language. This right is very important when trying to understand, in particular, the mode of transmission of some public health models in a country where the people speak a different language and whose model of prevention and support looks barbarous and colonial. Unfortunately, there is no common language universal to all countries.

Human rights violations disturb access to prevention and care, and we now know that prevention is very important to care. The human rights revisited by the AIDS epidemic now have more important meaning than before for the victims: the freedom of expression, the freedom of political expression, and the fight against torture, all these human rights in the age of AIDS become a question of life or death and a question of how to obtain access to care and prevention. If society excludes the people from vital information, education, and health promotion, the vulnerability to the infection by HIV increases dramatically. The conflicts arising between those working in public health on one hand and those who insist on the rights of the individual on the other have led to considerable problems by augmenting irrational fear of the epidemic and by giving rise to pseudomedical practices such as systematic surveys, resulting in violation of confidentiality or, even more, segregation of the patients and seropositives in many countries. Such criminalization drastically increases exclusion and vulnerability because, in prison, for example, one can be infected repeatedly. In prison everywhere in the world, one cannot obtain access to high quality care.

Everywhere and always exclusion from the society at large reinforces attacks on the conditions of daily life, especially on those who have only the minimum to live, to eat and to continue a life.

If there are some different degrees between the discrimination and the violations and if these violations indicate transgression of laws, it is very important for us all to reach a consensus on the action in fighting against the discrimination not to overlook the violations.

At the same time, it is important to note that discrimination and the violations exist in every country, developing and developed, and that we are always confronting the paradoxes of the developed countries which, for example, give important funds to fight against AIDS but which, at the same time, limit freedom, in particular, the freedom of movement.   I think, of course, this is the case in the USA and in Japan, and I am in deep despair to think that, in some countries, Patchworks commemorating the dead seem to circulate more easily than the victims themselves.   I hasten to add with all due respect that I love the Patchworks of the Names of the dead.

When we think about a problem of human right violations or rather the rights of the specific individual, human rights usually means the rights of men, women and children. We must create new laws, but creation of special laws is always dangerous because they could be utilized afterwards for discrimination.   It is very important, I believe, to know that there are various agreements, conventions and international laws to protect the virus-infected people and their neighbors, but the true question which we should raise all together is, "What can we do to carry out policies in order to respect or accept these laws?"

To fight against discrimination, I ask you to understand immediately that the mechanisms of denial, such as the denial of the very large impact of discrimination, denial of the epidemic and denial of the infected people, are based on some superficial ideas: believing that the danger comes from the exterior, particularly from foreign countries where the infection is prevalent; presenting the statistics but not the dynamic numbers of the epidemic in a reassuring fashion; disturbing the organization of virus-infected people and their neighbors; threatening them; using the police force and also they can give useless materials to these people.   Denying is ignoring and erasing the visibility and the expression of the people who live with the virus.

Another form of denial consists in discrediting prevention.   This is especially true in some countries where the use of condoms is discouraged, being equated as an incentive to premature sex.

Another way to disparage the expression of the people who live with the virus is the creation of para-governmental organizations which are more often connected to the authorities than to groups in the community.

Furthermore, we can also add betrayal of confidentiality.   Betraying confidentiality diminishes the rights of a person and it is quite contrary to aid for the visibility of the infected people in supporting their rights.   It also demonstrates ignorance of the existing laws and conventions.   There is no doubt in my mind that, in every country, discrimination and violations exist, even though a national program to fight against AIDS is in force.

Another very important point is the alliance of policy with culture and religion. Governments utilize cultural and religious excuses to reinforce the discrimination of virus-infected people.   Alliance with conservatism or a moral majority can increase exclusion. However, if religious people work in accordance with the support, tolerance and compassion that exists in all religions, it would go a long way to help.

We should talk about the violation of the rights of the persons, we should enumerate them, and we should make them known.   This is an extremely difficult task, probably as difficult as remembering close friends who died of AIDS since the beginning of the epidemic. Let me list violations which are augmenting in intensity:

• the situation of women exposed to violence, maltreatment, rape, sexual abuse, prostitution (claiming ever younger victims), drugs, migration, utilization of their bodies against their will but according to decisions made without their consent as seen in the decision to interrupt pregnancies, in the negation of symptoms, or in the disparagement of emotions, particularly when these emotions attract other women. The most popular form of violation of women's rights is certainly conjugal dependence in societies where their status does not allow them to protect themselves from the virus or to control the means of prevention.

• Children are increasingly exposed to organized prostitution and child labor. They are extremely vulnerable.

• Men are increasingly exposed today to infection in prisons, as I have told you, and in psychiatric hospitals. Homophobia exists everywhere and destroy relationships not only between man and man but also between man and woman, and, to have the best relations with women, many heterosexuals should consider changing their opinion against homophobia.

• I remember my deaf friends. As you know, the deaf suffer double discrimination: refusal and repression of sign language and, at the same time, a very big difficulty in obtaining access to prevention. I hope they are present with us today in this hall.

For all, in every culture, homosexuality might be a crime, and sodomy is a crime which is severely punished in India, for example, and in some American countries.

New risks appear in experimentation—I remind you that the only ethical basis for therapeutic experimentation is to bring about good results for those who receive the test— but we are far from such a situation, and in some cruel experiments there are human rights violations like non-inclusion in therapeutic protocols, exclusion from possible care, sexual act, behavior, or exclusion by prejudice, particularly in my country, against drug use and users.

Concerning drug users, the world should organize something different from the war against drugs, against the Mafia and other organized systems. However, is it possible that politicians get more money with the Mafia?

Speaking of human rights is also speaking of fundamental equity in relation to the means, the money, and the participation in the fight against AIDS. However, we have endured for long time a situation where 85% of the budget to fight against AIDS is spent in only 15% of the world, mostly in the rich countries.

What about our perspectives? Action or complicity? You are actors and sometimes patients in the fight against AIDS. You are witnesses of violations and daily discrimination. Some of you have come to every conference since the first one held ten years ago. Others do not come because they are sick, or because they are dead. I pose this question to you and to myself: "What are you doing today at the 10th Conference at Yokohama, with all your knowledge on the human right violations and discrimination?" I have looked at the posters: there are only five posters on the subject of human rights violations, and I want to know whether it is the Organizing Committee that has rejected other posters or it is yourself who has withdrawn them. In any case, it means that we cannot talk about the central theme of human rights by attending the international conference on AIDS, even though you are convinced that, without respect for the individual, no treatment could be given, no support and no prevention could be effective.

What level of self-regulation have we reached to think that a conference could be a science without a conscience?   We should all collect, at the same time, information on violations of individual rights.   For this purpose, we should, at the same time, provoke and support witnesses and guarantee that they will be able to testify what they have observed. The expression of personal rights violations is, so to speak, a litany which we repeat at each international conference on AIDS.   This needs true participation of local community groups such as NGOs of the people living with the virus.   The communication on personal rights violations should equal the communication of scientific themes, otherwise the gap between those countries which will be able to benefit by therapeutic progress and those countries which will be more and more relegated to a back seat and isolated by continuous violations will increase.

I propose that you promote a policy of reducing human rights violations.   What the epidemic taught us is that, even if we cannot find all the solutions for a problem, we can obtain short-term strategies for effective evaluation on limited aims which allow us, year by year, to measure our progress, instead of feeling, year after year, powerlessness and impossibility in managing the problems of human rights violations.

It is probable that economists will also be interested in evaluating the economic cost and impact of human rights violations.

It seems to me that the rapid increase in the epidemic curve in the last year is also comparable to the increase in human right violations, which are sometimes specifically organized as the large-scale genocides, in Serbia and Rwanda for example.

I will keep an eye on this curve as a witness of the increase or the decrease of such violations.

All of us have the possibility to assemble on December 1 at the Paris summit.   Forty ministers of health assembled in June to decide the themes of study: new basic researches.

I really hope that, on December 1, the subject of human rights can also be taken up, as in this conference, to throw light on all the difficulties facing us.

A Japanese poet, Yutaka Hirata, an AIDS patient, wrote a book of poems, entitled "I will love life a little bit more."   As a person who is also living with the virus under treatment, I too would like to adopt his golden words.   However, I believe that, if we still observe the slow progression of violations and barbarities until the next international conference to be held in two years at Vancouver, and if there is something which prevents me from attending, it will not be my disease, but the shame, the rage and the debt of survival in the feeling of the dreadful complicity with you that we did not do better in promoting human rights.

Thank you.

(Translated from French by Katsuhiko Ono, M.D., Ph.D.)

Ethical Issues on HIV/AIDS Care

Hakima Himmich

Medical School of Cassablanca, Faculty of Medicine, Casablanca, Morocco

Introduction

The number of people in need of care for HIV/AIDS will rise dramatically in the coming years, even if preventive efforts reduce the number of new HIV infections [1].   The majority of ethical problems raised in the context of HIV infection are not new, even though some issues are specific to HIV infection.   Moreover, problems are further complicated by the fact that HIV provokes a chronic, infectious disease with fatal issue.   Therefore, it is within the framework of existing legislation and rules that we have to consider HIV/AIDS patients' problems and inquiries.   Above all, the reinforcement of the rights of all patients is the implicit objective for those who fight for the rights of people with HIV/AIDS [2].

In this presentation, we will focus on the ethical issues of care and access to health care. These ethical issues vary not only from country to country, but also within each country according to socio-economic factors which determine the situation of HIV seropositive persons.   We will review the different ethical issues in HIV/AIDS care and access to health care in developing and developed countries, and we will discuss what has been done and could be done to solve these problems.

In this presentation, we will not discuss the problem of confidentiality because many presentations at this conference focus on this important ethical issue and this is a problem which comes up more frequently at the moment of diagnosis than during care.

Ethical Issues in HIV/AIDS Care and Human Rights

The right to health originates officially in governments' determination to adopt the 1948 Geneva Universal Declaration of Human Rights.   The United Nations enunciated in full the 'right to have a living standard sufficient to ensure one's and one's family's health and well-being as concerns food, clothing, housing, medical care and social services.'   The constitution of the WHO, adopted in New York in 1946, had already defined the right to health as 'the claim to the best possible health status, whatever be one's race, religion, political opinions, economic and social condition'[3].   Nevertheless, the principle of care itself for HIV seropositive persons is rejected by a significant part of the public and even considered debatable by some physicians, health care professionals, and policy-makers as well.

The realization that support for HIV/AIDS care is a worth-while investment is only beginning to appear and is still not obvious to everyone.   In 1987, however, WHO and the director of the Global Program on AIDS, Jonathan Mann, made significant progress when they established that discriminatory practices go against the fundamental objectives of public health and that it is essential to protect HIV seropositive people against discrimination.   In 1988, the Forty-first World Health Assembly called on all governmental, non-governmental and international organizations engaged in AIDS control programs 'to ensure that their programs take fully into account the health needs of all people as well as the health needs and dignity of people with HIV/AIDS' [4].

Nevertheless, not even the Universal Declaration of Human Rights, nor the clear position of WHO have convinced policy-makers in many countries and international organizations of the urgence to care for people living with HIV/AIDS.   These policy-makers and organizations are not convinced that care is an integral part of prevention. Unfortunately, the right to health remains unattainable not only under conditions of poverty, but also under a variety of circumstances which are beyond individual, and even, collective reach.

Inequality in Access to Care

Inequality Between Developing and Developed Countries

In developing countries, the right to health is more a theoretical right than a fact of life for all patients, and not just for those infected with the HIV virus.   In Sub-Saharan Africa, AIDS patients occupy nearly 75% of hospital beds leaving only a few available for all other patients.   These hospitalized AIDS patients are not receiving medicines like zidovudine or the less costly essential medicines [5].   International organizations refuse to fund the health infrastructure or provide drugs for the care of people living with HIV/AIDS.   They are willing to fund prevention programs only, while at the same time, they know that the governments of developing countries don't have the means to finance care for persons with HIV/AIDS.   For example, a Central African country estimated the cost per patient per year to be between US $13 and $38, using a very simple treatment regimen (excluding acyclovir, amphoterecin B and ketoconazole) [6].   Furthermore, it is estimated that the lifetime cost of treating a person with HIV from the time of infection until death is approximately US $119,000 in the U.S. [7].

Inequality in Developed Countries

Even when care facilities exist, they are not accessible to many people.   This is the case for people without social insurance (the majority of drug users, sex workers, illegal aliens). To these marginalized populations, we must add those who have lost their jobs.   For all these persons, there is a lack of continuity of care, prophylactic treatment and access to hospitals.   Finally, for those who know themselves to be seropositive, repressive laws, discrimination, and their own lack of prominence exclude them from the health care system.

In order to achieve accessibility to health care, we have to take on the fight against discrimination and promote the insertion of the marginalized population in society.   We also have to instill self-esteem in patients so that they will be able to recognize and protect their rights.

Physicians and Care for People with HIV/AIDS

The behavior of physicians and other health professionals allows for comments from an ethical point of view [8].   First of all, there are many testimonies concerning refusal of care reported by people living with HIV/AIDS.   According to a survey conducted in the US in 1990, 19.4% of the interviewed doctors think that a physician is not obliged to treat HIV seropositive persons, and 5.3% are not sure if they have the obligation to treat HIV seropositive persons [9].

The argument put forward by those, regardless of their professional ethics, who refuse to care for people with HIV and AIDS, is the risk of exposure to HIV transmission. Cumulative data from many studies on the continuous control of health givers exposed to the HIV virus indicate that the acquired risk of HIV infection from one exposure to a needle puncture is approximately 0.3% [10].   We cannot deny professional risk, but it has always been present, especially regarding hepatitis B and C, and the conclusions drawn by part of the medical profession concerning refusal to care are disproportionate.   In fact, the accepted custom is that physicians have the duty to treat any patient, even if it's exposing them to risk of infection.   The only conclusion that may be drawn from the risk of professional risk of infection is the obligation to assure good working conditions for health care givers by respecting international guidelines [11].

In fact, however, when good working conditions are available, health workers don't adhere to these guidelines.   In a study concerning mid-wives, it was reported that only 55% of them respected general precautions, although blood exposure during delivery is a constant threat [10].   The question gets even more complicated when hospitals don't have appropriate resources to offer constant and adequate protective supplies.   This is the case even in hospitals of large African cities.   This lack raises a question of a deontological nature which is difficult to resolve.

Furthermore, the fact that some physicians pass judgment and stigmatize people with HIV and AIDS, leads many patients to ask for care at a very late stage of the disease. According to a survey conducted in many French hospitals by the AIDES Association among patients with AIDS, more than 16% of those interviewed declared having observed among health care givers anti-AIDS attitudes and behaviors.   Nearly 20% of those interviewed have observed this intolerance toward seropositive intravenous drug users with physicians requiring that IDU's withdraw from drug intake as a condition for therapeutical care.   In most cases, the drug user finds himself, during hospitalizaition, experiencing withdrawal.   The recourse to product substitution is either absent or insufficient [12].

Another matter concerns pain.   The majority of physicians don't take into account or underestimate patients pain in general, and that of AIDS patients in particular.   In fact, even the existence of pain during AIDS was denied for a long time and pain-relieving drugs remain inadequately prescribed or prescribed too late.   However, it is well established that pain is often present at different stages of the HIV infection.

Another problem that people with HIV/AIDS were most prone to denounce is the fact that under the pretext of emergency and overwork, and sometimes under the pretext of a strictly technical concept of care, medical teams don't treat the patient as a person enjoying his fundamental rights.   He is more an object of care than an active subject in the therapeutical relationship. Because of their specialized training and knowledge, physicians have a powerful position vis-a-vis the patient who usually lacks the knowledge to immediately grasp the situation. That is why people with HIV/AIDS claim an ethical entitlement to full and objective health information from physicians [3].

On the other hand, a large part of physicians' negative behavior is related to the fact that physicians who give care need training to be able to provide not only medical treatment, but also support and comfort [13]. They also need training to be able to consider people living with HIV/AIDS as not only patients, but as partners involved in the entire care process.

But even among those who are used to giving care to HIV/AIDS patients, the depression that many physicians feel concerning AIDS makes them stop prophylaxis and treatment of complications [14]. The objective of all these remarks concerning the behavior of physicians isn't meant to accuse them. The objective is to underline what is wrong in view of improving the situation.

Critical Care of Patients with AIDS

Because the acquired immunodeficiency syndrome (AIDS) is up to now ultimately a fatal illness, the disease raises important and difficult ethical questions concerning the benefits and burdens of critical care. Sixty-seven percent to 90% of AIDS patients who require critical care do so because of respiratory failure caused by *Pneumocystis carinii* pneumonia (PCP). Early in the epidemic the indication for critical care for PCP was questionable because of the very bad prognosis with a survival rate of only 0% to 14%. Now this prognosis has improved to a survival rate of 36% to 56% and, with prophylaxis, relapses are less frequent [15]. The outcome is now better than that of other situations for which clinicians routinely offer intensive care unit care. Therefore, with rare exceptions, critical care for AIDS patients cannot be deemed futile unless we are willing to alter our concept of futility when caring for patients with other diseases carrying similar prognoses.

Another ethical issue regarding intensive care for patients with AIDS is that informed patient refusals of life-sustaining treatment should be respected. Such an attitude is consistent with the legal requirement of informed consent. However, the majority of patients with AIDS who receive critical care are, in fact, not given the opportunity to forgo such care. The legal designation of a close person for decision making, in case of the incapacitation of a patient, is also very important when the patient has a lover or a friend who, without this designation, could be excluded from decision making.

Over the past decade, the ethic has evolved, and it is now widely accepted, of allowing terminally ill patients to die with dignity. This allowance may involve withholding or discontinuing interventions [16], and, for some physicians, euthanasia [17]. I am not going to discuss in this presentation the problem of euthanasia. Euthanasia is the object of medical and philosophical debate, and patients with AIDS at the terminal stage wouldn't pose specific problems.

Palliative Care and AIDS

Not actually curable, AIDS, a chronic disease, poses the problem of palliative care at the end of life.   These problems are comparable in some aspects with those observed in cancer.   However, they may differ in other aspects.   Usually patients with HIV/AIDS are young.   They face exclusion and have difficulty in facing others.   Sometimes they suffer from the absence of their families and are forced to witness the death of many friends.   Dr. Salamagne, a physician involved in end-of-life care, vehemently denounces the condition of patients at the end of life in hospitals.   She says, 'the patient doesn't have the possibility to be cured; he often stops treatment; he is usually depressed, aggressive and anxious, and thus, transmits his anxiety to the physician.   He is rejected by everyone and is not considered a human being' [18].   The correct care during this phase should allow patients to deal with this moment in serenity, not in pain and anxiety, as is frequently the case.   Many community-based associations have been aware of this problem and have developed over the last 10 years, home care for those in the palliative phase and support for hospitalized patients.   They have also created housing to receive sick people at the terminal stage.

Ethical Issues in Drug Trials

Drug trials are necessary to determine the safety and the effectiveness of new drugs, but their implementation poses ethical problems.   The first is the ethical issue concerning the huge disparity in health resources between developed and developing countries which has long been the subject of a debate that has never come close to resolution.   The high prevalence of HIV in African countries makes research scientifically attractive.   Research in Africa is also attractive because it is less expensive and administratively easier to conduct than in developed countries.   Nevertheless, the selection of African people with HIV/AIDS as subjects of drug trials raises profound ethical concerns [19].   Indeed, African populations should not be subjected to a disproportionate share of the research risks.

A more critical question arises as to the fact that after a drug has been proven safe and effective, African people living with HIV/AIDS, including those who participated in the research, aren't receiving the drug because it is too expensive.   WHO and other international organizations have to ensure that the drug is made available and affordable to the people of the developing countries in which it was tested.

In developed countries, however, the willingness to be included in a drug trial is sometimes not a free choice.   Is it a free choice when a person can have, without charge, an experimental treatment only by participation in a drug trial?   When the only other alternatives are lack of treatment or the prohibitive cost of treatment?

Another ethical aspect concerns placebos.   Is it ethical to give placebos to a certain group of patients and, in doing so, prevent them from the possibility of improving their state?   The answer is not easy.

Concerning the acceleration of the rate at which new and experimental drugs and treatments have been made available, people with AIDS are not happy.   They wish to have, immediately, any treatment that is potentially effective.   However, it is necessary to keep a scientific approach and to respect protocols which permit careful testing so as not to deceive the hopes of patients.

Special Wards or General Wards for People with HIV/AIDS

Since there is no public health rationale for the isolation of people with HIV or AIDS, there is no justification solely on the grounds of their HIV status for the isolation of AIDS patients during hospital care.   When considering whether to care for AIDS patients in special wards or within general wards, policy-makers need to weigh the possible benefits against the risk that special AIDS wards might heighten stigmatization, and the risk that patients with HIV/AIDS would be concentrated in the hands of a few AIDS-care specialists.

Another argument against special wards is the enormous impact on physicians and, even more so, on nurses, who care for many AIDS patients.   The impact is responsible for the deleterious effect known as 'AIDS Burnout'[14].   But the choice between special wards and general wards is not easy.   Indeed, the conditions of reception and care are considerably better in special wards than in general wards.

What are the Solutions for Improving Care of Persons with HIV/AIDS?

To Recognize and Apply Hospitalized-Patient Rights [20].

For nearly half a century, deontologic codes, declarations and recommendations have promoted patient rights more and more according to fundamental ethical issues.   At present, with few exceptions, patient rights are completely ignored by governments.   They are subject to legislation in only a few developed countries: Switzerland, the US, Denmark and Canada.

Training and Improvement of Working Conditions for Health Workers

The requests of health workers who take care of persons with HIV/AIDS can be summerized as follows: safe conditions at work; educational training, including ethical issues; care systems which take into account hospital overload in terms of staff and means; and adequate opportunity to manage stress and to avoid AIDS-burnout [21].

Reinforce the Role of Community-Based Associations

These associations, in which persons with HIV/AIDS play a fundamental role, are vigilant against any threat of exclusion and have given very efficient and original answers to the problems posed by the epidemic.   These activities are conducted by volunteers who have received special training through the associations and whose work has had a substantial impact on patients as well as on health-care costs.   These associations should be financially sustained and be considered by care givers as real partners.   Unfortunately, this is in no way the case in many developing countries.

Encourage the Positive Initiatives Coming from Hospitals

In some hospitals, care groups have undertaken very positive initiatives, like in-hospital, multidisciplinary groups which include health professionals, volunteers and teams specializing in hospitalization at home.   Some of these initiatives can be adopted to the context of developing countries and should be encouraged.

Respect the Resolutions Adopted by the Forty-First WHO Assembly in 1988.
These resolutions insist on the respect of the human rights and dignity of HIV-infected people, avoiding discrimination and stigmatization, and taking fully into account the health needs of all people, as well as the health needs and dignity of HIV-infected people [4].

Help Developing Countries to Assure Care for People with HIV/AIDS
According to a report published in 1993 by the International Bank, health in developing countries should no longer be seen as a problem of consumption, but as an investment [22]. This should encourage international fundraisers to accept that investment in the field of health is important in economic, as well as human, terms.   Community-based associations and WHO should ensure that safe and effective drugs for AIDS and other endemic diseases in developing countries are availabale for people with HIV/AIDS.

Conclusion

The HIV/AIDS epidemic poses many ethical questions and necessitates that health professionals analyse the ethical aspects of their behavior.   It contributes to a redefining and strengthening of the societal approach to health.   Specifically, HIV/AIDS creates the obligation to 'lift up' the status and standards of existing health systems, rather than simply integrating HIV/AIDS prevention and care within inadequate existing health systems.

Policy-makers must be convinced that any public health decision cannot be effective if it is not achieved in collaboration with associations acting at the grass-roots level.

References

1   WHO: GPA promotes continuum of comprehensive AIDS care WHO.   Geneva 1994.
2   Lascoumes P: VIH, exclusion et luttes contre les discriminations.   Une épidémie révélatrice d'orientations nouvelles dans la construction et la gestion des risques.   Cahiers de recherche sociologique 1994; 22: 61 – 75.
3   Moulin AM: AIDS and the history of the right to health.   AIDS, health and human rights; Fondation Marcel Merieux, 1993.
4   The forty-first WHO Resolution, WHA41-24, Geneva, May 1988.
5   De Cock KM, Lucas SB, Lucas S, Agness J, Kadio A, Gayle HD: Clinical research, prophylaxis, therapy and care for HIV disease in Africa.   Ame J Public Health 1993; 83, 10: 1385 – 1389.
6   Katabira ET, Wabitsh R: Management issues for patients with HIV infection in Africa.   AIDS 1991; 5: S149 – S155.
7   Hellinger FJ: The lifetime cost of treating a person with HIV.   JAMA 1993; 270: 474 – 478.
8   Kelly, Laurence ST, Smith Hood, Smith Cook: Stigmatization of AIDS patients by physicians.   Am J Pub Health 1987; 77: 789 – 791.
9   Rizzo JA, Marder WD, Willke RJ: Physician contact with and attitudes towards HIV seropositive patients.   Medical Care 1990; 28: 251 – 260.
10   Grady C, Ethical issues.   In: Flaskerud JH, Ungivarski PJ: HIV/AIDS.   A guide to nursing care.   Saunders 1992; pp 484 – 501.
11   Bird AG, Gore SM: Revised guidelines for HIV infected health care workers.   BMJ 1993; 306: 1013 – 1014.
12   VIH á l'hôpital.   Etat des lieux.   AIDES-Paris 1993.
13   Planning of HIV treatment services and care.   Report of the working panel on treatment, services and care.   HIV/AIDS.   Department of community sevices and health 1989.
14   Zuger A: AIDS on the wards: A residency in Medical Ethics.   Hastings Center Report 1987; pp 102 – 106.

15   Bone RC: Critical care of patients with AIDS.   JAMA 1992; 267: 541 – 547.
16   Roy DJ: Ethiclal Issues in the treatment of cancer patients.   Journal of Palliative care 1989; 5: 56 – 61.
17   Moulin M: Le SIDA révelateur de la question de l'euthanasie.   Le SIDA un Défi aux droits.   Actes du colloque organisé á l'université libre de Bruxelles 10 – 12 Mai 1990.
18   Hirsch E, Salamagne MH: Accompagner jusqu'au bout de la vie.   Cerf, Paris 1992.
19   Ankrah EM, Gostin LO: Ethical and legal considerations of the HIV epidemic in Africa.   In: M Essex, S. Mboup.   AIDS In Africa 1994, pp 547 – 558.
20   Charrel J, Larher MP, Manuel C, Reviron D, San Marco JL: SIDA: droits des malades.   Santé Publique 1990; 3: 48 – 53.
21   Manuel C, Charrel J, Larger MP, Enel P, Reviron D, Sans Marco JL: SIDA: droits et devoirs des professionnels de santé.   Santé Publique 1990; 3: 54 – 58.
22   World Development Report 1993, the World Bank, Washington DC, June 1993.

Government/Community Partnerships

Dennis Altman

Politics at La Trobe University, Bundoora, Victoria, Australia

Let me begin by expressing my pride, my thanks and my humility at speaking to this plenary session of the Tenth International Conference on AIDS.

Ten years ago I attended the first of these meetings in Atlanta, and many of you here today have become friends and colleagues over the past decade in our fight against HIV/AIDS. Others who were friends, lovers, colleagues have died, and as always my pride is mingled with sadness at their loss. As a gay man I live in a community where death has become commonplace, and where the stress of our losses is compounded by the ignorance and the hostility with which too many people still view us. As a political scientist I seek to understand how these individual deaths and discrimination are shaped by larger economic and political forces. And as an Australian, a country which is part of the vast Asian/Pacific region, my greatest commitment is to expand the links and common purpose we have begun to forge with our co-workers across national and ideological boundaries.

But above all, I want to speak of those whose voices cannot be heard because they lack the resources to attend an international conference. I cannot speak for young girls forced into the sex industry in Burma and Thailand, for the terrified refugees of Rwanda and Bosnia, for the street kids in Rio de Janeiro and Bucharest, for the lesbians and gay men terrorized in Iran and Pakistan, for the Aboriginal people of my own country whose life expectancies are so much lower than those of the dominant population. But I can recall their presence, and remind us of our responsibility for those who, because of poverty, ignorance, persecution and neglect, are most affected by this epidemic.

I also speak with a deep commitment to the empowerment of those people and communities most affected by HIV/AIDS, above all of those who are positive, and whose bravery in fighting the disease and its stigma is a constant inspiration. The idea of 'community' is a complex one, but I am speaking of those people who share a common sense of purpose and all too often a common oppression, whether this be based on their gender, race, sexuality or HIV status. Whether in Uganda or the United States, in Poland or the Philippines, it has been the affected communities who have taken the lead in mobilizing the political will and energies necessary to deal with the impact of this epidemic.

We need to distinguish between different epidemics, both in terms of epidemiology and resources. We know that in Asia, as in the rest of the developing world, AIDS will spread rapidly, primarily through heterosexual intercourse, and that both education and care will be enormously hampered by the inequitable division of resources between and within nations.   We have all heard the rhetoric that only partnership between governments, health professionals and affected communities can meet this challenge.

Unfortunately while governments are more powerful and better resourced than community organizations they often lack the will to act effectively.   AIDS demands both economic and political resources, and relatively few governments have been willing either to take effective and sometimes unpopular decisions or to work in genuine partnership with those groups most affected by HIV.   At the same time we need recognize that neither the government nor the NGO sector is monolithic—there are divisions and possible alliances which cut across both sectors.   In many cases the perseverance and courage of government officials has pushed governments into action when their masters would have preferred silence.   Nor do all NGOs represent communities: some are created only to tap foreign donors, who too often support the well written application rather than the messier reality of grassroots organization.

Meaningful partnership between government and communities implies common goals, but also mutual respect and adequate resources.   Too often governments expect NGOs to rubber stamp their own programs, and fail to accept that partners have different interests and priorities.   Despite WHO resolutions to provide funding to the non-government sector too few governments are willing to enact this decision and make the funds available. Governments must avoid the temptation—not unknown in rich countries—to see the community sector as a source of cheap labor to disguise government inadequacies.

There are different as well as overlapping roles here.   Governments can mobilize resources and commitment, can accept responsibility for basic care and support, and can do much to combat ignorance and discrimination.   As the Director General of WHO, Dr. Nakajima, said in speaking to heads of government: 'Your influence is great and by your personal commitment, you can do much to allay fear and prejudice.   Set an example by visiting people affected by HIV/AIDS in their homes, hospitals and health centers; listen to them, and confront the reality of their needs, their sufferings and the difficulties they are going through'[1].

But CBOs too have certain real advantages.   My Thai colleagues, Jon Ungphakorn and Werasit Sittitrai, have identified three: flexibility; access to multidisciplinary skills; and most significant, development of participatory programs [2].   This last implies the empowerment of those affected, which means challenging the practice of most governments, who feel threatened by programs which seek to give control over their own lives to women, to young people, to homosexuals, to sex workers, to drug users, to those perceived as dying of a fearful disease.   We cannot hide the fact that the required empowerment and community development which this epidemic demands is subversive. To save lives governments need provide space and resources for unpopular and oppressed communities, and protect them against their critics.

Effective action to stop the spread of this epidemic, and to care for those already infected, is subversive because it disrupts existing power relationships.   Easier to organize another conference than to address the root causes of inequity, discrimination and poverty which underlie the rapid spread of the HIV virus across so many parts of the world.   As UNICEF has said: 'Containing the spread of the disease entails tackling deeply embedded traditions that encourage discrimination against young people (particularly young females), allow harmful cultural practices and preclude discussions of sexuality'[3].   It is impossible to underestimate the importance of addressing the interconnected questions of gender inequality, sexual ignorance and expoitation, and widespread poverty and discrimination.

Let me give an example: too often, the necessary stress on heterosexual transmission of HIV in Asia is used to deny the existence of homosexual men in every country, often at great risk of infection. The unwillingness of governments and health officials—indeed, of some NGOs—to acknowledge this means that these men are denied access to the basic information and recognition which could help save their lives. Equally many governments claim against all evidence that needle use and prostitution are not a reality in their countries. In face of HIV such denial is the most effective way of encouraging its spread.

Success against AIDS demands an honest discussion of sexuality, gender, political and economic power, the global maldistribution of resources, the monopoly of therapeutic drugs by a small number of powerful firms—honesty about all those obstacles which humans have created and thus have the power to change. Conferences such as this must go beyond medicine to explore factors such as the systematic denigration of women in many countries, and the economic structures which deny many people with HIV-related illnesses access to simple and effective therapies.

It is difficult for governments to be honest when this requires them to draw attention to realities unpalatable to powerful interests. Equally CBOs must never lose sight of their role as advocates because of the immediate need for service delivery. Particularly in the rich world too many CBOs have been co-operated by governments in return for resources, and are finding, perhaps too late, that in return they lose the capacity to speak for their community.

On balance Australia is an example of a successful decade of partnership between community, government and health professionals [4]. I recognize that ours has been a comparatively easy path: Australia is a small and rich country, and we have had a succession of federal Health Ministers committed to a partnership approach. This has meant government support for community based initiatives and programs working directly with PWAs, with gay men, with needle users, with sex workers, with people with haemophilia and with Aborigines and Torres Strait islanders. Partnership has meant the provision of needle exchanges, of safe sex information, of support for home based care programs and, most important, a willingness on the part of government to listen to AIDS organizations and to include them in the development of policy.

But there are traps in partnership of which we must be aware. Under pressure to co-operate with government the community sector can come to replicate the institutions of the state, with its 'leaders' being increasingly unelected, unaccountable and unrepresentative—those who buy the logic of government are those who survive the system. Thus despite the partnership our National Council on AIDS has become less representative of the communities most affected by AIDS. Our ability to resist government definitions of what's acceptable is constantly being tested, as the visionaries are replaced by the bureaucrats, the community leaders by the ambitious professionals and the accountants.

Yet the fight against AIDS in Australia has produced extraordinary alliances, friendships and mutual support. There are times when we join hands and tears in memory of those who have died, and I am reminded of the deep partnerships this disease has forged between unexpected allies. There have also been moments when the partnership has failed, and the interests of the most vulnerable and the most marginal are sacrificed to the short term interests of governments or AIDS organizations.

At times communities need stay outside the system—there is no doubt that ACT UP in the US had more impact by doing this.   While ACT UP's tactics may be inappropriate elsewhere, the basic lesson of retaining community independence and integrity is not. Once community organizations lose a process of open decision making and participatory involvement they cease to be able to empower their constituents, and however valuable their services something essential is lost.

Is this concept of community empowerment too western a concept?   Is advocating these principles a benign form of imperialism? (as has been said at previous conferences of some of the interventions from ACT UP).   These are legitimate questions, and I can only say that my own experience, and the testimony of others in this hall, suggests that the basic principles of the Ottawa Charter—which include 'empowering communities and assisting their ownership of their endeavors and destinies'—are valid in very different social, economic and cultural contexts.   Just as the virus cares neither about race or gender, so the need for voluntary and confidential testing, for humane case, for the provision of adequate information, is not limited by the religion or the economic system of any country.

In many countries governments will talk privately to affected communities while ignoring them in public rhetoric.   This is not enough: visible recognition is important as a way of legitimizing community development and challenging social stigma.   Even WHO has too often been timid in recognizing the leadership role taken by such communities as those of sex-workers or gay men.   As the President of the Western Australian AIDS Council said of this year's World AIDS Day theme of 'the family': 'In its press release…WHO identified feelings of trust, mutual support and shared destiny as essential constituents of a family.   It specifically defined family to include street kids, sex workers, injecting drug users, religious associations and even the corner store, but could not bring itself to acknowledge the existence of gay families.'   Too often WHO and other agencies treat gays as does the American soap opera 'Melrose Place'—both marginalizing and trivializing us.

Both justice and pragmatism demand that the voices of those most affected by HIV/ AIDS be heard, and that their expertise and their right to human dignity be acknowledged. While governments persecute sex-workers, drug users, street kids they merely compound their vulnerability to HIV.   Thus the tendency to view sex workers as 'vectors of infection', without any recognition of their very real oppression, is wrong, both morally and practically.   Unless and until we recognize the central role of empowering people who are in the sex industry—in the vast majority of cases because of social and economic pressures— we will fail many of those who are most vulnerable.

The concept of cultural difference is often invoked to claim that programs empowering sex workers or drug users or street kids won't work.   When this is said we need ask: in whose favor does this argument work?   Are there not Asian gays, African users, women forced into sex work in the Middle East and Europe?   The voices of those who claim 'cultural difference' makes frank discussion of sex or of drug use 'unacceptable' are too often the voices of those who would silence the poor and the weak in the interest of retaining their own power.

AIDS demands that we recognize the impact of political and economic systems, and identify governments and cultural institutions which create barriers to both effective prevention and care.   There is a basic human right to dignity, to adequate information, and to appropriate care which transcends cultures and ideologies.   To the extent that we are all vulnerable to the effects of poverty, torture and infection human rights are indivisible.   In the words of Secretary General Butros Butros Ghali: 'We must remember that forces of repression often cloak their wrongdoing in claims of exceptionalism.   But the people themselves time and again make it clear that they seek and need universality.   Human dignity within one's culture requires fundamental standards of universality across the lines of culture, faith and state' [5].

The great revolutions this century in Asia against external colonialism and domestic repression should remind us that the assertion that human rights or political self-determination are somehow 'not Asian' is itself a reverse form of colonial mentality which denies the history of the last century.   AIDS demands both legal/political and socio/economic human rights: the rights to freedom of speech, organization and expression are central, but so too are rights to basic care and survival.   This is not a case for western complacency: the impact of structural adjustment on many developing countries—and the misuse of resources by many governments—means that however many HIV projects are put in place they will merely be band-aids across the wounds created by economic injustice.

Partnership, too, applies to international agencies both government and non-government.   It means the creation of genuine networks and coalitions across borders which has been the mandate of both ICASO and the Global Network over the past few years.   Yet as we in the community sector have struggled to build genuine networks from the bottom up we find that too many agencies would rather pay consultants to discover what is already known than provide infrastructure for existing community groups.   There is a growing industry of well paid advisers making flying visits to 'the field'—while in some agencies you have to fill out three forms to buy a worker a cup of coffee or mail a letter. While ICASO, GNP etc. are fragile and incomplete networks they are the closest to representing those most affected at a global level.   Far better to support them than embark on the creation of yet more international organizations.

Research partnerships too are crucial, as in the extraordinary role which community groups have played in AIDS medical research (already beginning to impact on other diseases) [6].   One of the achievements in my own country was the early development of sophisticated collaborative research between academic and the gay community, in ways which have helped us develop effective educational interventions [7].   These examples suggest that researchers need show more humility in face of the enormous knowledge and experience of community workers [8].   As Jonathan Mann says: 'Each affected community, each community responding to AIDS, is a laboratory of discovery in HIV/AIDS prevention and care.   The capacity for accelerated global learning among communities is central to progress against AIDS, just as international sharing of scientific information from different research centers is fundamental to scientific advance' [9].

We need more economic/social/political analysis, but such analysis poses threats to government control and hence is dangerous.   AIDS is not primarily a matter of individual behavior and responsibility, but rather a disease of poverty, discrimination and ignorance, which requires an analysis based on political economy not more KABP studies.

Partnership means a sense of common purpose and respect for divergent tactics: too often we attack our allies while leaving the real enemies—ignorance, intolerance, false religious piety—to go unscathed.   The spread of HIV is hastened by the distortion of government resources into military spending and grandiose development projects, by denial and ignorance in the name of tradition and religion.   With HIV it is no longer possible to believe that Papal pronouncements against condoms or Hindu and Islamic prohibitions of homosexuality are 'merely' questions of personal values or traditional beliefs; people will live or die depending on how far traditional prejudices and superstitions are allowed to survive.   The rhetoric of taking responsibility for one's actions, so often applied to those with AIDS, must be applied to religion, government and business—religious inflexibility is as guilty of killing people as is the tobacco industry.

If this sounds harsh remember the devastation of this disease—in the cities of Newark and Paris; in the villages of Uganda and India; in the slums of Bangkok and Port au Prince. As Elizabeth Reid wrote:

"One story from the Kagera region in Tanzania is of a young girl sitting day after day at the edge of the yard, rocking on her heels and staring into space.   Both her parents are dead, brothers and sisters, aunts and uncles.   There is little food but she is not hungry.   She rocks, grieving" [10].

I remember today a young man from Goa who was incarcerated because he was HIV positive, and on his release fought discrimination against those with HIV in India until his death.   Dominic de Souza was young and fragile, but he spoke with such moral strength that senior officials exerted great efforts to keep him from the stage at international meetings.   Dominic played a role in the establishment of the Asia/Pacific network of community organizations, and he showed us that a sense of community embraces all those who are prepared to accept the realities of human diversity and fight against the realities of bigotry, injustice and inequality.   From him, and thousands like him, we can draw both the resolve to build real partnerships, and the strength to speak the truth, however politically inconvenient or embarrassing.

References

1   Press Release WHO/46 June 11, 1994.
2   Ungphakorn J, Sittitrai W: NGO and Community Responses to HIV/AIDS in Asia and the Pacific.   AIDS 1994 (Suppl).
3   AIDS: The Second Decade: A Focus on Youth and Women.   UNICEF; April 1993.
4   See Altman D: The Most Political of Diseases In: Tinewell E, et al: AIDS in Australia Sydney 1992 and Chalkley M, Fowler D & Young F.   Innovation, Tolerance and Pragmatism.   Paper presented at Tenth International Conference.
5   Ghali BB: Democracy, Development and Human Rights for All.   Int. Herald Tribune, June 10 1993.
6   See, eg, Epstein St.: The Critique of Pure Science.   In: Science, Technology and Human Values. Forthcoming.
7   See Kippax S., et al: Sustaining Safe Sex: Gay Communities Respond to AIDS, London, Falmer, 1993.
8   This is further explored in Altman D: Power and Community London, Falmer, 1994; ch. 6.
9   Mann J: A Global Epidemic Out of Control?.   AIDS Asia, Dec. 1993; p 5.
10   Reid E: The HIV Epidemic and Development: The Unfolding of the Epidemic.   UNDP; p 10.

The Impact of HIV/AIDS[1]

Stefano M. Bertozzi

Health Economist, Planning & Policy Coordination, WHO, Global Programme on AIDS, Geneva, Switzerland

As researchers, why do we study socio-economic impact? For one, to convince people to give higher priority to AIDS prevention. We have seen time and time again that policy makers are unwilling to commit significant human and financial resources to preventing AIDS until they are confronted with a lot of AIDS. So many places in the world, especially countries in Asia, are poised to experience a rapid rise in new infections that it is our job to advocate for immediate action. If we can use economic tools and arguments to help get this message across, especially to make the point to policy makers who do not usually deal with health problems, all the better.

To whom do we need to address our economic advocacy message?

• The private sector because when we convince them that a limited investment in prevention will avert future costs, then we have seen that they can undertake effective prevention activities with workers and their families.

• The public sector, especially ministries more familiar with economic rather than public health arguments (such as planning, finance, trade, commerce) or ministries that will have to deal with the epidemic's impact (such as social welfare, health, and the military)

• and finally, the international donor community to push AIDS higher on their agenda.

What do we need to study to be able to advocate more effectively? One approach has been to argue that society will bear a high cost if we delay starting large scale prevention efforts. For example, a Thai study argued that the total cost of AIDS by the year 2000 will be over 10 billion dollars [2]. If half of those cases could be prevented by an investment in the hundreds of millions, then we can use the argument that AIDS prevention is an investment with economic return, in addition to humanitarian return. In other words, that it costs more not to prevent AIDS.

Estimating the cost of HIV/AIDS

The most common approach typically estimates the cost of one HIV infection in two parts: the direct medical care costs and the indirect costs of lost production. The total cost per infection can then be multiplied by the expected number of infections to arrive at a projected cost to the national economy.

Many studies have been done estimating these costs both in developing and developed countries [3 – 14].   Typically these have shown high direct costs of care, as high or higher than most other causes of fatal adult illness which is understandable given the relatively long period of chronic disease preceding death; indirect costs have been estimated at many times the direct costs, 10, 15, or even 20 times higher depending upon the study.

But both direct and indirect costs have, as expected, varied with the wealth of the country.   In a low average income country, such as Haiti or Tanzania or Nepal, the average lifetime medical cost per AIDS patient is low, as is the average value of the person's lost earnings both are correspondingly higher in middle income countries such as Brazil, Botswana or Thailand and highest in high income countries such as the USA, Sweden and Japan.

The direct cost for one infection has typically been estimated as between 1 and 2 times the per capita GNP which, translated into US dollars, is hundreds of dollars for low income countries, thousands of dollars per infection for middle income countries and tens of thousands for high income countries with indirect costs correspondingly in the thousands, tens of thousands and hundreds of thousands of dollars per person infected with HIV—two orders of magnitude difference between rich and poor.

The other approach to estimating the cost of HIV infections uses more elaborate macroeconomic models of a national economy and examines the effect on national economic growth of reducing the labor force because of deaths from AIDS.   These models have been applied by Cuddington, Over, Kambou, Way and others to heavily affected countries in sub-Saharan Africa and have suggested that there will be significant, though not dramatic, decreases in economic growth under the assumptions used in the models [15 – 18].

McGraw-Hill has examined the projected effects of deaths due to AIDS using its global macroeconomic model and in doing so, highlighted a point that may be very useful for advocacy [19].   High income countries with a relatively small epidemic, such as Japan, are likely to experience the greatest economic impact not from infections in the Japanese workforce, but rather from a fall in trade because of infections in other countries.   This suggests that it may be in a country like Japan's self-interest to invest in HIV prevention in developing countries which are major trading partners.

However, we must be cautious about linking our advocacy arguments and even more cautious about formulating policy based on these crude estimates of macroeconomic impact.   At the Global Impact of AIDS Conference in London, a gentleman stood up and made a very unpopular observation.   He said that this talk of negative economic impact of AIDS was fine and well, but that he worked in New York City with persons who were injecting drug users and living with HIV and cautioned that if an economic analysis was done of the impact of deaths from AIDS amongst his clients, that it might show economic benefit for New York City.

David Bloom has pointed out that the per capita average income rose in Europe after the black death in the 1300s which killed an estimated 25% of the population of Europe and that it also rose in India following the 1918 – 1919 influenza epidemic [20].

There are many reasons why AIDS is different from those epidemics.   For example, influenza preferentially kills the elderly and chronically ill rather than society's most productive.   But Bloom also pointed out that though we have predicted important effects from AIDS on national economic growth, we have not yet been able to conclusively demonstrate such an impact even in the most heavily affected African countries.   So, caution is appropriate, before we argue too strongly that impact on economic growth is the reason to invest in prevention.

But is this not ridiculous?   Anybody who has visited Rakai in Uganda, Kagera in Tanzania, the Copperbelt in Zambia or even Northern Thailand knows that AIDS is having a devastating impact.   How could anybody suggest otherwise?   There is no attempt to deny the devastation weaked by AIDS, but rather to suggest that change in the national economic growth rate may not be the best way to measure it.

If we have learned anything from the last two decades, it is that national wealth may increase at the same time that the number of poor increases; if some people get richer while others get poorer.   Perhaps because we don't like to think about it, we have almost no information about how the epidemic may be improving the welfare of some non-affected households.   Consider, for example, that a job lost because someone falls ill is a job opportunity in the eyes of someone who is unemployed.

Breakdown of Vulnerable Structures

Many studies have observed that if AIDS affects a moderately well-off household, it may join the ranks of the poor, a poor one may be pushed to the frontier of survival.   There is strong evidence that the epidemic is both exacerbating existing poverty and creating new poor [21,22].   Thus it may be that if we want to best capture the impact at the national level, we need to study the epidemic's impact on the magnitude and severity of poverty, rather than on national economic growth.

Consider another possibility.   Suppose that the most important economic impact of AIDS is not a result of its incremental effect in reducing the labor supply, but rather the result of concentrated impact on vulnerable structures causing them to break down.

If someone took a blowtorch and heated the railroad track as the train rolled from Tokyo to Yokohama, the heat would be absorbed and dissipated and nobody would notice. But if the same time was spent heating one place, the rail could be cut and the train derailed—what an economist might call a discontinuity.   The train doesn't gradually slow down.   Instead, it runs along just fine until all of a sudden it ends up in the Bay.

Similarly, a family, community or even nation may be able to adopt a number of coping mechanisms that help to absorb and thus conceal the impact of the epidemic until that household or community is no longer able to cope and breaks down.   The vulnerability of a structure to breakdown obviously depends upon how strong it was before.

A vulnerable household [23], as Barnett and Blaikie and others have described, may be poor, have few working-age adults, minimal extended family or community support and have a rigid division of labor and skills by sex.   A vulnerable community may be poor, marginally food secure, and dependent on crops with high peak seasonal labor demand.   A vulnerable country may be poor, land scarce and politically unstable.

Vulnerability is not only a function of how weak the structure is, but also a function of how much the impact is concentrated.   We are all familiar with extreme differences in HIV prevalence between countries, between communities within a country, and most strikingly, from household to household — where this particular virus, because it spreads between couples and from mother to child, often affects multiple members of the same household.

We have seen AIDS breakdown households around the world, from the Bronx to Santo Domingo, from Milan to Ouagadougou and Chiang Mai. We have watched it wreck communities in places like northwest Tanzania and southern Uganda.

When David Bloom remarked in August 1993 that in no country could he yet find clear evidence of a macroeconomic impact from AIDS. One possible exception came to mind, Rwanda. It was poor, land scarce and beset by decades of ethnic tension. To that AIDS added worsening poverty and thus increasing social inequity. But perhaps more importantly, Rwanda faced an HIV prevalence in the general population that was among the highest in the world; among the military personnel it was almost certainly higher still.

Nobody knows the ingredients of the glue that holds the thin veneer of peace on society. But our concern about our long-term future and that of our children must be one important element. HIV robbed many, many of the young men in the military of their dreams for a long term future. While we will never understand the relative importance of all of the factors, surely HIV contributed in an important way to the breakdown of a country.

Resource Allocation

If we succeed in convincing policy makers with our advocacy message, and obtain the needed funds for HIV/AIDS prevention, then how useful are these economic cost estimates for helping local, national and international policy makers allocate funds for prevention?

If the impact of an HIV infection and therefore the benefit of preventing one is measured in direct and indirect cost as described above, then the economic benefit of preventing an infection in, for example, Uganda would be in the thousands, in Thailand in the tens of thousands and in the USA in the hundreds of thousands of dollars. All else being equal, that suggests that the greatest benefit from preventing one infection would be in the USA.

Consider a completely different approach for example, using a hypothetical HIV hunger index to measure impact. On average, for every case of HIV infection, how many people who would have been able to meet their nutritional needs are now hungry? And how many that would have been hungry are now acutely malnourished?

Using such a hunger index, all else being equal, the greatest benefit from preventing one HIV infection would probably be in Uganda. This suggests that there are clear value implications in the choice of methodology that is used to measure impact. And it suggests that when we measure the impact of AIDS, we have an obligation to develop and use methods that capture not only changes in production, but also changes in broader measures of welfare.

Impact Alleviation

Suppose that instead of studying socioeconomic impact for advocacy, that we have been asked a completely different kind of question by a ministry of social welfare: Should it focus on improving access to primary education? On developing support groups for caregivers? On protecting property rights of widows and orphaned children? Or on helping infected military personnel learn how to live positively with HIV? Estimates of average direct cost and indirect cost won't be of much help.

The primary impact of AIDS is to increase poverty [24]. That statement may be true, but it doesn't help the ministry figure out who is becoming poor or help them figure out how to modify their poverty alleviation program.

For example, Shaeffer has argued that AIDS has an important impact on the education sector, in part because the demand for education will decrease as children from affected households are less able to go to school [25]. While this is certainly true, we know very little about the magnitude of this problem relative to other problems — even in the most heavily affected areas.

Why is that? Partly because we know so little about the socio-economic characteristics of the households affected by HIV. If a relatively well-off household in a developing country is affected, the effect on education may be minimal because the household can protect its investment in education at the expense of other consumption. In a poor affected household, there may also be no effect on education because there was no money for school fees even before AIDS.

The team doing a major household survey in the Kagera region of Tanzania reported preliminary data on the correlation between parental death and school enrolment rates of children. The striking finding was that parental death seemed to be a relatively minor determinant of whether a child was in school. For example in the seven to ten year old age group it was difficult to show an effect of adult death, but less than 40% of all the children in that age group were in school regardless of orphan status [26].

A study from Zaire in a population with a much lower seroprevalence was unable to demonstrate significant differences in morbidity, mortality, or socioeconomic status between children whose mothers had died of AIDS, those whose mothers were living with HIV and those whose mothers were not infected [27].

Neither of these studies suggest that a parental death is not a catastrophe for a child—that is incontestable—but they do suggest that there is likely to be a large variation in socioeconomic status across the children in a community and that the average difference between children who have and children who have not lost a parent to AIDS may be much smaller. Thus, we cannot assume that orphan status is the best way of identifying the children in a community most in need of material support.

However, a caveat is also appropriate, if the hypothesis about the importance of collapse of social structures, in this case the household, is correct, then these studies may have missed some of the most affected children because they dropped out of the sample.

Research Priorities

Hypotheses repeated often enough in the literature and at conferences have a way of appearing to become facts. We now need to collect data to find out which of the hypothesized impacts are the most important, especially in countries where the epidemic is shifting from a rapid growth phase to a major endemic problem. Only in that way can we base alleviation policies on more solid ground than the conjectures of armchair economists.

Fortunately such efforts have begun. Major quantitative studies designed to understand the impact on households have been completed by teams in Tanzania and the Cote d'Ivoire and should be analyzed within the year [28,29]. Smaller qualitative studies on household coping mechanisms supported by the World Health Organization (WHO) are underway in five countries.   The Food and Agriculture Organization (FAO) supported an important series of studies of the effect of AIDS on smallholder agriculture in Uganda, Tanzania and Zambia which demonstrated the usefulness of using available data to map the relative vulnerability of different farming systems to labor loss—in essence creating an early warning system.

A study being finalized in India has surveyed households in an attempt to map the most important determinants of vulnerability to the impact of an adult death [30].   A large scale population-based household survey is planned for next year in Thailand that expects to collect data on HIV prevalence as well as socio-economic data.

However, in countries poised to experience rapid growth in HIV prevalence, like many of those in Asia, that do not yet have major epidemics, let us not concentrate our economic research on predicting the scale of economic impact.   The numbers will be disappointingly low for advocacy and premature for impact alleviation.   Rather, let us concentrate on understanding how economic factors fuel the spread of HIV and on learning to spend our prevention dollars more wisely.   The results of those studies will not only help to slow the epidemic, but will also prove to be more effective tools for advocacy.

Regardless of the stage of the epidemic in a country, there is one step that needs to be taken whether to improve our understanding of how economic factors fuel the epidemic or how they determine its impact.   More socio-economic data need to be collected with the data on HIV prevalence.   This far into this epidemic we are still guided far too much by conventional wisdom about the socioeconomic distribution of infection.

Impact on the Individual

Why is it that whenever we talk about impact of AIDS, we jump right to survivors, households, or communities, just as this paper has done?   The focus seems very different than for other serious or fatal diseases of young people, like sickle cell anaemia, or Huntington's chorea.   For those diseases the primary concern seems to be impact on the affected individual, not his or her household.

It is worrisome to think that it has happened because the primary use of 'impact' has been as an advocacy tool and consciously or sub-consciously people have decided that policy makers are more likely to pay attention to the impact on 'innocent' survivors than the impact on the 'guilty' persons infected with HIV.

If that is true, then it forces us to ask ourselves about how much our own thinking about the problem has been influenced by our approach to advocacy.   Now that increasingly we are doing advocacy for alleviation of impact, our biased reporting of impact will result in inattention to the needs of the people affected most, those who are infected.

As economists, we have largely ignored this area.   Yet we have been ringing alarm bells for years about the increasing expenditures for medical care that can be expected with the epidemic.   Medical care is part of what we can do to alleviate the impact on people living with HIV/AIDS, but only part.   If we do not understand what the most important aspects of the impact are from the perspective of the infected person, how, as economists can we pretend to be optimizing the expenditure of resources to minimize the impact?

Permit me a personal perspective.   I am much more afraid of dying than I am of being dead.   Thus it makes a big difference to me what I die from and what the circumstances of my death are.   I want the illness that leads to my death to be short.   I am not especially worried about the number of days from work I will miss (indeed this may be the only benefit), but I am very concerned about pain, nausea, chronic diarrhoea, shortness of breath, and incontinence.   I'd want to avoid them all, and if I lived in circumstances where it was a twenty-minute walk to clean water, or where I couldn't cook unless I went out and collected firewood, I would be even more concerned about avoiding those problems.

If I tell people that I'm dying, I want them to worry about how I'm doing, not about who I've been sleeping with.   I want them to help me, not avoid me, appreciate me, not fire me. To avoid all of these problems, I would be willing to pay an awful lot of money.   I haven't mentioned postponing death—I assume that we would all be willing to do that.   I'm talking about willingness to pay to avoid all the disease-related problems mentioned above.

How is this personal perspective related to economics?   Economics is the science of making choices; of making choices that maximize benefit.   Sometimes the most difficult part is figuring out how to define benefit.   Most economists are defining benefit of an intervention to a person living with HIV/AIDS in terms of years of life gained and months of disability averted.   And those measures don't begin to capture all of the things I would be willing to pay to avoid.

This poses a serious problem for economic analysis.   If interventions are evaluated only on the basis of disability reduced and death postponed, then many developing countries with severely constrained resources could conclude that they are relatively impotent at alleviating the impact on a person living with HIV/AIDS because reducing this impact requires expensive drugs and diagnostics.   This would be an unfortunate conclusion, because interventions to reduce many of the types of impact mentioned above are within the means of all communities.

Pain control is not expensive.   Discrimination, stigmatization, and isolation cost money to maintain.   Support groups for people living with HIV/AIDS and for their caregivers are not expensive.   Helping people with the activities of daily living can be done inexpensively because the cost of interventions like these is largely determined by the cost of labor and that is correspondingly lower in low income countries.

If we use a resource allocation model that values the benefit of treating *Cryptococcal meningitis* but not that of pain relief or a clean bed then we will end up purchasing amphotericin at the expense of morphine and sheets.   And if that does not reflect the priorities of the people living with HIV/AIDS in that community then we have not been helpful.

AIDS has once again forced us, physicians and economists alike, to recognize our weaknesses.   It has taught physicians that they cannot assume that they know what is best for their patients and it has taught economists that they cannot assume that they know what patients want.   We won't know until we ask.

Conclusions

• Abrupt changes or discontinuities in social structures as a result of the impact of HIV may be more important determinants of the magnitude of the impact than the incremental changes we are accustomed to measuring.   At the individual level this is certainly true, disease is often abrupt and death is the ultimate discontinuity.   The larger the structure, as one goes from household to community to economic sector to nation state, the greater the capacity to distribute and thus absorb the impact. We must develop a better understanding of what makes structures at all levels vulnerable to collapse — so that we can intervene before breakdown occurs and catastrophe ensues.

• AIDS will push affected households down the poverty scale, pushing some into poverty and aggravating the poverty of others.   Thus we must address household impact in the context of poverty alleviation more generally in that community, targeting the neediest, not necessarily those who joined the ranks of the poor most recently.

At the same time, we can recongnize that the particular characteristics of this epidemic offer opportunities for designing and targeting interventions to households in new ways. For example, households often have years of warning before children become orphans.   If coping mechanisms can be strengthened during that time, the household is more likely to be preserved.   Similarly, because we have the opportunity to identify those at risk of becoming poor, we may be able to develop poverty prevention interventions such as facilitating access to credit.

• To design comprehensive care approaches for infected individuals that are appropriate for different settings with different cultural and resource constraints we must learn more about how people living with HIV/AIDS in those settings perceive the impact so that we can prioritize interventions by using yardsticks that measure what they perceive to be their most important needs.

References

1 Adapted from a plenary presentation made at the Tenth International Conference on AIDS, Yokohama, Japan, August 1994.
2 Bloom DE, Lyons JV, eds: Economic implications of AIDS in Asia, United Nations Development Programme, Regional Bureau for Asia and the Pacific, HIV/AIDS Regional Project, New Delhi, India.
3 Hassig SE, Perriens J, Baende E, Kahotwa M, Bishagara K, Kinkela N, Kapita B: An analysis of the economic impact of HIV infection among patients at Mama Yemo Hospital, Kinshasa, Zaire. AIDS 1990; 4(9): 883 – 7.
4 Hellinger FJ: The lifetime cost of treating a person with HIV. JAMA 1993; 270(4): 474 – 8.
5 Postma MJ, Leidl R, Downs AM, Rovira J, Tolley K, Gyldmark M, Jager JC: Economic impact of the AIDS epidemic in the European Community; towards multinational scenarios on hospital care and costs. AIDS 1993; 7(4): 541 – 53.
6 Tan ML: Socio-economic impact of HIV/AIDS in the Philippines. AIDS-Care 1993; 5(3): 283 – 8.
7 Cordeiro H: Medical costs of HIV and AIDS in Brazil. In: Fleming AF, Carballo M, FitzSimons DW, Bailey MR, Mann J, (eds): The global impact of AIDS. Proceedings of the First International Conference on the Global Impact of AIDS. New York, Alan R. Liss, 1988, pp 119 – 22.
8 Scitovsky AA, Over M: AIDS: costs of care in the developed and the developing world. AIDS 1988; 2 (Suppl 1): S71 – S81.
9 Over M, Bertozzi S, Chin J, N'Galy B, Nyamuryekunge K: The direct and indirect cost of HIV infection in developing countries: the cases of Zaire and Tanzania. In: The global impact of AIDS. AIDS 1988; 2 (Suppl 1); 123 – 35.
10 Shepard DS, Bail RN: Costs of care for persons with AIDS in Rwanda. Development Discussion Paper No. 411, Harvard Instute for International Development, Cambridge, Massachusetts, 1991.
11 World Bank, Tanzania: AIDS assessment and planning study. A World Bank Country Study. Washington, DC, 1992.
12 Bloom D: The social and economic implication of AIDS in China. Beijing Institute of Information and Control, June 1993. [manuscript]
13 Hanvelt RA, Ruedy NS, Hogg RS, et al: Indirect costs of HIV/AIDS mortality in Canada. AIDS 1994, 8: F7 – F11.

14   Hanson K: AIDS. What does economics have to offer? Health Policy and Planning: 7(4): 315 – 328, 1992.
15   Cuddington JT: Modeling the macroeconomic effects of AIDS, with an application to Tanzania. World-Bank-Economic-Review, May 1993; 7(2): 173 – 89.
16   Way PO, Over M: The projected economic impact of an African AIDS epidemic 1992 [Manuscript].
17   Cuddington JT: Further results on the macroeconomic effects of AIDS. The dualistic, labor-surplus economy. World-Bank-Economic-Review, September 1993, 7(3): 403 – 17.
18   Kambou G, Devarajan S, Over M: Les effects economiques de l'épidemic du SIDA en Afrique subsaharienne: Une analyse d'équilibre général (with English summary). Revue-d'Economie-du-Developpement; 1993; 0(1): 37 – 62.
19   DRI/McGraw-Hill: Measuring the global economic impact of the AIDS epidemic. Nariman Behravesh, Jan 1993.
20   Bloom D: Presentation, Manila, 1994.
21   Panos Dossier, The Panos Institute: The hidden cost of AIDS-The challenge of HIV to development. Panos Publications, London, 1992.
22   Barnett T, Blaikie P: AIDS in Africa: Its present and future impact. London, Belhaven Press, 1992.
23   Ibid.
24   Barnett T: The effects of HIV/AIDS on farming systems and rural livelihoods in Uganda, Tanzania and Zambia. A summary analysis of case studies from research carried out in the period July-September 1993. Overseas Development Group, University of East Anglia, Norwich, UK., Food and Agriculture Organization (FAO) Final Report, February 1994.
25   Shaeffer S: Background Paper for Experts' Seminar on the Impact of HIV/AIDS on Education, International Institute for Educational Planning, 8 – 10 December 1993.
26   Ainsworth M, Over M: The economic impact of AIDS: shocks, responses and outcomes. The World Bank, Africa Technical Department, Population, Health and Nutrition Division, Technical Working Paper No. 1, June 1992.
27   Ryder RW, Kamenga M, Nkusu M, Batter V, Heyward WL: AIDS orphans in Kinshasa, Zaire: incidence and socioeconomic consequences. AIDS 1994; 8(5): 673 – 9.
28   Ainsworth, Martha et al: Measuring the impact of fatal adult illness in Sub-Saharan Africa: An annotated household questionaire. Living Standards Measurement Study Working Paper, No. 90. Washington, DC, World Bank, 1992.
29   Report of a workshop on the economic impact of fatal adult illness in Sub-Saharan Africa. September, 1992. The World Bank and the University of Dar es Salaam.
30   Basu AM, Gupta DB, Krishna G: The household impact of adult morbidity and mortality. Institute of Economic Growth, University Enclave, New Delhi, 20 July 1994.

Tenth Anniversary Special Sessions

AIDS Research Towards the Future

Robert C. Gallo

Laboratory of Tumor Cell Biology, National Cancer Institute, NIH, Bethesda, MD, USA

AIDS research is at a juncture point. The current pessimism of patients and frustration of scientists is due in part to the enormous progress of the early period (roughly 1983 – 1985). Initial success led to expectations for a quick and final solution for the end of the problem by development of preventive vaccines and successful anti-HIV forms of treatment for people already infected. The plateau of progress has fostered discussion on what should be done.

Here I have selected several questions and areas of research which I think merit special targeted programs. Though most of them involve studies from my laboratory, I am aware that there are many results from others which I will not be able to include and which are equally or more important. The topics I will briefly cover are: (1) select questions on HIV-induced immune pathogenesis and some concepts on therapy and vaccines from them; (2) recent advances in our understanding of Kaposi's sarcoma (KS); and (3) some new therapeutic approaches against HIV and against KS.

Some Critical Issues on HIV-induced Immune Impairment

We have known for a decade that only a small percentage of T-cells are infected at any one time. Consequently, many studies have been carried out to explain the steady decline of the CD4$^+$ T-cells by invoking the idea that some indirect mechanism(s) of HIV (as well as direct cell killing) must be involved. We know that direct infection of these cells can result in their death and studies of infected infants and of SIV-infected monkeys indicate that the thymus tissue is harmed by HIV. Consequently, the capacity for regeneration of the T-cell population must be impaired and contribute to the decline in immune function. We also know that the lymph nodes degenerate and that this is correlated with the amount of virus. Many of the so-called indirect effects of HIV are thought to be due to HIV proteins, e.g., the gp120 envelope binding to the CD4 cell surface protein of uninfected cells and causing premature death of such cells when they are triggered to proliferate by some antigen (as may occur from other infections). We have also known since 1985 that these uninfected T-cells of an HIV-infected person do not proliferate normally even when removed from an internal environment of gp120 or other HIV proteins. Some have argued that this is a long-term effect of some cytokines circulating in high amounts in the

263

patient and producing lasting effects, even evident after culturing these cells in the laboratory. Remarkably, in vitro 'correction' of this incapacity for appropriate proliferation has been reported now by several groups but each by different means, e.g., by treating the cells in vitro with antibody to alpha interferon (α-IFN) (Zagury et al., 1985), or interleukin 12 itself (Shearer and colleagues, 1994), or gamma IFN (γ-IFN) itself (Turano et al., 1994). There is also the controversial issue of HIV infection of stem cells (see for instance the studies of Chermann and colleagues). If stem cells are confirmed to be an early significant target of HIV (or some strains of HIV), it would have major bearing on our thinking about HIV immune pathogenesis. If confirmed, what is needed of these cytokine and stem cell results is an explanation of the mechanisms involved. More broadly, we also urgently need many more attempts to determine which of the many laboratory in vitro results are relevant in vivo.

Other questions, self-evident in their importance to HIV immunopathogenesis, concern the apparent resistance of some people to infection (e.g., F. Plummer's results from studies of Kenyan prostitutes), and the ability of some to survive much longer and with less pathology once infected. In other words, we need very intensive studies of the long-term non-progressors now described by many groups. Is it the genetics of the person? Or is it genetics of HIV—some strains being less virulent? Or do other environmental factors account for these differences? It now seems safe to say that all three contribute. Exposure to the same HIV-1 strain produced very different outcomes in some groups and some reports (e.g., Dean Mann and colleagues) have correlated this with genetic patterns (HLA). This area of research is another example for targeted intense research as well as very basic immunochemistry. Yet, other results argue just as strongly that the particular HIV strain is important (consider the difference in pathogenicity of HIV-2 and HIV-1 and the recent Australian report showing that several individuals infected with the same HIV-1 strain are all doing well). Despite an enormous wealth of information on the genes of HIV, the molecular basis for these differences in virulence remain disappointingly unclear. As for environmental factors (co-factors)—there are both conceptual and laboratory results as well as epidemiological results which support the notion that many kinds of chronic infections with other microbes or any chronic general stimulation of the immune system might favor progression to disease, at least in part by activating more HIV expression. I have also suggested that one particular herpesvirus, human herpesvirus type 6 (HHV-6), is one of the more likely candidates for enhancing HIV-induced progression to AIDS based on several different in vitro results. However, this suggestion remains speculative.

One other aspect of HIV-induced immune impairment which I have selected for emphasis is the longstanding, still ongoing, and often confusing discussions of whether humoral (antibody) or cell mediated immunity is the more important in preventing HIV infection and in controlling HIV after infection has occurred. Which is the more important? What should we try to induce for these purposes? These questions are much more than of academic interest because increasing one arm of the immune system may involve approaches (including therapies with some cytokines and inhibition of other cytokines) which inhibit the other. Some vaccine studies with diverse animal retroviruses and some, but not by means all, vaccine studies in animals with HIV (chimps) and with HIV-2 and SIV (monkeys) have correlated protection with prior induction of neutralizing antibodies, and most recently some evidence (e.g., M. Murphy-Corb) has correlated protection with specific types of neutralizing antibodies, namely those which are conformational, i.e., not targeting one linear region of the HIV envelope but directed to a three-dimensional configuration of the envelope involving multiple different non-linear regions.   On the other hand, some SIV and HIV-2 monkey vaccine studies of protection and others showing control of spread of the virus to local regions, e.g., to the inguinal lymph nodes after infection with low dose SIV (studies of David Pauza) argue strongly for cellular immunity and, in particular, for CD8$^+$ cytotoxic T-lymphocytes (CTL).   Similarly, Shearer et al. and others have provided evidence tht exposed people who have controlled, prevented and, in some instances, perhaps even eliminated a low dose HIV-1 infection have developed cellular immunity and not neutralizing antibodies.   Still other results (from my laboratory by G. Franchini and M. Robert-Guroff in collaboration with E. Paoletti and J. Tartaglia of Virogenetics in Troy, New York and Pasteur Merieux) have shown protection against HIV-2 in monkeys without correlation with any measured immune function, i.e., neither CTLs nor neutralizing antibody.   One explanation is that CTLs are involved, but detectably present in tissues (lymph nodes) not in the blood cirulation.   Another, and not mutually exclusive possibility, is that protection is due to an immune response not usually measured in vaccine studies, e.g., the CD8 T-cell soluble factor of J. Levy, which inhibits replication of various strains of HIV by unknown mechanisms.   If there is any area of HIV research which screams for more intense and targeted research this is it.   For instance, are there CTLs in the lymph nodes of protected monkeys?   When CTLs do correlate with protection what segment(s) of HIV protein(s) do they target?   Can we grow such cells in vitro and after re-infusion of the expanded population back into an individual early after HIV infection—will this help control disease?   And what about using Levy's factor? Several years after its discovery we still do not know what it is.   It is of obvious interest to identify, mass produce, and use this factor in early treatment trials.

We badly need much more information on the immune response of uninfected people to candidate vaccines.   However, such trials were recently stopped because the candidate vaccines employed purified HIV-1 envelope proteins alone, and there are few results that indicate that this approach will work.   As noted above, our recent results with Virogenetics and Pasteur Merieux show that protection against infection of monkeys with different strains of HIV-2 can be achieved using modified vaccinia virus as vectors carrying the gene for the virus envelope.   Even the HIV-1 envelope protein carried by the modified vaccinia protected some animals against HIV-2.   Due to its limited ability to replicate, it is no doubt easier to protect against HIV-2 infection of monkeys (and presumably also in humans) than it is to protect against HIV-1.   However, since HIV-2 can cause AIDS (even if less efficient than HIV-1), since it is endemic in West Africa, since protection in monkeys occurred with an HIV-1 vaccinia based vaccine, and since HIV-1 is now epidemic in West Africa I think it is reasonable to argue for vaccine trials in West Africa now for two reasons: (1) in the hope of reproducing the experimental primate results and achieving protection against HIV-2; and (2) the possibility that in using HIV-1 reagents there may also be protection against HIV-1.   At a minimum—important new information would be obtained.

KS Pathogenesis

KS remains the most important tumor associated with HIV-1 infection both in terms of frequency and in the suffering it produces.   Its greater incidence in males, and especially homosexual men, suggest to many that another microbe, working in concert with HIV-1, must be involved.   However, no such microbe has been found and our results on studies of KS pathogenesis suggest to us none may be needed to explain this phenomenon.   In 1986 we began to develop systems for the experimental (laboratory) study of KS.   Several concepts and a few conclusions have come from experiments with those new laboratory systems.   Early KS is a complex tumor, consisting of many cell types and resembling an inflammatory response.   The tumor cell was believed by pathologists to be a spindle-shaped cell.   We have been able to culture these cells obtained from KS lesions.   We also find these spindle cells in the peripheral blood of KS patients and also in a substantial number of HIV-1-infected homosexual men prior to the appearance of overt KS.   It is possible that these circulating cells are responsible for the multiple and often widely separated lesions.   We showed that these cells have properties of normal vascular endothelial cells—but ones in a state of chronic activation.   We think inflammatory cytokines like γ-IFN and tumor necrosis factor induce their activation.   These cytokines are increased in HIV-infected people, perhaps due to the suppression of glutathione levels which occurs after HIV infection and the resultant stimulation of gene controlling elements for inflammatory cytokines.   We do not believe KS results from immune deficiency.   Paradoxically, our results suggest that the origins of KS arise more from chronic immune activation in a setting of an impaired immune system.   Activated endothelial cells have a propensity for growth, migration, and for the production and release of other cytokines.   Among the cytokines prominently produced by the early stage KS spindle cell is basic fibroblast growth factor (bFGF).   For many reasons, among them being the ability of bFGF to promote new blood vessel formation, we think bFGF is critical to the development of the early KS lesions.   Indeed, we can show that most of the growth of these cells is due to bFGF effects.   Inhibitors of bFGF (like with antisense to bFGF or with molecules that complex bFGF) inhibit the growth of KS spindle cells in vitro.   As I have noted in the past, these cells will produce transient KS-like tumors in immune deficient mice.   But these tumors are of mouse origin.   The human KS spindle cells produce cytokines, like bFGF, which produce the mouse lesion.   Indeed, we recently found that bFGF alone will mimic this effect.   Futher, we have shown that the HIV protein, Tat, is released by acutely infected T-cells, can enter these spindle cells, and synergizes with bFGF in promoting cell growth in vitro and the KS-like lesion formation in mice when acting on activated endothelial cells which have receptors for Tat.   Other new results show that Tat mimics the effect of extracellular matrix molecules such as fibronectin.   These molecules, which hold cells in a local environment, when 'cut' by specific proteases (released with signals that indicate an inflammatory response should occur) can cause cell migration and adhesion as well as inducing growth.   Tat has the same properties and shares an important region of homology with these extracellular matrix proteins.

    To summarize, we believe most of the cells of a KS lesion are hyperplastic—not malignant cells, and that their origin lies in the chronic overproduction of inflammatory cytokines.   These cytokines activate endothelial cells, inducing them in turn to produce large amounts of other cytokines, in particular bFGF.   The activated spindle cells also develop receptors for extracellular matrix molecules, but these receptors are also recognized and used by the HIV protein, Tat, and Tat synergizes with bFGF in promoting new blood vessel formation and continued proliferation of these cells.   Control of the growth of the hyperplastics cells then seems to lie in inhibition of the effects of bFGF and Tat and/or in reversing the overproduction of inflammatory cytokines like γ-IFN.

Until very recently we had no evidence that HIV-associated KS contained any neoplastic cells, i.e., we did not know if the hyperplastic cells ever transformed into malignant cells.   One recent result from Levinton-Kriss in Israel indicated that classical KS cells can sometimes become neoplastic because she and her co-workers have obtained an immortalized cell line from one such patient.   Below I will describe our development of the first such cell line (KS Y-1) from HIV-1-associated KS.   The characteristics of KS Y-1, like the hyperplastic cells from KS lesions described above, resemble activated vascular endothelial cells, but differ from the hyperplastic cells in that KS Y-1 cells induce metastatic malignant sarcoma in immunodeficient mice, contains abnormal chromosomes (both in number and type), and grow continuously in the absence of any growth factor.   In short, they are malignant cells.   These results were obtained with the first passage of KS Y-1 cells in culture.   Therefore, they did not develop while in culture in the laboratory but were present in the primary KS tumor.   Therefore, we can now safely conclude that KS can evolve into a true malignancy.   It is possible that KS even begins with such malignant cells, but that these cells are masked by an abundance of the hyperplastic spindle cells responding for unknown reasons to the neoplastic clone.   These hyperplastic cells in turn promote angiogenesis.

KS Y-1 cells do not produce bFGF and are not responsive to it or other cytokines or to Tat.   The fact that these cells are not influenced by factors that promote growth of the hyperplastic vascular endothelial cells is not surprising since KS Y-1 cells are autonomous and may be growing at maximum capacity.   Inhibiting bFGF, Tat, or blocking inflammatory cytokines will have little effect on these cells.   However, we have found that these malignant cells are totally controlled by a hormone of pregnancy.   (1) Sera of pregnant humans and mice block growth of these cells in vitro and tumor formation in mice.   (2) We have identified the active factor as the beta chain of human chorionic gonadotropin (βhCG).   (3) The mechanism involves binding of hCG to a cell surface receptor which is followed by apoptotic death of the tumor cells.   (4) These findings should not be limited to this single case because assays of biopsy clinical specimens from tumor lesions of other KS patients show evidence for cell surface receptors for βhCG.   To our knowledge this is the first evidence of a potent anti-tumor effect of hCG.   Since hCG is not toxic at concentrations over the range used here or even much higher, these results point to a treatment of KS.   Of course, appropriate clinical trials are required to demonstrate safety and effectiveness.   Since βhCG shares strong homology with the β chains of luteinizing hormone (LH) and less but significant homology with follicle stimulating hormone, and since these hormones rise to levels during a phase of the menstrual cycle of females, which are far above levels in males, these results may also provide clues for the greater frequency of KS in males.

Blocking HIV Replication (The Quest for Inhibitors from Which HIV Will Not Escape)

Some health officials have emphasized that a preventive vaccine is the priority for AIDS research, and since there has never really been success in treatment of a serious viral disease, i.e., not after infection has taken place, we have another good reason to emphasize vaccine development. The counter response to these arguments, of course, is: first, we cannot ignore the millions of infected people; and second, we never really made a devoted effort to develop antiviral therapy against a serious viral disease, and certainly not with all the information avilable that we have on the molecular biology of HIV and on its replication cycle. It is, however, necessary to ask whether blocking HIV will be sufficient to halt progression to AIDS. It is not possible to give a definitive answer to that question. It is possible that the continued presence of integrated HIV DNA proviruses, even if not expressing virus, will impair immune function. However, the vast majority of clinical and laboratory studies indicate that AIDS progression correlates with HIV replication. Also, blocking HIV infection should reduce the indirect pathological effects of HIV such as from its proteins or their induction of unwanted cytokines. Therefore, it is reasonable to argue that one sine qua non of all therapy should include attempts to block HIV replication and do it as early as possible.

The biggest obstacles to effective therapies are toxicity and virus mutations with resultant resistance to therapy. Most testing for new anti-HIV therapy today is based on targeting the enzymes of HIV (reverse transcriptase, protease, integrase, and ribonuclease H). These programs now seem to be well established in the pharmaceutical industry and ultimately I expect that the proper combination of some of them will make for significant therapeutic advances.

Inhibiting HIV Replication

Strategies for controlling HIV replication are a top priority in AIDS research. The most common approaches available for the immediate future will be a combination of inhibitors of HIV enzymes, such as protease inhibitors coupled with reverse transcriptase inhibitors. These are being chiefly pursued by the pharmaceutical companies.

Our efforts are aimed at inhibiting HIV for prolonged periods, i.e., trying to overcome HIV mutations which escape drug effects. We are studying four approaches to this end.

Blocking HIV Entry into Cells

Blocking HIV entry into cells by using another virus which binds to the same cell surface receptor (CD4) as HIV. We have recently reported that HHV-7 utilizes CD4 as its receptor for infection of $CD4^+$ T-cells. Consequently, it competes with HIV for this receptor and in so doing inhibits infection of every strain of HIV we have tested.

Infection of primary T-cells, primary macrophages, and T-cell lines is blocked with HHV-7. The current main objective is to identify, purify, and test the effects of the HHV-7 envelope protein responsible for this effect, and then to study the toxicity and efficacy of this protein in the SIV macaque animal model by delivering active peptide components in liposomes.

Targeting Cellular Factors

Because viruses require cellular factors for their replication and since cellular factors are not hypermutable like HIV, it seems reasonable to add such cellular factors to our list of drug targets. The chief target of HIV infection is the 'resting' $CD4^+$ T-cell. But HIV is blocked after entry of these cells due at least in part to the insufficient amounts of deoxynucleotides in those cells.   As a result viral DNA synthesis is incomplete.   The pools of these nucleotides are increased when T-cells are activated, and this leads to successful completion of HIV replication.   The increase in deoxynucleotides is dependent on the induction of an enzyme, ribonucleotide reductase.   If this enzyme is inhibited HIV DNA synthesis remains impaired and virus replication is inhibited.   Hydroxyurea is a well studied, simple, inexpensive, and orally administered drug which inhibits this enzyme. Our results show that hydroxyurea inhibits HIV in vitro.   Last year I suggested that hydroxyurea might synergize with AZT, ddI or other nucleoside analogues.   By reducing the pools of deoxynucleotides more nucleoside analogues should be incorporated into the viral DNA being synthesized.   This hypothesis was verified.

Hydroxyurea is inexpensive, can be given orally, and crosses the blood-brain barrier. Although it has been safely used in clinical medicine for some chronic leukemias for over 30 years, we must remain vigilant for unexpected toxicity.   We suggest that after appropriate pre-clinical evaluation, clinical trials with combinations of hydroxyurea and nucleoside analogues be initiated.

Antisense

In collaborative studies with S. Agrawal of the Hybridon Co., P. Zamecnik of the Worcester Foundation for Experimental Biology, and G. Zon of Lynx Co., we have shown that short stretches (20 – 30) of oligodeoxynucleotides complementary to some conserved segments of HIV-1 can inhibit replication of the virus.   The potential of antisense therapy, of course, is not limited to AIDS.   Targeting messenger RNA molecules of specific genes is one goal of some other viral diseases, some cancers, and genetic diseases.   The advantage of this approach in AIDS is that regions of the HIV-1 genome which do not change (because they are vital to the virus for replication and do not tolerate significant change) can be targeted.   For example, specific long-term inhibition of a number of HIV-1 strains was achieved in vitro with antisense to a region of the HIV-1 genome called the Rev response element (RRE) needed for the interaction of a key HIV protein, Rev.   The antisense to RRE complexes with RRE and blocks the binding of the Rev protein.   Similarly, the Hybridon Co. antisense, known as GEM 91, complexes to a region of HIV-1 needed to make structural proteins of the virus core will also inhibit replication of various HIV-1 strains.   GEM 91 is the first antisense to enter clinical trials.   It is now in phase-one studies in France and the U.S.   The chief obstacles of antisense therapy are its cost, current difficulty of production, and getting sufficient amounts across the cell membrane.   These problems do not appear insurmountable, and the next phase of clinical studies with GEM 91 should determine whether the in vitro cell culture studies, which showed strong inhibition of HIV-1 replication, will be reproduced in patients.

Gene Therapy

This approach to the treatment of AIDS is a method of delivery and does not say what the given therapy will be.   For example, an antisense molecule can be given as gene therapy.   In general, the concept of gene therapy in AIDS is to deliver any gene which inhibits HIV infection to an uninfected cell.   Preferably, we wish to target a stem cell.   A protected stem cell will produce progeny, like $CD4^+$ T-cells, that also contain the inhibitory gene and be protected from HIV infection.   The stem cells (and T-cells) are obtained from bone marrow or blood, cultured, and the inhibitory gene transduced into those cells and then re-infused back into the HIV-infected patient. In order words, the goal is to ultimately reconstitute the immune system by protecting cells from infection. There are almost innumerable ideas to achieve this end. Two are almost ready or, in fact, already in phase-one clinical trials.

In collaboration with Gene Therapy, Inc. (GTI) we have been comparing the inhibitory effects of five different inhibitory genes. One is a fragment of the gene for an antibody to the HIV-1 reverse transcriptase. Another utilizes a gene for antisense to the HIV-1 Tat sequence. A third is a polymer of the sequences Tat binds to—known as Tar. This works as a molecular decoy, i.e., when the cell is infected the poly-Tar is expressed and binds the Tat formed (and needed) by the infecting virus. A fourth approach, similar to the poly-Tar, is to use an altered HIV gene, the product of which dominates the normal gene product in competing to form a virus particle. However, the virus particle with the altered gene cannot form proper. The fifth approach is to use HIV-2. S. Arya in our laboratory discovered that components of HIV-2 (insufficient to form virus) interfere with HIV-1 infection. The mechanisms by which genetic components of HIV-2 inhibit HIV-1 is unknown.

We have found that all the above approaches strongly inhibit HIV replication in laboratory culture systems, that inhibition works against all the strains of HIV-1 tested, and that a combination of a few are better than any one alone. The chief problem faced in gene therapy for AIDS is the difficulty of obtaining a sufficient number of successfully transduced stem cells. We are also uncertain of the long-term safety of these genes. Nonetheless, I agree with the argument that clinical trials in HIV-1-infected people are needed to have information on their in vivo efficacy.

There are principles for controlling progression to AIDS that do not involve antiviral therapy that also should not be forgotten. For example, there has been evidence available since 1985 that chronic T-cells activation (e.g., as from other infections) will promote more HIV infection. Needless to say, prevention and treatment of other infections is also a useful goal in its own right.

Summary and Concluding Remarks

One major argument is to increase and broaden the definiton of basic AIDS research. This notion, in its extreme and simplest version states that since we know so little and since we do not know which basic research will produce a positive application to AIDS therapy, it is reasonable to increasingly fund almost all areas of basic research. In so doing there should be positive spinoffs, not only to AIDS but also to other areas of medicine. The opposite point of view is that we know a great deal or at least that we have sufficient information to mount a major highly structured, planned and targeted research program sometimes called a mini-Manhattan-like project but with an important difference, e.g., no secrecy. I have argued that despite the increased cost that will incur, it is not logical to argue one versus the other. To solve the AIDS problem will take time, effort, and money, and resolution will be accelerated not only by an increase in basic research but also very likely by highly targeted 'crash' programs. I suggest that a few areas of obvious importance and ripe for targeting could be selected as pilot programs for intense and planned research. There is considerable information on HIV pathogenic mechanisms which suggest urgency for answers to certain questions.   I selected a few for discussion—particularly those that have therapeutic or vaccine implications.   For example: studies of cellular immunity in long-term survivors; studies of the nature and role of the soluble factor from $CD8^+$ T-cells which inhibit HIV replication (described by Levy); studies to determine which of the many laboratory findings concerning the many ways HIV impairs the immune system are important in vivo; the reason for the impaired proliferation of even the uninfected T-cells in an HIV-infected person, and quick confirmation and clarification of the different claims of overcoming this defect by modulating different cytokines in vitro.

Specific new systems for the study of KS were described, and results showing that much of the KS tumor mass is composed of non-malignant but nonetheless proliferating endothelial cells of spindle shape.   Our results indicate that some cytokines, like γ-IFN, involved in inflammation (e.g., in wound healing), and known to be elevated in HIV-infected people, promotes the activation and proliferation of these spindle cells.   We found that these activated vascular endothelial cells then produce substantial amounts of other cytokines; among them bFGF is notable because it promotes formation of new blood vessels (angiogenesis) as shown earlier by others, and angiogenesis is a prominent feature of KS.   Moreover, our new results show that bFGF synergizes with the HIV-1 Tat protein in producing these effects and in promoting self-growth of these spindle cells.   These findings indicate that control of some of the tumor mass of KS (and perhaps of the entire tumor lesions in early stages) might be achieved by inhibiting bFGF.   The partial success of α-IFN in treatment of early KS may be due to its known ability to inhibit bFGF.   We have also obtained results in collaboration with Tikva Vogel and Amos Panet in Israel that a naturally occurring molecule, Apolipoprotein E (Apo-E), involved in cholesterol transport and known to interfere with the normal presentation of bFGF to its receptor, inhibits KS cell growth in vitro and tumor formation in our mouse model.   Consequently, we think that clinical trials with Apo-E in early stage KS are warranted.

Other new and more exciting information obtained over the past year in our laboratory has revealed that at least some KS tumors contain neoplastic cells.   This is the first evidence that HIV-1-associated KS can be a true malignancy.   Our evidence suggests that these cells may 'recruit' the hyperplastic (non-malignant but proliferating) endothelial cells and the latter in turn still other cell types.   We do not know if these malignant cells are present in all KS but usually not detected because of an over-abundance of hyperplastic but otherwise similar cells.   But we now have an immortalized cell line (KS Y-1) of these cells which in time should provide specific molecular probes to evaluate this question.   A remarkable finding is that the KS malignant cells are under the control of a hormone, hCG. Specifically, the β chain of this molecule prevents tumor formation and destroys pre-existing KS tumors in a mouse model. βhCG is homologous to the β chain of LH which rises to high levels in each menstrual cycle of women.   I think these results are both provocative, for their possible contribution to an understanding of the much greater incidence of KS in males than females, and have immediate therapeutic implications.

I have also argued that there is sufficient information available now on the HIV replication cycle to mount more intensive research into development of anti-HIV agents and to strategize in approaches to avoid resistance.   I suspect that the pharmaceutical companies will steadily advance our treatment approaches by developing new and better combinations of compounds which target enzymes of the virus, like reverse transcriptase and the viral protease, which others focus more on newer concepts.   I breifly reviewed progress in our laboratory in collaboration with others on four approaches: Antisense therapy, e.g., GEM 91 from Hybridon is in phase-one clinical trials and efficacy studies will soon begin.   Clinical trails with genes (gene therapy) that inhibit HIV replication are beginning by Gary Nabel (using an HIV molecular decoy approach) and by Flossie Wong-Staal with a gene for a ribozyme which 'cuts' the HIV genome.   R. Pommeranz is approaching the problem with a gene for an antibody to an HIV protein.   We developed a series of inhibitory genes which also inhibit HIV replication in laboratory culture tests, and comparison of their effects was summarized.   The strategy in all these studies is to obtain bone marrow or blood from an HIV-infected person, and to transduce the HIV inhibitory gene into uninfected cells (preferably stem cells) in a laboratory cell culture system and then to re-infuse these cells back into the patient.   There is awareness in this field that the problems are not so much the development of genes which inhibit HIV, but in adequate delivery of these genes to a sufficient number of stem cells in order to protect such cells against infection so that they can reconstitute the impaired immune system.

Two other novel anti-HIV approaches were described.   Last year we reported that a common and seemingly innocuous herpesvirus (HHV-7) uses the CD4 molecule as its receptor, like HIV.   Consequently, HHV-7 can block HIV infection at the cell surface in vitro.   Our objective is to identify the protein of HHV-7 responsible, to purify it and to use its active factors (peptides)—perhaps in liposomes, in testing for its safety and efficacy in the SIV monkey model.

We are also trying to avoid HIV-escape mutants by targeting cellular factors rather than viral because cell proteins do not mutate like HIV.   Cell factors, which HIV needs for its replication, are selected.   This approach has led us first to a study of hydroxyurea, a simple compound, available as an oral drug and used in clinical medicine for over 30 years, e.g., in the treatment of some chronic leukemias.   Hydroxyurea inhibits an enzyme needed for synthesis of deoxynucleotides, precursors for DNA synthesis.   Relatively low doses inhibit HIV replication and synergize with ddI and AZT (presumably by lowering the pools of deoxynucleotides more of the nucleotide analogues, namely AZT or ddI can be incorporated into the newly forming viral DNA and block its further synthesis).   The side effects (e.g., possible bone marrow toxicity) would have to be monitored.   This approach (hydroxyurea and ddI or AZT) is currently being tested in the SIV monkey model.

Finally, in collaboration with Virogenetics and Pasteur Merieux—our recent results on preventive vaccines in HIV-2 monkey studies (HIV-1 does not infect these monkeys) show that prevention can be obtained against different HIV-2 strains with the HIV-1 (or HIV-2) envelope gene carried by a safe modified vaccinia virus (a mutated human vaccinia or the avian vaccinia).   These vaccinia vectors enter cells, express the HIV envelope gene—forming the envelope protein which is then presented at the cell's surface.   This occurs without replication of the modified vaccinia.   Apparently, the manner or presentation is critical because the same experiments with the gene carried by the bacterium Salmonella or as the envelope protein alone (not carried) did not work.   It is important to determine the immune basis for these results, but to date we have found no correlation.   I think an intensification of these studies is now warranted as is a consideration of using this approach for vaccinating against HIV-2 in HIV-2 endemic areas of the world.   It is likely that beyond expanded and broadened basic research and in addition to select targeted and intensive research programs, substantial progress will also depend upon many more independent minded clinical trials.

Acknowledgments

I wish to acknowledge colleagues and collaborators chiefly responsible for this work.

KS Studies
Barbara Ensoli was key to all the studies on the hyperplastic cells with contributions from Valeria Fiorelli, Hsiao Chang and Giovanni Barillari of our laboratory, and Mark Raffeld of the Pathology Branch of NIH.   Philip Browning performed most of the work on identifying KS spindle cells in the blood.   He is now at Vanderbilt University.   He also performed the Apo-E studies in collaboration with Tikva Vogel and Amos Panet in Israel. Yanto Lunardi-Iskandar developed the KS Y-1 cell line and was also critical to the hormone studies.   He was helped by Victor Lam, Robert Zeman, Alain Theirry, and Felipe Samaniego, all also in our group.   Joseph Bryant of NIDR, NIH was central to all our animal work, and our clinical collaborators included Parkash Gill of USC in Los Angeles, Philippe Hermans of Brussels, and Jacques Besnier of Paris.   bFGF antisense came from Gerals Zon of Lynx Laboratories in San Diego.

Vaccine Studies
Genoveffa Franchini and Marjorie Robert-Guroff were the main contributors with help from John Benson and Alash'le Abimiku, all of our group.   The studies depended upon collaboration with Enzo Paoletti and James Tartaglia of Virogenetics, Inc. in Troy, New York and with Pasteur Merieux in France.

Anti-HIV Studies
The antisense studies mostly by Julianna Lisziewicz and Mary Klotman in our group with collaboration with Sudhir Agrawal and others at Hybridon in Massachusetts and with Gerald Zon of Lynx Laboratories in San Diego.

Gene Therapy
Mostly by Julianna Lisziewicz, Daisy Sun, Frank Weichold, and Suresh Arya of our group.   Collaborators include GTI in Rockville, Maryland.

HHV-7
Mostly by Paolo Lusso and Paola Seccherio of our laboratory.

Hydroxyurea
Mostly by Franco Lori with input and help from Julianna Lisziewicz, Andrei Malykh and Andrea Cara, all from our laboratory.

HIV 10 Years on: Research Finding and Future Prospects

HIV: A Decade of Research

Jay A. Levy, M.D.

School of Medicine, University of California, San Francisco, CA., USA

The human immunodeficiency virus, or LAV, HTLV-III, or ARV as it was first known, has with time demonstrated to the scientific community its great diversity, its ability to infect a variety of cell types and its ability to remain present in many different tissues of the body [1]. This heterogeneity of HIV is reflected in two different types of AIDS viruses, HIV-1 and HIV-2 [1, 2]. The diversity results from the replicative nature of the virus in which its error-prone reverse transcriptase [3], making up to ten genetic mutations per replication cycle, can yield a variety of different virus subtypes or strains.

HIV can be transmitted as a free virus, or as probably the most challenging component in this infection, the virus-infected cell. On transmission, the virus finds targets in not only T cells and macrophages, but also in the mucosal lining cells of the bowel, cervix, and endometrium [4, 5]. Initially considered only T lymphocyte-tropic, a large number of cells have now been recognized as being susceptible to HIV from the hematopoietic system, the skin, the brain, the bowel and other tissues of the body [1] (table 1). It is important to note, however, that while HIV is polytropic, its effects on various cell types differ. In some cells, it may exist as a reservoir in the body from which low levels of replicating virus can spread to other cells; in others, it can show substantial detrimental effects as noted in the immune system, the brain and the bowel [1].

Furthermore, over the past decade, the scientific community has learned that CD4 is not the only cellular receptor for virus entry. In the brain and bowel, galactosyl ceramide can serve as an alternative receptor for HIV [6, 7]. Or, when virus is complexed with antibody, the Fc or complement receptor can be entry sites and cause enhancement in the infection process [8, 9]. The discovery of still other cellular receptors for HIV is expected.

These accumulated observations reflect the great diversity of HIV strains that can be distinguished by their cellular host range, their replicative properties (replicating slowly to low titer or rapidly to high titer), and their extent of cell killing, in which both multinucleated cells or syncytia formation and cell death can be observed [1]. These kinetics of replication and viral growth have been used by some investigators to refer to viruses as having a slow/low or rapid/high phenotype [10] (table 2).

Virus Heterogeneity

The heterogeneity of viral isolates can also distinguish HIV strains that grow well in macrophages or T cell lines [1, 2]. Many macrophage-tropic viruses do not directly kill cells nor do they induce syncytia. In contrast, the T cell line-replicating viruses are highly

Table 1. Human cells susceptible to HIV

Hematopoietic	Brain	Other	
T lymphocytes	Capillary endothelial cells	Myocardium	Cervix (epithelium ?)
B lymphocytes		Renal tubular cells	Prostate
Macrophages	Astrocytes	Synovial membrane	Testes
NK cells	Macrophages (microglia)	Hepatocytes	Osteosarcoma cells
Megakaryocytes		Hepatic sinusoid endothelium	Rhabdomyosarcoma cells
Dendritic cells	Oligodendrocytes		
Promyelocytes	Choroid plexus	Hepatic carcinoma cells	Fetal chorionic villi
Stem cells	Ganglia cells		Trophoblast cells
Thymic epithelium	Neuroblastoma cells	Kupffer cells	
Follicular dendritic cells	Glioma cell lines	Dental pulp fibroblasts	
	Neurons (?)	Pulmonary fibroblasts	
Bone marrow endothelial cells	Bowel	Fetal adrenal cells	
	Columnar and goblet cells	Adrenal carcinoma cells	
Skin		Retinal cells	
Langerhans cells	Enterochromaffin cells	Cervix-derived epithelial cells	
Fibroblasts	Colon carcinoma cells		

Summary of studies examining the sensitivity of human cells to HIV infection.   Results reflect data from cell culture experiments as well as the evaluation of tissues removed in vivo

cytopathic and usually syncytia-inducing—the reason some researchers term them SI viruses [11].   Nevertheless, the non-cytopathic, or NSI (non-syncytia-inducing), strains may cause cell death indirectly, most likely by apoptosis [1].   We have observed this phenomenon in studies with Don Mosier using the immunocompromised SCID-hu mouse system in which human peripheral blood mononuclear cells (PBMC) have been used to repopulate the hematopoeitic system of the animal [12].   HIV-1$_{SF162}$, a non-cytopathic macrophage-tropic virus, induced a faster CD4$^+$ cell loss in these animals than did the highly cytopathic, T cell line-tropic HIV-1$_{SF33}$ strain.

The biologic properties of HIV can also be linked to clinical disease in humans.   For example, the macrophage-tropic strains appear associated with disease in the brain [13].

Table 2. Classification of HIV strains by host range and replicative properties

Biologic subtypes
• Virulent versus non-virulent strains
• Macrophage-tropic versus T cell line-tropic viruses
• Syncytium-inducing versus non-syncytium-inducing strains[1]
• Rapid/high versus slow/low strains[2]

Viruses have been classified by their replicative properties and their ability to cause cytopathology in cultured cells [1]
1. Cytopathology as defined by cell kiling or induction of syncytia via cell-cell fusion.
2. Replication as defined by how quickly virus is released from the cell (kinetics, e.g., rapid versus slow) and to what levels it is produced at peak virus replication (titer, e.g., high versus low).

The cytopathic, SI-type viruses rapidly kill CD4$^+$ cells and have been linked to a fast progression to AIDS [1, 14].

Furthermore, studying these varying features of HIV has indicated that, with time, viruses can change in their biologic and serologic properties to have characteristics associated with induction of disease in the host [14, 15]. These include an increased cellular host range, rapid kinetics of replication with high virus production, induction of alterations in cell permeability resulting in syncytia induction and increased cell killing. These viruses also do not readily induce a silent (or latent) state in cells. Moreover, they are resistant to neutralization and can be sensitive to antibodies that enhance their infection (table 3).

Table 3. Characteristics of HIV strains associated with virulence in the host

- Expanded cellular host range
- Rapid kinetics of replication
- High titers of virus production
- Alteration of cell membrane permeability
- High level of syncytium induction
- Increase in cell killing
- Failure to enter a latent state in vitro
- Sensitivity to antibody-mediated enhancement of infection

This brief overview of HIV indicates that the ability of the virus during its replication in different cells to change its genetic make-up can determine whether it takes on highly cytopathic properties that affect the immune system or those that are destructive to other tissues in the body, such as the brain (fig. 1).

The approach then is to arrest virus replication before selection or mutations result in the emergence of the pathogenic viruses or those with specific tropism for tissues (fig. 1). In this regard, both neutralizing antibodies and cellular immune activity are part of the host response to HIV infection.

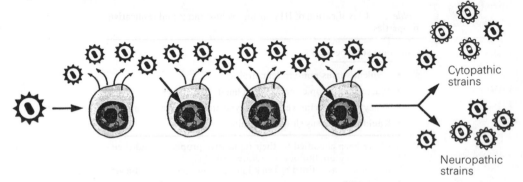

Cytopathic strains

Neuropathic strains

Fig. 1. HIV replication permits genetic mutations. Continuous HIV infection and replication in cells can lead to genetic mutations that bring about the emergence of viral strains with different pathogenic properties or tropisms for certain tissues (e.g., brain). Up to ten mutations per replicative cycle have been estimated [3].

Table 4. HIV isolation from peripheral blood of a clinically healthy infected man

Date	Virus isolation	Date	Virus isolation
10/84	+	8/88	−
11/84	+	2/89	−
1/85	+	8/89	−
2/85	+	2/90	−
4/85	−	8/90	−
8/85	−	2/91	−
11/85	−	8/91	−
2/86	−	2/92	−
8/86	−	8/92	−
2/87	−	2/93	−
8/87	−	8/93	−
2/88	−	2/94	−

The peripheral blood mononuclear cells (PBMC) of an asymptomatic HIV-infected individual were evaluated for virus production. No virus has been detected in the cultured PBMC after February of 1985. By removal of $CD8^+$ cells, virus can be recovered. The clinical course and laboratory studies, however, indicate that under standard virus detection procedures, HIV replication in the PBMC is blocked.

Anti-HIV Cellular Immune Responses

Cellular immunity can involve NK cells and $CD8^+$ cells with antiviral cytotoxic activity, such as CTLs which kill virus-infected cells [16]. We have concentrated on another antiviral function of $CD8^+$ cells: suppression of virus replication without killing the infected cell [17]. These studies began 10 years ago with observations on a clinically healthy homosexual man. After five months of study, we could no longer isolate virus from his PBMC by conventional techniques (table 4). Recognizing that these white blood cells consist of T lymphocytes of the $CD4^+$ helper and $CD8^+$ suppressor/cytotoxic cell type, we investigated whether the $CD8^+$ suppresser cell, responsible for inhibiting replication of other viruses such as Epstein-Barr virus, might play a role in suppressing HIV production by the $CD4^+$ lymphocyte.

In these initial studies, we demonstrated that, whereas virus was not detected in cultured PBMC from these healthy individuals as measured by the reverse transcriptase activity in the cell culture supernatant, we could demonstrate the virus after removal of the $CD8^+$ cells from the blood sample [18]. This procedure was achieved through the process of panning by which monoclonal antibodies to CD8 were attached to the bottom of a petri dish. When the PBMC from the infected subject were added to the dish, the $CD8^+$ cells bound to the bottom surface. The non-adherent CD8-depleted cells were recovered in one tube and the $CD8^+$ cells, removed by vigorous pipetting, were placed in a second tube. When the $CD8^+$ cells were returned to the culture at the same level as in the blood, at a 50% level, or at a 25% level, HIV replication was either completely suppressed or partially

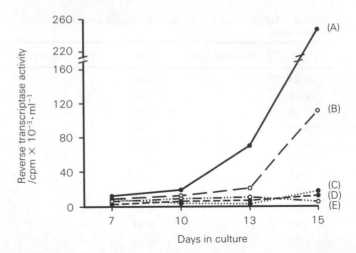

Fig. 2. CD8⁺ cell anti-HIV response. Peripheral blood mononuclear cells (PBMC) from an asymptomatic individual were placed in culture to examine for HIV replication. No virus was detected (E). When the CD8⁺ cells were removed by the process of panning, HIV replication took place (A). When CD8⁺ cells were returned at the same level as in the blood (D) at 50% (C) or at 25% (B), the extent of suppression of virus replication was observed in a dose-response pattern [18].

inhibited in a dose response pattern (fig. 2). The data indicated that CD8⁺ cells were responsible for this antiviral response and a certain number of CD8⁺ cells was necessary to suppress HIV replication.

This inhibition of HIV by the CD8⁺ cells did not involve CD4⁺ cell killing nor a block in their proliferation. Thus, this cellular immune response represented a new type of antiviral activity with the properties noted in table 5.

The mechanism of this antiviral activity was found to involve a cellular factor. The evidence for this antiviral factor was demonstrated through the use of a transwell device in which infected CD4⁺ cells were placed in the top chamber and CD8⁺ cells were placed in the bottom chamber. With the cells separated by a filter, a product of the CD8⁺ cells could be detected that suppressed HIV replication [19]. This finding has been confirmed by others [20]. We have since shown that this CD8⁺ cell antiviral factor, or CAF, is unlike any known cytokine including the interferons and interleukins [21]. We have found as well that CAF suppresses virus replication at the transcription level. This latter point was demonstrated by showing a block in HIV RNA and protein production in the presence of

Table 5. Properties of the CD8⁺ cell antiviral suppressing activity

- Observed with activated CD8⁺CD28⁺ cells
- Active against HIV-1, HIV-2 and SIV
- Non-lytic mechanism
- MHC unrestricted
- Blocks HIV RNA expression
- Does not block activation or proliferation of CD4⁺ cells
- Mediated by a novel factor

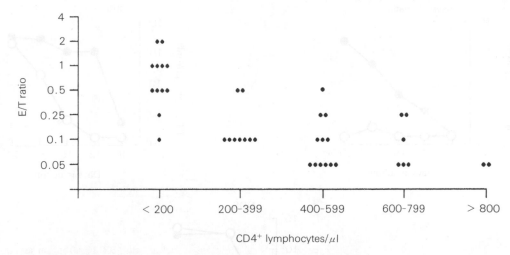

Fig. 3. CD8$^+$ cell antiviral response and CD4$^+$ cell number. CD8$^+$cell antiviral responses measured by suppression of HIV replication in cultured PBMC correlates directly with the number of CD4$^+$ cells present in the peripheral blood of individuals. E/T ratio: effector CD8$^+$ cell/target infected CD4$^+$ cells. Each dot represents a single subject. Reproduced from ref. 23 with permission.

CD8$^+$ cells and CAF as well as a block in the expression of reporter genes linked to the viral LTR [17, 22]. In the latter studies, reductions in CAT expression in CD4$^+$ lymphocytes (unpublished obs.) and in luciferase production in a Jurkat cell line were demonstrated [22].

In several studies, we have shown that the extent of this CD8$^+$ cell antiviral response is reflected by the clinical state [23]. Those healthy individuals with high numbers of CD4$^+$ cells have a strong CD8$^+$ cell antiviral response, whereas CD8$^+$ cells from patients who have lost CD4$^+$ cells show poor antiviral activity (fig. 3). Individuals who are asymptomatic may show that as few as one CD8$^+$ cell per 20 CD4$^+$ cells is needed in culture to block virus replication; the opposite is true for those progressing to AIDS.

Production of CAF also correlates with the clinical state (fig. 4). Individuals who are asymptomatic with strong CD8$^+$ cell anti-HIV activity show production of the factor that suppresses virus in culture for several days. In contrast, CAF production by CD8$^+$ cells from symptomatic individuals (ARC) is either at relatively low levels that do not persist (e.g. ARC patients), or there is an absence of this antiviral activity (AIDS patients) [19].

Many of these studies were performed with asymptomatic individuals initially seen in my laboratory over 10 years ago. They have evolved, along with others we are studying, as long-term survivors—defined as individuals infected for more than 10 years, clinically healthy with a stable CD4$^+$ cell count above 500/μl, and not receiving antiretroviral therapy. They can be distinguished by several characteristics from infected individuals progressing to disease (table 6).

This CD8$^+$ cell antiviral response is observed readily in the peripheral blood of long-term survivors, and also mirrored in the lymph node. For example, many CD4$^+$ cells were present in the lymph node (a helper/suppressor ratio of 1.6) and blood from a long-term survivor (table 6). And, about a 100-fold greater number of virus-infected cells was detected in the lymph node compared to the amount present in the PBMC. That

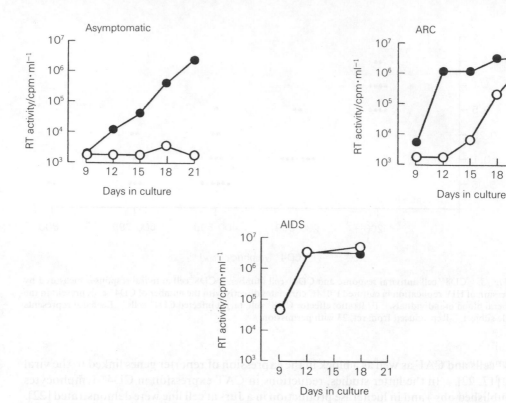

Fig. 4. Levels of CD8$^+$ cell antiviral factor (CAF) production correlate directly with clinical state. RT, reverse transcriptase; ●—●, control infected CD4$^+$ cells cultured alone; ○—○, infected CD4$^+$ cells cultured in one chamber of a transwell device with CD8$^+$ cells in the other chamber [19].

observation on virus load has been made by others [24, 25]. Most importantly, we noted that, similar to findings with the peripheral white cells, virus could not be isolated from the lymph node of this infected individual unless the CD8$^+$ cells were removed. Moreover, the antiviral response was similar and strong with CD8$^+$ cells recovered from the lymph node as well as the peripheral blood. The results are encouraging and suggest that both peripheral blood and lymphoid tissue can reflect the effects of a CD8$^+$ cell antiviral response. Virus is blocked in replication without the killing of CD4$^+$ cells.

The CD8$^+$ cell anti-HIV activity can be found quite early in infection as we have observed in studies of acutely infected individuals. This cellular immune response, not

Table 6.   Characteristics of long-term survivors vs. progressors

---

- Have low virus load in blood
- Infected with less cytopathic HIV strain
- Have no enhancing antibodies
- TH-1 response > TH-2 response
- Strong CD8$^+$ cell antiviral response

Table 7. Comparative studies of peripheral blood and lymph node of a long-term survivor

	Peripheral blood[1]	Lymph node
CD4$^+$: CD8$^+$ cell ratio	.8	1.58
Virus isolation:		
Total cells	–	–
w/o CD8$^+$ cells	+	+
CD4$^+$ cell		
Viral load	.001%	.1%
CD8$^+$ cell		
Anti-HIV activity	+++	+++

The presence of viruses is found to be 100x greater in the lymph node than in the peripheral blood. The virus in the blood and lymph node cannot be recovered unless CD8$^+$ cells are removed (w/o, without). Evaluation of the CD8$^+$ cell response in the lymph node and PBMC indicates strong anti-HIV activity. Thus, in the lymph node as well as in peripheral blood, virus replication is controlled by this CD8$^+$ cell antiviral response
1. Peripheral blood CD4$^+$ cell count=1078/µl.

neutralizing antibodies, is associated with a reduction in virus titer (fig. 5) [26]. This immune response can be maintained for several years as observed with long-term asymptomatic individuals. A similar observation on virus control by CTL activity in primary infection has recently been reported [27].

TH1 and TH2 Responses
A major question is why CD8$^+$ cell anti-HIV activity is lost in many infected individuals

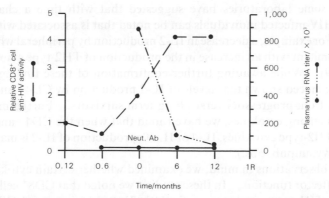

Fig. 5. CD8$^+$ cell anti-HIV response in primary infection. CD8$^+$ cell antiviral activity measured by suppression of HIV replication in culture can be noted even before the presence of antibodies in individuals acutely infected with HIV-1. 0 time=seroconversion. No neutralizing antibodies (neut-Ab) are noted. CD8$^+$ cell anti-HIV activity is expressed as a relative amount of response with 4 – 5 being the highest (*y* axis, left). Plasma virus RNA titer was measured by QC-PCR (*y* axis, right). In this case, the cellular immune response is associated with a drop in virus levels in the blood [26].

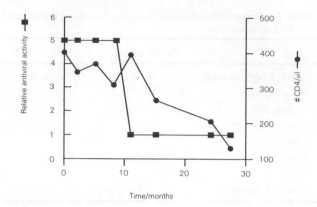

Fig. 6.   CD8⁺ cell anti-HIV activity in a healthy infected individual followed over time.   CD8⁺cell antiviral suppressing activity can be observed to decrease prior to loss of CD4⁺ cells in an infected individual who subsequently progressed to disease (reprinted from reference 28 with permission).

over time.   As shown in figure 6, the CD8⁺ cell antiviral response decreases prior to the loss of the CD4⁺ cells, which mirrors a return of high virus production and progression to disease.

A recent insight into this question on the cause of the loss in CD8⁺ cell responses is the possibility that the type of cellular factors or cytokines produced by peripheral white cells determine progression to disease [28].   Cytokines made by CD4⁺ lymphocytes (or T helper, TH cells) have been classified into two major subgroups, TH1 and TH2.   The TH1 type cells appear to preferentially support cell-mediated immunity.   TH2 type cells are associated with increased antibody production.   The distinction between the two cell types, however, is not always that clear.   The TH1 and TH2 cytokines can cross-regulate one another so that production of TH1-type cellular factors can suppress production of the cytokines produced by TH2-type cells [1, 29].

Results in some laboratories have suggested that with time a change in cytokine production in HIV-infected individuals can be noted that is associated with progression to disease [29].   For example, a decrease in IL-2 production by peripheral white cells has been observed concomitant with an increase in the production of TH2-type cytokines such as IL-4 and IL-10 [29].   While awaiting further confirmation of these findings, studies in our laboratory have indeed shown that levels of IL-2 production by CD4⁺ and CD8⁺ cells are reduced in cells from progressors versus long-term survivors.   Furthermore, recognizing the interactions among cytokines, we have found that when the CD4⁺ and CD8⁺ cells are exposed to the TH2-type cytokines, IL-4 or IL-10, production of IL-2 is markedly decreased (Barker and Levy, unpub. obs.).

With these observations in mind, we examined whether certain cytokines might affect the CD8⁺ cell effector function.   In these studies, we noted that CD8⁺ cells, cultured in the presence of the TH1-type cytokines particularly IL-2, had increased CD8⁺ cell antiviral activity, whereas CD8⁺ cells exposed to the cytokines associated with TH2-type cells (e.g., IL-4 and IL-10) inhibited this antiviral response [28].   Based again on the known interplay of TH1 and TH2 cytokines, we examined whether IL-2 might change the inhibitory effects of IL-10.   IL-2 was added in equal amounts to IL-10 in cultures of CD8⁺ cells.   The results

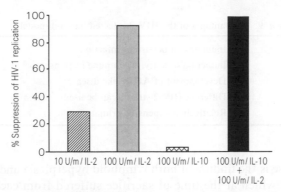

Fig. 7.   Effect of IL-2 on the inhibition of CD8⁺ cell suppressing activity by IL-10.   CD8⁺ cells cultured for three days in the presence of IL-2 show enhanced antiviral activity.   In the presence of IL-10, the CD8⁺ cell response is reduced.   When both IL-10 and IL-2 are mixed, the strong CD8⁺ cell antiviral response is maintained. Studies by E. Barker, unpublished observations.

showed that IL-2 can prevent the inhibition of CD8⁺ cell activity by IL10 (fig. 7).   These findings suggest that similar effects may be seen when cytotoxic or CTL activity is examined in the presence of cytokines.   These observations on the benefit of IL-2 to cellular immune responses could have relevance to recent clinical trials with this cytokine [30].

Baboon Animal Model

Finally, some new observations show promise that an animal model is available with which we can examine directly some aspects of HIV pathogenesis and develop approaches at controlling it.   We have been studying the effects of HIV-2 in baboons [31].   This virus replicates readily in cultured PBMC from these animals.   Our results have revealed that not only is persistent infection by HIV-2 established in the baboons, but also an AIDS-like syndrome can develop 2 years after the infection.   It consists of CD4⁺ cell loss, lymphoid depletion, lymphocytic interstitial pneumonia (common in children with HIV infection), skin lesions (e.g., alopecia), and extensive fibromatosis (table 8).   The latter condition exists as tumors within the skin of the animal or as fibrous lesions in other tissues, such as the lymph node.   These hyperplastic cells appear to be derived from the musculature of the vascular endothelium [31].   Thus, conceivably, the fibrous tumors are the baboon counterpart to Kaposi's sarcoma in humans.   A similar tumor has been found associated with SRV-2 infection in rhesus macaques [32] but baboons are not infected with this virus [31].   The cause of these tumors in baboons is under study.

In the lymph node of these animals, the loss of follicular dendritic cells and B cells can be demonstrated with specific immunohistochemical markers.   What is remarkable and

Table 8.   AIDS-like disease in HIV-2-infected baboons

- CD4⁺ cell loss
- Lymphoid depletion
- Lymphocyte interstitial pneumonia
- Skin lesions
- Fibromatosis

Table 9.   Advantages of the HIV-2-infected baboon model

- Induction of persistent infection
- Induction of antiviral immune responses
- Development of AIDS-like disease
- Different HIV-2 strains can be used
- Relatively inexpensive primate

important in this case is the finding of both lymphoid hyperplasia and lymphoid depletion in the same animal, which at the time of sacrifice suffered from cachexia and end-stage disease [31].   These different observations on two distinct lymph nodes in the same infected baboon suggest caution to those who believe a prognosis can be made for an individual after examination of just one lymph node.   Pathologists remind us that a full spectrum of infection can be observed in lymphoid tissue of infected individuals even those with AIDS, ranging from the hyperplasia of early infection to end-stage destruction [33].   Thus, perhaps the virologic findings in the blood reflect the sum-total of immunologic events occurring in all lymphoid tissues.   This possibility merits further evaluation.   The advantages of the HIV-2 infected baboon model are obvious, particularly because there is persistent infection and induction of an AIDS-like disease in a relatively inexpensive primate host (table 8).

Conclusions

Over the past ten years, a great deal about HIV has been learned in terms of its heterogeneity, its ability to enter cells by different receptors, and to replicate and mutate in the cells into strains that give rise to immune pathogenesis and diseases in tissues such as the brain [1].   The virus, by its evolution in the host, can escape immune response [34, 35] and it can kill CD4$^+$ cells by both direct and indirect means.   It also differs in its sensitivity to neutralizing or enhancing antibodies that can influence the clinical state and viral transmission [1].

In terms of the host, we have observed that cellular immunity can be a major mechanism for controlling HIV, even more than neutralizing antibodies.   Known cytokines, including CAF, can influence these immune responses against HIV.   In this regard, the HIV-2 baboon model could provide us with an approach to look at these various viral and immunological features that influence pathogenesis and uncover directions at developing antiviral therapies and a vaccine.

A reasonable approach to HIV infection is to reach a state of balanced pathogenicity in which the virus is held in check by a strong host immune response.   This state is directly linked to a balance in the immune system in which CD8$^+$ cell production of the CD8$^+$ cell antiviral factor prevents virus replication in CD4$^+$ cells and permits continual production of IL2 by these cells (fig. 8).   This cytokine, as we have seen, can maintain the CD8$^+$ cell antiviral response.   If an inhibitory event occurs either to block IL2 production or CAF production, a loss in control of HIV would take place with subsequent emergence of replicating virus and development of disease (fig. 9).

This decade of research on HIV further emphasizes a key concept recognized in the beginning—the importance of the CD4$^+$ cell in long-term survial with HIV infection.

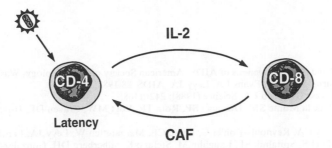

Fig. 8. Balanced immunogenicity.   In this model, CD4⁺ cells are infected with the virus but are prevented from releasing HIV through the action of the CD8⁺ cell antiviral factor (CAF).   IL-2 production by the CD4⁺ cells maintains the production of CAF (reprinted from ref. 1 with permission).

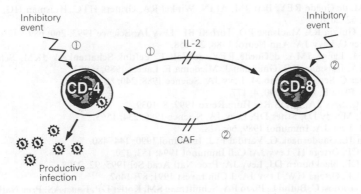

Fig. 9. Immune pathogenesis.   CD4⁺ cells producing cytokines such as IL-2 maintain the production of CAF by CD8⁺ cells.   HIV production is therefore blocked.   If IL-2 production is compromised or CAF production is reduced, the suppression of virus in the CD4⁺ cells is inhibited.   Virus replication presages advancement to disease (Reprinted from ref. 1 with permission).

Approaches should be directed at inhibiting replication of HIV to prevent its emergence as a pathogenic agent.   If TH1-type cells, or the IL-2 they produce, are maintained in the host, CD8⁺ cell anti-HIV function with production of the antiviral factor will be maintained and virus production inhibited.   Toward this objective, my laboratory is concentrating on defining the CD8⁺ cell antiviral factor and its function.   An important direction has been defined and the means of getting there remains our major challenge.

Acknowledgments

The research by the author and his coworkers was supported by grants from the National Institutes of Health, the University of Califormia Universitywide Task Force on AIDS, and the American Foundation for AIDS Research.   Christine Beglinger and Ann Murai are thanked for their help in preparation of the manuscript.

References

1   Levy JA: HIV and the Pathogenesis of AIDS, American Society of Microbiology, Washington, DC, 1994.
2   Castro BA, Cheng-Mayer C, Evans LA, Levy JA: AIDS '88 1988; 2: s17.
3   Preston BD, Poiesz BJ, Loeb LA: Science (1988); 242: 1168.
4   Pomerantz RJ, de la Monte SM, Donegan SP, Rota TR, Vogt MW, Craven DE, Hirsch M: Ann Int Med 1988; 108: 321.
5   Nelson JA, Wiley CA, Reynolds-Kohler C, Reese CE, Margaretten W, Levy JA: Lancet 1988; i: 259.
6   Harouse JM, Bhat S, Spitalnik SL, Laughlin M, Stefano K, Silberberg DH, Gonzalez-Scarano F: Science 1991; 253: 320.
7   Yahi N, Baghdiguian S, Moreau H, Fantini J: J Virol 1992; 66: 4848.
8   Homsy J, Meyer M, Tateno M, Clarkson S, Levy JA: Scinece 1989; 244: 1357.
9   Robinson WE, Jr, Montefiori DC, Mitchell WM: Virol 1990; 175: 600.
10 Fenyo EM, Morfeldt-Manson L, Chiodi F, Lind B, von Gegerfelt A, Albert J, Olausson E, Asjo B: J Virol 1988; 62: 4414.
11 Tersmette M, de Goede REY, Bert JM, Al IN, Winkel RA, Gruters HTC, Huisman HG, Miedema F: J. Virol. 1988; 62: 2026.
12 Mosier DE, Gulizia RJ, MacIsaac PD, Torbett BE, Levy JA: Science 1993; 260: 689.
13 Cheng-Mayer C, Levy JA: Ann Neurol 1988; 23: s58.
14 Tersmette M, Lange JMA, deGoede REY, deWolf F, Eeftink-Schattenkerk JKM, Schellekens PTA, Coutinho RA, Huisman HG, Goudsmit J, Miedema F: Lancet 1989; i: 983.
15 Cheng-Mayer C, Seto D, Tateno M, Levy JA, Science 1988; 240: 80.
16 Walker BD, Plata F: AIDS 1990; 4: 177.
17 Mackewicz C, Levy JA: AIDS Res Hum Retro 1992; 8: 1039.
18 Walker CM, Moody DJ, Stites DP, Levy JA: Science 1986; 234: 1563.
19 Walker CM, Levy JA: Immunol 1989; 66: 628.
20 Brinchmann JE, Gaudernack G, Vartdal F: J. Immunol 1990; 144: 480.
21 Mackewicz CE, Ortega H, Levy JA: Cell Immunol 1994; 153: 329.
22 Mackewicz CE, Blackbourn DJ, Levy JA: Proc Natl Acad Sci 1995; 92: 2308.
23 Mackewicz CE, Ortega HW, Levy JA: J Clin Invest 1991; 87: 1462.
24 Pantaleo G, Graziosi C, Butini L, Pizzo PA, Schnittman SM, Kotler DP, Fauci AS: Proc Natl Acad Sci USA 1991; 88: 9838.
25 Embretson J, Zupancic M, Ribas JL, Burke A, Racz P, Tenner-Racz K, Haase AT: Nature 1993; 362: 359.
26 Mackewicz CE, Yang LC, Lifson JD, Levy JA: Lancet 1994; 344: 1671.
27 Koup RA, Safrit JT, Cao Y, Andrews CA, McLeod G, Borkowsky W, Farthing C, Ho DD: J. Virol. 1994; 68: 4650.
28 Levy JA, AIDS 1993; 7: 1401.
29 Clerici M, Shearer GM, Immunol Today 1993; 14: 107.
30 Kovacs JA, Basseler M, Dewar R, Vogel S, Davey RT Jr, Falloon J, Polis MA, Walker RE, Stevens R, Salzman NP, Metcalf JA, Masur H, Lane H-C: New Engl J Med 1995; 332: 567.
31 Barnett SW, Murthy KM, Herndier, Levy JA: Science 1994; 266: 642.
32 Stromberg K, Benveniste RE, Arthur LO, Rabin H, Giddens WE Jr, Ochs HD, Morton WR, Tsai C-C: Science, 1984; 224: 289.
33 Hawrawi SJ, O'Hara CJ: Pathology and Pathophysiology of AIDS and HIV-Related Diseases, The C. V. Mosby Company, St. Louis, 1989.
34 McKeating JA, Gow J, Goudsmit J, Pearl LH, Mulder C, Weiss RA: AIDS 1989; 3: 777.
35 Phillips RE, Rowland-Jones S, Nixon DF, Gotch FM, Edwards JP, Ogunlesi AO, Elvin JG, Rothbard JA, Bangham CRM, Rizza CR, McMichael AJ: Nature 1991; 354: 453.

HIV 10 Years on: Research Finding and Future Prospects

For a Coherent and Global Strategy of AIDS Research

Luc Montagnier

Institut Pasteur, France and World Foundation for AIDS Research and Prevention

More than eleven years after the first isolation of HIV, we need to ask ourselves: are we on the right track, are we getting close to a treatment able to eradicate HIV infection in seropositive patients, are we getting close to a practicable vaccine?

Knowledge of the virus, its genes, its replication is abundant, although not complete: HIV is certainly one of the best known viruses, but it is still necessary to continue and expand its studies. However, AIDS is more than an infectious disease, it is a complex pathology of the immune system with some degenerative aspects, and these aspects should be studied as thoroughly as the virus itself.

I propose in this short presentation three new lines of research of interest, which might lead to new therapeutic approaches and a vaccines.

Apoptosis in AIDS

In recent years, new concepts in the mechanisms of CD4$^+$ lymphocyte depletion have emerged. Besides the direct cell killing by HIV, programmed cell death (apoptosis) appears to be an important cause of cell destruction in AIDS, and consequently of decline of the immune system.

A large fraction of circulating CD4$^+$ and CD8$^+$ lymphocytes seems to be primed in vivo for death by apoptosis, which is triggered in vivo by culture in the absence of lymphokines. Activation by calcium ionophores (ionomycin) or bacterial superantigens further increases the fraction of apoptotic cells. This phenomenon is well correlated with AIDS pathogenesis and occurs early following HIV infection. It has been observed in HIV-1 and HIV-2 infected asymptomatic patients and increases at the clinical phase of the disease. It is also present at the time of seroconversion, in primary infections [1, 2].

A recent technical improvement (use of an actinomycin D derivative and monoclonal antibodies coupled with fluorescent dyes) has allowed to distinguish between apoptotic CD4$^+$ and CD8$^+$ lymphocytes [3]. Both populations are concerned but the mechanisms underlying their apoptotic death are probably different.

The apoptotic death of CD4$^+$ lymphocytes is probably linked to virus replication. Non-infectious viral particles, virus glycoprotein gp120 free or complexed to antibodies

287

could bind to CD4 receptor, and induce, a signal leading to apoptosis or anergy, when the cells are further stimulated (by antigens or superantigens) [4, 5].

This could lead to clonal deletion of CD4 cells involved in the control of intracellular infectious agents.

There is reported evidence that indeed masking of CD4 receptors can occur in patients' lymphocytes [6].

Other mechanisms are obviously involved in the priming of CD8+ lymphocytes for apoptosis. These cells bear some activation markers and might reflect a chronic activation of the immune system against the virus and other infectious agents.

However, a more general factor could be the oxidative stress which occurs early following HIV infection.

This is another new line of research which may yield important insights in AIDS pathogenesis. The group of Dröge in Germany and the Herzenbergs in the USA have produced evidence that glutathion content was decreased in the lymphocytes of patients and also in SIV-infected macaques [7, 8].

The serum level of some antioxidants (vitamin E, selenium) is also reduced in such patients, and likewise, there is an increase of peroxidized lipids.

In collaboration with Dr. G. Piedimonte and his colleagues from Parma University, we have studied the oxidation of lymphocyte proteins. Indeed there is a 3.0 fold increase of proteolytic degradation of proteins in the PMCs of HIV-infected asymptomatic individuals, as shown by pulse-chase experiments. This group has also studied the fate of some particular proteins, such as Mn-superoxide disimutase (involved in the clearance of superoxides) and interleukin 2.

The half-life of such proteins is indeed significantly shortened. This phenomenon may in part explain the defect of circulating H in the blood of HIV-infected patients. Such an oxidative stress may also contribute to the induction of apoptosis in patient lymphocytes, and also activate HIV in cells in which the provirus is latent.

What could be the origin of this oxidative stress? Infected macrophages, neutrophils, the secretion of inflammatory cytokines (TNFα, ILσ) may mediate the release of oxidation products, intestinal malabsorption of nutrients (vitamins) may also reduce the level of antioxidants. Among infectious agents, opportunistic microbial and viral infections should also be considered.

Antioxidants are often taken regularly by HIV-infected patients in an empirical way.

We have conducted in collaboration with our colleagues of the Hospital La Pitié-Salpétrière, a preliminary trial with N-acetylcysteine. Six months treatment with the compound could achieve a complete decrease of apoptotic death in lymphocytes of such patients, who were HIV infected but asymptomatic [9]. Other markers such as the CD4+ cells number are now being studied.

More recently, another study using a protein extracted from milk (whey) has also shown promising results in reducing in vitro the apoptotic death of patient lymphocytes [10].

One should recall also that apoptotic death of lymphocyte can be prevented by a mixture of interleukin 2 and interleukin 1.

Another line of research which should not be overlooked is that of infectious cofactors, particularly mycoplasmas. In the last 4 years, two laboratories, that of S. Lo and ours have been involved in the isolation and characterization of mycoplasma species from HIV-infected patients.

Several species have been isolated, including *M. pirum, M. fermentans* and *M. penetrans,* a new species isolated by Lo and collaborator from the urine of HIV-infected homosexuals.

All three species have in common the property of fermenting glucose and arginine, and invade the cells by penetrating the cytoplasm.

PCR studies have shown that in around 10% of HIV-infected individual's blood, lymphocytes contain the *M. fermentans* genome.   But a similar proportion has also been found in HIV negative individuals.

By contrast, serologic studies have shown a highly significant correlation between HIV infection and the presence of antibodies against membrane extracts of *M. penetrans..*

Around 40% of HIV-infected homosexuals have been found to harbor such antibodies, against 1% or less in HIV negative subjects [11].   We have been able to essentially confirm this correlation and to extend it to some African subjects [12].

This antibody reaction (by LISA and Western blot) is specific, and we have recently cloned the major antigen, a p35 protein, which has no known sequence homology with cellular proteins.

These results suggest that *M. penetrans* infection (in the genital and intestinal tracts) could be a cofactor of HIV transmission or progression to AIDS.

Longitudinal studies are now in progress.   If *M. penetrans* (and perhaps some species yet to be discovered) are strongly associated with HIV and involved in AIDS pathogenesis, they deserve appropriate treatment (antibiotics) and preventive immunization (vaccine). A mycoplasma mucosal vaccine may be easier to design than an HIV vaccine.

Our results point to the use of a global therapeutic approach to HIV infection as early as possible.   Appropriate combinations of antivirals, antibiotics, antioxidants and immunotherapy should be tested.

We can even foresee in the future a complete cure (eradication) of HIV infection, if we are able to activate latently infected cells which could then be eliminated by the immune system.

References

1   Gougeon ML, Montagnier L: Science 1993; 260: 1269.
2   Gougeon ML, Garcia S, Heeney J, Tschopp R, Lecoeur H, Guétard D, Rame V, Dauguet C, Montagnier L: AIDS Res and Hum Retrov 1993; 9: 553.
3   Gougeon ML, et al: Manuscript in preparation.
4   Banda NK, Bernier J, Kurahara DK, Kurrie R, Halgwood N, Sékaly RP, Finkel TH: J Exp Med 1992; 176: 1099.
5   Di Rienzo AM, Furlini G, Olivier R, Ferris S, Heeney J, Montagnier L: Eur J Immunol 1994; 24: 34 – 40.
6   Carrière D, Vendrell JP, Fontaine C, Reynes J, Atoui N, Pau B: Tissue Antigen 1993; 42: 426.
7   Dröge W, Eck HP, Mihm S: Immunol Today 1992; 13: 211.
8   Roederer M, Staal FJT, Osada H, Herzenberg LA: Int Immunol 1991; 3: 933.
9   Olivier R, Lopez O, Mollereau M, Dragic T, Guétard D, Montagnier L: In: Oxidative Stress, Cell Activation and Viral Infection (Pasquier C, et al, eds.), Birkhäuser Verlag Basel, Switzerland, 1994, p. 323.
10   Baruchel S, Olivier R, Wainberg M: Anti-HIV and anti-apoptotic activity of the whey protein concentrate: Immunological™ Abstract presented at the Tenth International Conference on AIDS, Yokohama, Japan, August 1994.
11   Wang RIH, Shih JWK, Weiss SH, et al: Clin Infect Dis 1993; 17: 724.
12   Grau O, Slizewicz B, Tuppin P, Launay V, Bourgeois E, Sagot N, Moynier M, Lafeuillade A, Bachelez H, Clauvel JP, Blanchard A, Bahraoui E, Montagnier L: Association of Mycoplasma penetrans with human immunodeficiency virus infection. J Infect Dis, in press.

HIV 10 Years on: Research Finding and Future Prospects

A Brief Note as a Moderator

Masakazu Hatanaka

Institute for Virus Research, Kyoto University, Kyoto and Institute for Medical Science, Osaka Japan

From December 26, 1984 to February 7, 1985, within the 44 days, the complete nucleotide sequences of a putative causative agent of AIDS were reported for the first time to the world. The sequences of LAV isolated by Luc Montagnier, HTLV-III by Robert Gallo, and ARV by Jay Levy, demonstrated clearly the existence of a new human retrovirus that was coined later as human immunodeficiency virus, of HIV. From that time on, the real AIDS research in a scientific term, started based on solid genetic information obtained from the viral sequences.

We were personally acquainted with each other from our younger ages, because all of us have been studying the same cancer-causing viruses in animals called retroviruses since 1960s. Consequently Luc, Bob and Jay have been very familiar and well-experienced with retroviruses for a long time.

I visited each person in 1994, and asked them to participate in the tenth International Conference on AIDS at Yokohama and commemorate the tenth anniversary of the HIV discovery and to present their new research findings and discuss future prospects on AIDS.

All agreed to join this special session together for the future.

Current Concepts of Care and Prevention

AIDS in 1994: The Personal and Global Challenge of Renewal

Jonathan M. Mann

François-Xavier Bagnoud Center for Health and Human Rights, Epidemiology and International Health, International AIDS Center, Harvard School of Public Health, Cambridge, MA, USA

This is an exciting and in some ways unsettling period in the history of our confrontation with AIDS. There is a curious mixture in the air: of new energies and action in Asia, stirring and impressive. Yet there is also, beneath the smooth surface of a state-of-the-art air-conditioned conference center, a distinct, although muted sense of unease, a persistant and palpable discomfort, difficult to identify precisely, as if something central had somehow slipped out-of-focus.

Indeed, today, something vital is in grave danger of being lost: the coherence and cohesion and credibility of the global effort against AIDS. This global effort—the first in history—belongs to us all. Yet now, in 1994, we can feel and hear and see it slipping away from us. Our global effort—our solidarity—that mixture of vision and ideas, experience and knowledge—has become dangerously fragile.

For the coherence of the global effort erodes when pretense—empty gestures, thoughtless promises or public posturing—substitutes for hard analysis, honesty and courage to confront difficult truths. Do we really understand enough? Are we really doing enough? Is our course for the next years really clear enough? And most importantly, do we believe in it? Where is the clash of ideas? Have you been surprised by anything you have heard about prevention at this Conference—have you not heard it all before? Have we not become comfortable—too comfortable—with our analysis of the pandemic and the response? Are we not too content with the correctness of our approach, with our position on the issues? And thus, despite hearing reassuring words about the global effort, our inner compass tells us we are losing direction, our inner sense of tone detects—with unfailing fidelity—the difference between false and true notes. At night, alone, or with friends, we listen to the inner truth, feel our collective unease, and ask, what has happened?

I realize that in saying this, I may be speaking mainly to those involved in this work for some time. For we have lived through a remarkable period. We witnessed the birth of an authentic impulse of solidarity; our credo was tolerance; the scope and span of our communication was breathtaking. We helped to open a new era in history, and as we stormed the gates of the status quo, we knew we would prevail. What has happened?

Of course, it is tempting to dismiss the earlier years of the global effort as simply a period of naivete: quaint and in retrospect, faintly amusing. And of course, the guardians of the status quo will always label efforts to make important changes—especially changes which threaten them—as either naive or utopian.   But we know better: we know that while maturity—personal or collective—means change, there is also a way of evolving which remains true and authentic.   We must pity the person who dismisses their youth as folly; as if we are not all guided throughout our lives by ideas, symbols and, yes—dreams of what may be.

Therefore, to find a way forward in the global effort against AIDS, we must start by looking first within ourselves.   For just as we learn about life by living, so we have learned about HIV/AIDS through real experience and hard work, pain and understanding.   There is nothing peripheral or superficial about what we have done.   For this reason, the path of revitalization and genuine renewal of our efforts against AIDS will be found—once again— through honesty, authenticity, and the strength to believe in the reality of our experience and our discovered truths.

In the mid-1980s, together, we constructed the first global AIDS strategy, based on what we knew at the time—both about AIDS and about public health.   We defined the problem of prevention as follows: AIDS is a new, serious global health threat; since HIV spreads through personal behaviors, individuals must change their behaviors; accordingly, programs are needed to help people accomplish this task.   In turn, these programs were based on a three-part model: two parts were from traditional public health practice and one part was new.   The two standard parts of this 'prevention triad' were information/ education, and health and social services.   The third element, not part of the standard lexicon of public health, was the need—discovered through practical experience—to prevent discrimination towards HIV-infected people and people with AIDS.

The period of global mobilization from 1986 - 89—the most dramatic and remarkable public health response in history—had two major elements: first, countries and communities were supported as they mobilized to create programs to deliver the 'prevention triad', adapted to local settings.   And secondly, a powerful set of ideas about the meaning of the HIV pandemic was articulated and expressed in global policy.   HIV/AIDS was the first epidemic identified as both a global scientific and societal challenge; the narrow biomedical paradigm of disease was broadened to include its societal impact and meaning; and a coherent, clear global strategy was developed which respected and fostered diversity, while still providing common ground for local, national and global efforts.

While this was very good public health, built to modern specifications, it was still essentially only a new and improved, global expression of the traditional public health paradigm.   For precisely this reason, paradoxically, the collective work during this period was—at the same time—both highly successful and inadequate.

First consider its successes.   It became possible for virtually all countries to acknowledge the existence of AIDS; then, at least at the national level and at least to some extent, countries advanced along the path of providing programs for HIV prevention. While many differences existed, most national efforts took shape with reference to the Global AIDS Strategy.   In turn, global policies were remarkably effective in helping to block the adoption of many useless and poorly thought-out proposals for prevention and control of HIV at the national and international level.   Solidarity involved people; there was nothing quite like the feeling of walking into the opening plenary of the first, or second, or sixth International Conference on AIDS.   Regardless of how 'international' we may have felt before, the experience of being part of a global movement energized and changed us all.   And, the strategy was also impressively effective: at the small-scale of pilot or demonstration projects, when the 'prevention triad' was applied actively and adapted sensitively to local conditions, it worked extremely well to slow HIV spread—in different populations literally around the world.   HIV prevention—done properly—has a record of effectiveness as great or greater than for any other health issue which relies principally on behavior change.   And all this despite the negativism of those who claimed that individual behavior could not and would not change; and despite those who believed (or still believe) that societies are monolithic and static.

And yet we have a fundamental problem—a dilemma.   For the gap between the expanding pandemic and the global response is growing—rapidly and dangerously; pilot projects fail to be sustained; the lessons painfully learned from hard global experience are ignored and not widely applied; community and political commitment to AIDS is plateauing or even declining; the disparity between rich and poor, within and between nations, grows ever larger; and HIV remains disconnected and isolated from broader health concerns.   Most importantly, it is now evident that while the first period, the first global AIDS strategy and all our work based upon it, was courageous, extremely important and necessary, it is also manifestly insufficient to bring the pandemic under control.

Yet the first Global AIDS Strategy and the global mobilization were in many ways so successful, and there is such an intense universal desire to escape from AIDS realities, that the public and even some of us have come to believe that if only governments would do what the current global strategy requires, the pandemic would be brought under control.   Sadly, we know all too well that this is not true!   For example, if countries thus far relatively less affected by the pandemic—such as Indonesia—do indeed follow the current global AIDS strategy, we can predict that the impact of their work on the shape of the coming epidemic in that country will be relatively small.   Precisely because of what we have learned and discovered during the first decade, today the global strategy has become a source of false and tragic reassurance.

For others, or at another time in history, this might well have been the end of the story. But to allow our global effort to dissipate and fragment, to watch passively—would neither be true to ourselves not to our own history.

Recall what we have done!   During the past decade, people around the world, facing specific, immediate problems with prevention and care, or struggling against exclusion and discrimination, responded with a creativity and courage which had no historical precedent, and which the world had no right to expect.   This is the essence of our collective achievement: that through many thousand individual actions—in our words and deeds—we refused to accept the status quo, when it was unacceptable.   This real experience, this honesty and commitment, now equips us to understand AIDS as no other disease had ever before been understood, and thereby to renew our global effort against the pandemic.

We are a generation which has—because it has earned—the privilege of seeing beneath the surface manifestations of AIDS—tragic and painful—to grasp the roots of the problem.

One way to see these roots is to do the following experiment.   Take any specific component of HIV prevention—for example, STD control.   If we ask 'what should be done to control STD in the community?'—the experts can readily provide us with a list of activities which together constitute the public health approach, such as: establishing STD clinics, training clinicians, ensuring accurate and rapid diagnosis, making treatment readily accessible, providing information through media and pamphlets, educating in the schools. All of these activities are important, must be taken seriously, and must be performed conscientiously. Yet, curiously, if we then ask these same experts—our colleagues, ourselves—whether doing all these things will control STD control in the community, the answer is a clear 'no!' If we then ask what would be required to achieve control, a short list of deep societal issues will be proposed, such as: gender inequality, cultural barriers to open discussion of sexuality, and economic inequity. These are precisely the kind of issues we so often refer to, usually in a phrase at the end of a speech or an article, as 'vital cultural, economic and political factors'.

Then, if we repeat this process for each of the specific elements of HIV prevention— condoms, a safe blood supply, injecting and other drug use—the same result occurs. For each specific problem there will be a list of traditional public health activities—different for each—along with a shorter list of deeper, underlying societal issues. Each time, we will conclude that our public health based work is useful, but not sufficient to get to the heart of the problem. Then, we discover that the short list of deeper, societal problems is remarkably constant and similar; the specifics vary widely yet the deeper issues are common denominators.

This is actually a re-discovery. For public health has long recognized the fundamental importance of societal factors for health. The problem is the difference between recognizing and responding; we have been trained to see but not how to act. This large gap between our appreciation of the deep causes of ill-health and the limited definition and scope of most health work, helps explain the frustration and subtle lack of self-confidence characteristic of public health. This hesitancy, this timidity shows itself when we defer reflexly, as if it was right and natural and just, to a political, or an economic, or a loosely defined 'social' reason when some health goal is dismissed as impractical or impossible.

What is new in AIDS is that we are resolutely determined not to stop at the traditional boundaries. We respect—and need—the standard public health approaches, but we are not willing to stop at the level of clinics, educational programs, treatment and technology— the domain we know best, in which we are most comfortable, and for which we have been trained. We are seized by the need to uproot the pandemic by addressing its deeper causes.

The epidemic and hard experience have shown us where these roots lie. We have seen the epidemic follow the path of least resistance within each society. This pathway is highly specific within each society and yet fundamentally similar around the world. The major societal risk factor for vulnerability to HIV is to belong—before AIDS ever appeared—to a group which is discriminated against, marginalized, stigmatized by, and excluded from society. Most often this discrimination involves race, gender, ethnicity, religion, age or sexual preference.

We are not speaking here about discrimination directed against HIV-infected people and people with AIDS—which is a vitally important and terrible effect of the pandemic. Rather, we are identifying discrimination as a cause—at the very root of the pandemic.

To illustrate this further, compare the characteristics of adults in your society who are at the lowest and the highest risk of becoming infected with HIV. Assuming that the epidemic has existed for at least a few years—for its entry point into society may be quite varied—the least vulnerable adults are those who are in possession of their basic human rights; accordingly, their life choices are real, and their dignity is protected. In contrast, those at highest HIV risk are those whose rights are least realized and whose dignity is least protected by society; their choices are often not real but illusory—as in the so-called choice to become a sex worker or starve; or when practical barriers block genuine access to education, regardless of what the laws or national constitution might promise.

No matter how hard we try, traditional public health programs cannot make up for the negative impact of this difference in societal status and realization of rights.   Public health activities cannot, by themselves compensate for the vulnerability to disease, disability and premature death created by society.

As one of the architects of the first global AIDS strategy, I share pride in what was accomplished.   I am not ashamed of what we did not know or could not see, nearly a decade ago.   Yet it is clear that the first strategy—innovative and powerful in its time—is now terribly incomplete and therefore outdated and inadequate—and it is not surprising that it no longer has the conceptual power to mobilize people and resources: standing now in the way of progress, it must be replaced.

A new strategy, seeking to reduce vulnerability to HIV infection, would involve a dual approach in which current, public health based efforts are strengthened and in which the societal causes of the pandemic are also directly addressed.

Yet how can we approach the societal causes of vulnerability to HIV in a coherent manner?   Frequently, when we list 'social, cultural and economic factors', we are actually disempowering ourselves; for example, as soon as we identify poverty as the problem, we become paralyzed, for eliminating poverty seems insurmountable, and what specific actions does it call forth from us—today and tomorrow?   So we mention these factors—for completeness' sake—and then, with some important exceptions, we go back to our usual sphere of work and leave the big picture to others.

Fortunately, there is a language we can use, which can be translated sensitively into words and ideas we can share: the language and concepts of modern human rights.   Let us not fall into the easy rhetoric of East versus West: recall that the courageous HIV-infected speaker at the opening of this Conference identified human rights as a principal mission of his Japanese organization; recall that Aung San Suu Kyi, Burmese Nobel peace prize laureate, declared from her house arrest that Asians also want human rights; recall that governments around the world, from my own to yours, prefer to talk about human rights in other countries, while violating them at home.

Human rights can offer us a guide for practical action, a coherent framework for 'acting locally and thinking globally', and a common basis for a global strategy to reduce vulnerability to HIV/AIDS.   First, we can use the framework provided by international human rights to identify the forms of discrimination—and other systematic violations of human rights and dignity—which are most critical in each society.   Next, we can identify how the violation and lack of respect for these rights increases vulnerability to HIV/AIDS. Then, we can work with others concerned with these social issues and human rights in each society—our goal being to promote and protect the human rights of those in society whose rights are least realized and respected.

This work is as concrete as any work in public health—with definable short, medium and long-term actions and goals.

Example
In the United States, millions of people lack access to health care and social services. We can identify how this tragic situation increases vulnerability to becoming HIV infected and to receiving poor care if infected or ill.   We must rectify this violation of the right to health care.

Example

Injecting drug users and commercial sex workers in most Western European countries and sexual minorities in many, if not all countries, are persecuted and harrassed by the police.   The violation of the right to peaceful assembly and association interferes critically with the ability to form effective support groups and to participate in HIV/AIDS policy and program development, resulting in increased vulnerability to HIV.   We can work with others to change laws and practices to permit drug users, sex workers and members of sexual minorities to organize and associate.

Example

When men are hired to work at locations distant from home, their right to 'just and favorable conditions of work' is violated; in this situation, vulnerability to HIV increases, both for the men and for their families at home.   We must bring forward these issues and their related downstream social costs, and help business and government find ways to arrange for families to accompany or be near the men, or to otherwise ensure ways to help maintain and support family relationships.

Example

Worldwide, women's role and status is associated with vulnerability to HIV.   There are many rights which lead towards reducing HIV vulnerability: the right to education, the right to 'take part in the government…directly or through freely chosen representatives' and the right to non-discrimination are important examples.   Increasing the proportion of girls who receive an education is a practical objective, and has also been identified by the World Bank—not known for its primary emphasis on human rights—as one of the most important interventions for improving health in developing countries.

Example

Racism in many countries—from the US to France to Japan—results in diminished access of stigmatized groups—whether African-American, or Arab, or Korean—to health services, education and information.   We can help combat these concrete forms of discrimination, which increase vulnerability to HIV infection and poor care.

Starting, therefore, with an analysis of the status of respect for human rights and dignity in our own society, we can uncover vulnerability to HIV/AIDS which can then be addressed both through AIDS-specific programs and services, and by working to improve realization of those rights.

This means that our work seeks to transform society to deal with AIDS, rather than transforming—or deforming—what AIDS is about to fit society.   It is also essential to note that the societal vulnerability which underlies HIV/AIDS is common to many, if not most of the major health problems of the modern world, including cancer, heart disease, violence, maternal and infant mortality, and accidental injuries.

Our collective insight—that there is an inextricable, fundamental linkage between promoting and protecting human rights and promoting and protecting health—ranks as one of the major discoveries in the history of society; it connects HIV/AIDS to a broad new vision of health and it promotes health as a central societal value.

Can this lead to a global ethic of caring, the lack of which interferes with HIV prevention and AIDS care around the world?   Modern human rights is based on a single fundamental idea: that 'all human beings are born free and equal in dignity and rights.' This calls forth an ethic of caring based on solidarity and mutual respect—not on charity or convenience.

Are we prepared to commit ourselves to the goal articulated in the Constitution of the World Health Organization, which states boldly that '...the highest attainable standard of health is one of the fundamental rights of every human being...'

In a decade of work against the global pandemic, we have struggled to change the status quo of others' attitudes and institutions.   But we should not forget how much our own ideas and inherited beliefs have been shaken and have had to change; and how painful a process this can sometimes be.   Now we must do it again—once again we must confront our own status quo and the status quo of our institutions—international, governmental and nongovernmental: for we are all now threatened by rigidity, inertia, defensiveness or fatigue.

Two paths lie before us, and we must choose.   To one side is the holding fast to ideas and approaches which are necessary but not sufficient; to strategies which we know will be useful and even professionally rewarding, but which will not sufficiently control the pandemic; in other words, to a traditional and useful public health approach.   On the other side is a more difficult, complex and challenging path—requiring that we transform our approach, to include, yet go beyond traditional public health, in order to bring our actions into closer harmony with what we know must be done to prevent HIV infection and care for those who are affected.

The challenge to us today—personal and collective—should not be under-estimated. Do we have the confidence—in our knowledge, our experience, our discoveries?   Do we have the necessary courage, strength and imagination?

The epidemic—our special responsibility—will not wait.   We find ourselves— unexpectedly and awed—at a great intersection of world history. The challenge of solidarity, respect for diversity and an ethic of caring is not ours alone, but pervades every aspect of our world.   Our responsibility is great, for we are the women and men who have the confidence and the historic opportunity to stand before both a pandemic and injustice and say—'we will prevail'.   Mere survival is not our goal.   Let us choose the path of self-examination, rigorous honesty, and tolerance.   Let us revitalize and rekindle the effort against AIDS, drawing on the spirit and inspiration which—a few short years ago—ignited an unprecedented global response.   Then we can truly say, when our time comes, that we did what we could.   And when the history of AIDS and of our time is written, this may well be our most important contribution: that we resisted the temptation to be lulled into complacency; that we chose instead to prevail by expressing through our work our belief— our spiritual conviction—that our lives have meaning, that we are connected to each other and within a larger world, that we can make a difference, and ultimately, that we are all worthy—and equal—carriers of the spark of life itself.

Confronting Reality: a Personal Perspective on the First Decade of HIV Prevention

Juan Jacobo Hernandez

Chavez Colectivo Sol, Mexico

I want to dedicate this presentation to a person and to a people. The person, Marco Antonio Osorio, GNP + management committee member for Latin America and the Caribbean, human rights fighter and pioneer in the struggle for gay liberation and AIDS work in the continent, who presently struggles for his life in Mexico.

And to the people of Rwanda, who besides striving in the midst of horror and war, hunger and disease, are also stricken by more than a decade of the HIV epidemic—an issue that seemingly nobody wants to even mention.

When I received the invitation from Dr. Jonathan Mann and the conference organizers to participate in this session, I experienced an initial sensation of terror and pride. The responsability implied in sharing points of view, experiences, successes and failures in prevention with such a rich and diverse audience, and the opportunity to share—however modest—a joint reflection on what the work on HIV prevention has meant for thousands like myself in Mexico, swiftly transformed my fear and insecurity into an acceptance of the challenge. My comments are an attempt to represent not only my own views, but also those of my colleagues working in the community unable to be here with us and whose voice I will try to articulate.

To speak out of personal and community experience, implies speaking of the relevance in HIV prevention, of the stories behind the epidemic, and of the parables within the epidemic. For me, these stories are closely linked with the assertion that the personal is political, which has led us to discover challenges, acknowledge obstacles, accept errors, appraise achievements and establish a vision of the future concerning what still lies ahead.

The reference points of the present presentation are necessarily associated to the prevention experience in Mexico, which is the country where I live and work. Yet, along the years we have discovered that despite national, local, and cultural differences, there are universal aspects to our work similar to those we share—as nations, communities, families and individuals, due to the impact of HIV and its consequences.

Preparing this paper has meant a necessary exercise in humility regarding many limitations of my personal performance, and I haven't stopped thinking that maybe—as we say in Mexico—I am only bringing a *taco* to this magnificent banquet. Nevertheless, I hope it will be a very tasty *taco*, just as there may well be thousands of other *tacos* which many of my peers have also brought along to share, which will serve a purpose: to illustrate the personal insights which color with light and shadow the fabric of the epidemic.

For more than a decade now, and following the discovery of HIV as the cause of AIDS, during nine previous international conferences such as this one and perhaps hundreds of smaller meetings, we have been talking about the millions of men, women, children, young and old struck by the epidemic—the majority of whom have already died.   We have heard over and over that 40 million people will be infected by the year 2000.   These statistics transcend our ability to grasp their significance, and they force us to confront an inescapable reality: HIV infection is advancing at a frightening and unstoppable pace.   A vaccine is not likely in the near future, thus ensuring the continued vulnerability of individuals, families, communities, and nations.

We have known a great deal about HIV for some time now, and I was particularly struck by the level and sophistication of information being presented at this conference, including David Ho's talk about long term survivors (see p. 65).   More is understood about HIV than any other virus in history and in such a short space of time.   The narrow parameters of the biomedical approach have been surpassed and the human capacity of response has been challenged in all fields.

We know and sense that HIV has infected the whole of our collective body politic, and no community or nation has escaped its impact, nor been able to stop it.   For years we have known about its silent and latent nature, a knowledge that will be increased with all the new information that we are learning from this conference.

At several of the past few conferences, we have realized that international funding against AIDS is decreasing proportionately to the rate that the infection is spreading.   We know and are feeling the enormous disproportion that exists between funds available to fight AIDS in rich countries and poor countries and the possibilities of accessing funds in one or the other.   For example, the difficulty for Mexican NGOs to get funds increases as the government promotes an international image of economic self-sufficiency and of not needing international cooperation: remember, we are members of NAFTA now...this is not only happening in Mexico, but other countries such as Chile and Malaysia come to mind.

We have also accumulated proof over the years of the increase in the violation of human rights of people living with HIV and AIDS around the world.   As far as Mexico is concerned, there are many areas where this occurs, prisons, for example, and paradoxically, the health care setting where a very high percentage of complaints concerning human rights abuses, mistreatment and refusal of care have their origin.   Forgotten and neglected communities are experiencing an increase in the spread of HIV.   Men who have sex with men—outside of two or three well-intended research projects based in the national AIDS program—, is a completely neglected community, with no real programs that cater specifically to them.   The unwilligness of senior health authorities to deal openly with the issue of homosexual behavior among Mexican males is an obstacle to open and direct prevention campaigns from government with its expected consequences: men who experiment sexually with others and do not identify themselves as homosexual continue infecting themselves and both their male an female sexual partners.

The provision of information is one of several crucial components of a comprehensive prevention program.   For example, we have been involved and the production and distribution of an international newsletter that provides reliable, practical and accesible information for Spanish-speaking Latin America.   Despite very positive feedback, we know that, on its own is insufficient to prevent infection or change behavior.   In Mexico, as in any other Latin American or Caribbean country, the perception that publishing series of pamphlets and producing posters that we rarely see on any other walls than those of our offices and which convey information that fails to hold meaning to anyone in particular, is mistakenly assessed as preventive education.

I remember Ana Filgueiras—a Brazilian educator who works with street kids—saying in one of these conferences three or four years ago, that children must receive sexual education in order to protect themselves from infection before they become sexually active. Conveying information on AIDS to children is an issue so difficult to tackle that excellent materials produced in Mexico for children in elementary and secondary schools by the National AIDS Program are not distributed in the public health system for fear of the conservative backlash, thus depriving Mexican boys and girls with the opportunity to learn at an early age the facts about HIV and putting them at potential risk of HIV infection, STDs or unwanted pregnacies.   The decision to surround children with silence around these issues puts them in an extremely vulnerable position.

When so many obvious truths about HIV are repeated over and over without action, and in the absence of any change, a paradoxical effect sets in whereby we begin to doubt. It is true that we know many things about HIV, but there are equally many more questions to answer.

What is the significance to those of us engaged in the prevention of HIV that the magnitude of the pandemic has increased more than 100 times since the discovered of the virus in 1981?

How do we respond when the speed and silence of the spread of HIV affects new communities and more individuals every day?

In light of our increasing understanding of the complex profile of the epidemiology of the epidemic, what impact does this have on the design of strategies to prevent infection among individuals families and communities?   Trying to read and interpret the data in Mexico, we never understand them.   I am always confused when I am told that one woman for every three men with AIDS is the ratio of heterosexual transmission.   How, I wonder, is this possible when we are told that man to man and man to woman are the most effective ways of sexually transmitting HIV.   When we know that it is socially accepted and expected that men have more sexual partners than women?   Perhaps the problem is partly because of the way an HIV positive man is questioned about his sexual behavor just after receiving a positive antibody test result.

What future does prevention have when we know that the devastating impact of HIV is yet to come?   And how do we cope when each time we think we have a small victory, we discover that HIV has surged ahead yet again.

When and where epidemiological data exists, it indicates an ever increasing rate of infection.   Prevention programs and campaigns exist in every nation—at least on paper—, but we must ask ourselves whether these are succeeding or failing and why.   As far as our experience shows—and I must refer to men who have sex with men because this is where we work the most—no campaign is having any impact among men who have sex in public bathhouses, where unprotected anal sex takes place at an astounding rate everyday, not only in Mexico city, but in at least 15 or 20 other Mexican cities in the provinces.   Bath-houses are traditional places where males gather to socialize and occasionally have anonymous sex. Many of those bath-houses cater almost exclusively to men who want to have sex with men and who do not necessarily identify themselves as gay or homosexual, or are closeted gays. What we witness in those general steam rooms provides us with sufficient evidence to strongly suggest that HIV infection is on a constant rise among those men and, consequently, among their sexual partners outside those settings.

This situation also relates to official resources. Let us concede that many NAP officials are extremely liberal and avant-garde, and would like to promote an intervention in those place where men have sex with men. Can the heads of national AIDS programs or others attending this conference honestly share with us the level of support they would receive from their government for such a project? Is their budget and support sufficient to carry out effective programs in other areas, ensure access to care and treatment for people with AIDS, and to guarantee the protection of human rights for all affected by HIV?

We have heard once and again how important it is that leaders—especially heads of state address their citizens to do everything possible to prevent HIV, to join in the global effort, and to stand in solidarity with those affected by HIV. How many heads of state take AIDS seriously and have personal plans of action to protect themselves?

The HIV epidemic as a new and complex phenomenon has put into question the prevailing ways we had of understanding health and human development; it has forced us towards new ways of knowledge and its unstoppable spread demands for holistic responses; HIV forces us to perceive new issues; to see old issues with new eyes.

The issues HIV has raised make us go back to the decisions we have or have not taken, promoted or hindered, during the epidemic years and the effect this has had in the number of people infected and, as a consequence, in the number of people that die or have survived. In this respect we can say without hesitation that the community experience has been a very rich one which has increased our sense of responsability, knowing that HIV affects more and more those most vulnerable.

In my country, as in most in the region, a goal of prevention is to promote risk awareness to precisely reduce vulnerability and advance towards a change of attitude and—ideally—of behavior. How can we do this in Mexico, I ask myself, when the concept of 'high risk group' is still deeply imbedded within the health system? When resources for care and treatment are extremely scarce, when compared with the immoral expenditures of, for example, official party campaigns to win elections in states they already had assured their triumph, as in the case of Veracruz in 1992 when they spent more than 40 million dollars while at the same time, not spending one single dollar to educate their own party memebers on HIV?

When talking about personal vulnerability the least we can do is to recognize the central role played by people with HIV who tell the stories, which of course can only be possible if the social environment is an enabeling and supportive one. Toishiro Oishi moved us last Sunday with his personal testimony before the crown prince and princess, and the prime minister, who also delivered a message of concern and committment with HIV and the Japanese people.

This made me wonder if in Mexico we will be forced to organize International AIDS Conferences in order to convince President Sailinas de Gortari—or his successor—to speak out about AIDS and not only to read the three or four lines that someone in the health ministry writes for his annual report. And, moreover to express a personal committment and courageously speak against mandatory testing and about people living with HIV and the protection the constitution grants them.   In my own wild imagination, it would be extraordinary to know that he has a personal plan of action to protect himself and his family from HIV.   That a head of state in any of our countries does this would mean an important step forward for enhancing prevention.   We don't have to wait as in the case of Zambia, to have a personal tragedy move a president into action.

Let me close this presentation urging you not to think that the examples I have given somewhat erratically on HIV in Mexico are only valid for my country.   I am convinced that they reflect many situations in your own communities, in your own national experiences.   I decided to focus on my country because I am convinced that I am talking not only about me but also about you.   The same that can be said when a person living with HIV, who speaking out of his or her experience, is not only talking of his or her infection, but of the impact it has upon us all.   Let us reflect on our future actions and hope— wholeheartedly—that we may gather enough strength among ourselves to resist and, in the end, defeat HIV.

Thank you.

Current Concepts of Care and Prevention

Report

Junsuda Suwunjundee

Wednesday Friends' Club, Program on AIDS, Bangkok, Thailand

My name is Oom.   I am 23 years old.   I sold heroin before I, myself, became a drug addict at the age of 17.   After three years I tried quitting my habit.   However, I became addicted once again.   Then, with emotional support from my mother and other relatives who had looked after me ever since I was born, I was finally able to kick my drug habit.

Two years after kicking my habit, I began to relax and began thinking about starting a new life.   I applied for a new job and had my blood tested for HIV.   I prayed for my own sake to not have the virus because I wanted a new start on life.   When the doctor gave me the results of the test, they showed that I had HIV.   It served me right, I told myself, and lost all hope and desire to continue living.   To make it worse, the first people to know that I had HIV were my older brother and my mother, neither of whom had very much information on AIDS.   They were afraid to have me live in the same house.   My family was also worried that I would be rejected by the neighborhood and other family members. I was also terrified that other villagers would find out.   I didn't want anyone I knew to see me dying of AIDS so I decided to leave home for the Clinic where I believed other people with AIDS were kept.

The staff at the clinic suggested that I join the Wednesday Friends' Club where I could meet other people like me.   I began to feel better because I met friends who had been infected with HIV for a much longer time that I and most of them were in good condition. Because the Club was only set up for the purpose of providing a place for people with HIV to meet and to organize, no housing could be provided.   I continued to have difficulty finding a place to stay and rotated between friends who did not know that I had HIV.   I would stay with one person for two days and then with another person for three days and so forth.   Later, another member of the Wednesday Friends' Club helped me out.   He saw me carrying my bags back and forth and in sympathy, invited me to live with him.

Once I joined the Club, I began to make a distinction between people with HIV and those without HIV.   The titles, 'person with HIV', 'person with AIDS', and 'AIDS victim' now separated me from being a full human being.   The media campaigns were some of the reasons why I was so nervous about my fate.   Campaigns using awful pictures and headings such as 'no cure but death' were no small factor to why people became frightened and victims rejected.   People were more frightened of people with AIDS than the virus itself.   Out of fear created from the media, people with HIV are out of work, looked at as worthless, and are left without hope and without a future.   Yet I want to tell everybody that we are not without hope and we are planning for the future.   We won't wait for the end of our lives but we do accept that we will get sick someday in the future.   Except for those of us, whose need for medical care has been denied, we rest our hopes in the doctors' hands. Unfortunately, the signs of contempt can be seen in many of the health care providers' eyes, only helping to diminish our hopes.

I would like to tell you more about the different problems which we face.   Many people will not give their consent to be tested for HIV.   Some doctors, however, secretly test for HIV.   Then, if the patient has HIV they will refuse to treat that patient.   Many of the patients are not even given the test results.   They eventually find out, they are still unaware of the support available to them.   The result is that some of these people are not really convinced that they have HIV.   Others remain uncommitted to a change in risk behavior.   And, sadly, others commit suicide.

As we are not welcome in some hospitals, we must go to the few hospitals that will accept us.   Bed space, however, is limited.   In Chulalongkorn hospital, for example, it is common to find not enough medicine, beds and other services.   I would like to thank the good doctors and blame the careless ones.   Those of us who are ignored by the doctors, some time turn to 'black magic' treatments as a last resort and are cheated.   We always get excited about any new information on treatment but, time after time, we are disappointed.

Our problems are not limited to medical treatment only.   Even though there is a law to prevent AIDS testing it is not effective.   To enter some schools, for example, depends on the results of the test for HIV.   Also, all government institutions test.   Before you can be employed in most any public or private job, you have to be tested.   There seems to be no way to avoid being tested.   People with HIV need to work.   When you are ill, you can't work.   When you can't work, you have no money for treatment.   When you have no money for treatment, it is difficult to get well again and then no one else will employ you. Then we become a burden on the society.

Death no longer frightens us.   What frightens us is how we can continue to live in society.   We have found many ways to help ourselves continue living in society.   From our religion we have learned that meditation helps us to focus.   Some Buddhist temples now provide us with special help in meditation.   Others such as Wat Phrabath Nam Phu, for example, provides hospice care for people at the end.

We can still live and work like people who are not infected.   Sometimes, though, we need a little more care and emotional support.   The Wednesday Friends' Club was set up for mutual support and to follow up on each other's health.   The Club provides a quiet place where we can meet and find support for our thoughts.   With others, we are now playing a significant part in the fight against the spread of AIDS.   We begin to realize how useful we still are even though in revealing ourselves to others we may be exposing ourselves to many different forms of hate.   We want to let all people see real and clear pictures of AIDS.   We take the risk of rejection because we do not want anyone else to suffer as we have.   We need to gain more acceptance from people so that the next time someone is infected with HIV, they will not have to suffer society's hate as we have.

Every staff member of the Club is teaching others from their experiences to help them learn.   We are glad of all the support we receive but, unfortunately, we have been used by some organizations which take advantage of us.   So, we have to be careful of the activities in which we participate.   We have made our own project for providing AIDS information to students.   The objective is to provide youth with correct information and help them develop positive attitudes about AIDS so that they will be able to live together with people with HIV and AIDS.   We have achieved this in two provinces.   I am pround of this work and thank Dr. Praphan Panuphak, Director of the Program on AIDS, Thai Red Cross Society, and Mr. Kamoneseth Kengkanrua, at Chalulongkorn Hospital.

What we are trying to do might not be completed before we die.   But we are proud that we have tried to improve the world by supporting ourselves and encouraging others to make good decisions so that we may continue living together.

My thanks to all who have offered me this special opportunity to speak my mind today.

Thank you very much.

International Cooperation in the Fight against AIDS

'What is an Expert?'

S. E. Mellors

Global Network of People (GNP), Cape Town, South Africa

It surprises me that 10 years after these conferences were first started, people with HIV/AIDS are not still not seen as able to 'expert input' This brings me to a crucial question, which I do not think any of us have the answers to — what and who are the experts?

In the beginning of the epidemic, the 'scientific experts' were confident of finding a cure, and did not see the need to include people with HIV/AIDS, as they would be dead in a few years anyway. Ten years on, however, the scientific world is confused, desperate and in disarray, and there is still no sign of a cure or an effective vaccine.

The prevention campaign for various reasons has failed. Part of the reason is I believe because people with HIV/AIDS have not been included in the prevention campaigns. After all who knows more about being vulnerable in situations that would lead to unsafe sex practices than the people who were there before?

Governments and bureaucratic organizations either believed that they did not have a problem or believed that they could control the epidemic without the help and input of people living with HIV/AIDS.

Who has however, proven to be the so-called experts in the last 10 years? We, the people living with the virus, who have outlived our initial diagnosis, who are still struggling and fighting, we who are teaching educators and the scientific world something, and we who have changed the face of medicine as we thought we knew it. Yes, we are still alive, we are still going to be around for a while yet, but does this make us 'experts', or does it basically make us human beings, fighting for our lives and survival. Fighting for our right to be accepted as contributing members of society, and fighting for our right to be acknowedged as equal partners in the struggle against this disease.

I challenge us all here today, to define what we mean by the term expert, and who the real experts are. According to me the only thing qualified to be called an expert is the virus. The virus in my blood, the virus in your blood, your country, your community. The virus that has the scientific world confused, educators scrambling and society frightened, and we need to work together as equal partners, if we have any hope of making an impact on this virus.

If the last 10 years has proven anything it is this. You can no longer afford to fight this battle alone, because it has become clear that without us, you are fighting a loosing battle. You can no longer to afford to exclude us, or pay us lip service, as we *are part of the solution*.

So in the hope of international cooperation, let the scientific world take a hard look at what they are trying to achieve, and admit to not having all the answers.   Let international agencies work in cooperation instead of competition, and let us commit ourselves to finding a solution to this disease, with the same energy and passion that we all had at the beginning of the epidemic.

For if we want any hope of making an impact on this very demanding virus we *have to do it together*, and then maybe just maybe at the end of it all our children would turn around and say, 'they did it, because they were prepared to do it together...'

International Cooperation in the Fight against AIDS

Bilateral Response

Helene D. Gayle

Centers for Disease Control and Prevention, Atlanta, GA, USA.

Bilateral assistance, the direct provision of technical or financial assistance from one country to another, is increasingly playing a major role in the international response to the human immunodefficiency (HIV) and acquired immunodeficiency syndrome (AIDS) pandemic. At the start of the epidemic, donor nations were not anxious to develop bilateral assistance programs for HIV/AIDS. This was probably based on multiple factors including reluctance to become involved in an issue that might stigmatize and detract from ongoing projects and relationships and the lack of an obvious, simple intervention that could be depended on to produce tangible outcomes and demonstrate effective use of resources. Because of the sensitive nature of the epidemic, most traditional donor countries were quite willing to have the Word Health Organization (WHO) play the lead role in addressing this issue with developing countries.

HIV research was one of the first arenas in which bilateral assistance developed in the early stages of the epidemic. The first international HIV/AIDS research collaboration, Projet SIDA, was started in 1984 in Kinshasa, Zaire and was a collaboration between the Government of Zaire, the United States' Centers Disease Control and Prevention (CDC), National Institutes of Health (NIH) and the Belgian Institute of Tropical Medicine. Project SIDA has served as a model for collaborative research in Africa and beyond. The CDC has since developed two additional projects, located in Abidjan, Cote d'Ivoire and Bangkok, Thailand, that focus on epidemiologic, laboratory and prevention research. NIH has funded clinical, laboratory and epidemiologic research, and training in multiple sites throughout the world, with the goal of developing vaccines and treatments for HIV that can benefit the whole world. Also, the United States Department of Defense, through a long-term research collaboration with the Thai Army, has been working on preparing for HIV vaccine trials in Thailand.

In 1986, the United States Agency for International Development (USAID) began providing funds to the Global Programme on AIDS (GPA). Since 1987 USAID has played a major role in international HIV/AIDS prevention efforts, providing direct bilateral assistance to more than 70 countries. The United States assistance to developing countries in both research and prevention has continued to grow over time.

Several reasons for the growth in bilateral funding and involvement in the international effort can be postulated. First, in the area of research, it was clear that knowledge gained from research done in developing countries could benefit the world broadly including, the country in which the research was conducted and the country providing funds and technology. An important example can be given of the contribution that research in Africa has had on our understanding of mother-to-child and heterosexual transmission which were both less prevalent in countries funding research than in many African countries. Much of what the world knows today about these modes of transmission came from these international research collaborations.

In the area of prevention, the experience gained and lessons learned through these activities have been shared widely with many countries. Second, the evidence increasingly showed that HIV/AIDS would reverse many of the improvements in health and socioeconomic development of previous decades. If bilateral investment in health and development were going to realize their expected gains or even maintain existing ones, HIV and AIDS had to be addressed.

Also, it became increasingly clear that many bilateral development assistant organizations, such as USAID, had considerable field experience and strength in program development and program management that could be advantageous for developing effective country programs.

At the same time there are certain limitations in the role played by the United States and other countries providing bilateral support. A first limitation is the influence of bilateral politics. One can give multiple examples of countries for which, it has not possible to provide much needed assistance because of strained or non-existent diplomatic relations. In such situations, multilateral organizations are less constrained by the political relationships of any one particular government and can fill important gaps.

Second, bilateral financial support and technical assistance may come with certain conditionalities, for example the need to purchase products for programs, such as drugs, condoms, and equipment, from the donor country. These may be more expensive, take longer to get to program sites and may not be suitable for local circumstances.

Third, because there are often multiple different countries providing bilateral assistance within a given country, coordinating of activities can be extremely challening and ineffective. Problems of coordination can lead to duplication of efforts and even compertition among bilateral donors within a country. Donor competition can manifest itself by using assistance as a way of gaining influence or capitalizing on the opportunity to work in a 'desirable' country.

Finally, agencies of donor countries often have specific mandates that fit the priorities of the particular agency but may not necessarily correspond to the highest priority needs of host governments or complement activities of other donors. An example of this is preference for donor nations to fund prevention activities exclusively, leaving a major void in funding for care of HIV-infected persons in countries that are being overwhelmed by these costs.

Despite these limitations, bilateral assistance has been very effective in many regards and has provided many positive examples upon which to build.

The future role and direction continues to evolve. There seems to be a tendency towards relatively more bilateral compared with multilateral assistance. This may be because many donor countries prefer to have more control, more accountability and greater domestic and international visibility than can be achieved through support to multilateral organizations alone. The following are considerations for continued bilateral assistance for HIV/AIDS programs, but are relevant for all actors in the international response.

Greater intergration of HIV/AIDS activities into other related activities is critical. Faced with growing domestic economic demands and constraints for donor countries, greater cost-effectiveness and demonstration of impact are critical requirements of bilateral assistance. This coupled with a greater understanding of the HIV/AIDS epidemic, its root, socioeconomic causes, means that HIV/AIDS programs must be better integrated and better coordinated with other health and development activities.

More emphasis must be placed on improved coordination as more organizations and individuals become involved in HIV/AIDS. Better coordination can not be achieved without acknowledging the central role of the host government in developing national priorities and ultimately being responsible for the coordination of all players at the country level.

Additionally, new partnerships are important to optimize the effectiveness of external support. In the past, bilateral support was often provided to or channeled through host governments. While, the role of the host government as mentioned is fundamental, new partnerships with the nongovernmental and the private sectors must continue to growth. New partnerships between donor nations should also be encouraged. An example of this is a recent agreement developed between the United States and Japanese governments to build collaborative projects with developing countries.

Last, but not least, as expertise and knowledge is gained on the part of developing countries and their communities, support from donor nations should evolve towards greater reliance on host country and regional expertise. In other words, besides the direct goal of decreasing HIV infection and its impact, our assistance should also aim at decreasing dependency and redefining traditional relationships of power and inequity. Patterns of assistance and project development must take all of this into considertion if we expect our assistance to stay relevant to the need of the people it is intended to benefit.

International Cooperation in the Fight against AIDS

Multilateral Cooperation

Lars O. Kallings

National Institute of Public Health, Stockholm, Sweden

AIDS is perceived as one of the major threats to the survival of mankind along with population growth, pollution of the environment and nuclear war. It is unique that a single disease is considered to have such dimensions. The enormous and historical dimension of the AIDS pandemic calls for a correspondingly forceful international response. Internationalization and interdependence are two key words that describe current world trends. AIDS stands out as an illustration of a global dramatic problem where the interdependence between nations is very prominent and which can only be successfully dealt with in a global context. There is also a shared understanding that the course of the pandemic is very much influenced by the efficiency of multilateral actions.

I am going to talk about the multilateral cooperation channeled through the UN system, the efforts of the secretariats of the various UN agencies and the efforts of the member countries, be it recipient or donor countries. However, multinational cooperation cannot be seen as separate from bilateral cooperation or from activities of non-governmental organizations, they are all interrelated. The same donor agency is often involved in multilateral, bilateral and NGO support and the recipient country needs to coordinate support of different kinds. As this is a tenth anniversary session I will start with a short review of how it all started in order to give the proper perspective, then mention the Global AIDS Strategy as the main policy framework to deal with the pandemic. Then I will emphasize the future, the new joint and cosponsored UN Program on AIDS and what that means in terms of opportunities to strengthen the global response.

The need for a multinational approach was obvious already in 1984 when the global scope of the AIDS epidemic was realized. The issue was in particular politically sensitive and inflamed at that early stage and unbiased scientific analyses were called for. As a first step, WHO started consultations to assess the size of the epidemic, modes of transmission and preventive measures. The objective, authoritative and competent advice of WHO as a UN specialized agency was especially important in relation to the highly charged issue of AIDS. It should be emphasized that multilateral cooperation contains an essential element of research, training, technical advice, transfer of technology and normative work in addition to logistic and financial support.

As insight into the magnitude of the HIV/AIDS problem developed, a special WHO Program on AIDS was established in 1986, later renamed the Global Program on AIDS (GPA). An unprecedented mobilization of funds and activities was unleashed. WHO raised public and political awareness and effectively counteracted discrimination and panic. National AIDS programs were rapidly established.   As a result, in less than ten years time most individuals on the globe know about AIDS and almost all countries in the world have a national mechanism to prevent HIV/AIDS and to deal with the consequences.

After the first years' frantic efforts to start preventive activities, the social and economic causes and consequences of HIV/AIDS came into focus, in particular AIDS as a threat to further development in developing countries.   AIDS on top of the already existing economic difficulties threatens to reverse gains in development and deepen the economic crisis of poor countries.   A WHO-UNDP alliance was established in 1988 to provide a broader base for interventions.   Subsequently, other UN agencies contributed within their areas of expertise and comparative advantages, for instance UNICEF in relation to mother-to child transmission, orphans and youth, UNESCO in education, FAO on the consequences for agriculture and ILO on AIDS in the workplace.   The World Bank stepped in as a major actor, analyzing and demonstrating the economic consequences of AIDS and granting substantial loans to developing countries to finance national AIDS Control Programs.

The main policy framework for the global response to the pandemic including multilateral cooperation is the Global AIDS Strategy.   It was initially endorsed by Ministers of Health from over 160 countries at the World Health Assembly in 1987.   It was adopted as a common UN strategy by the UN General Assembly which again shows that AIDS has political charges and implications beyond a separate health issue.   The strategy as upgraded in 1992 is comprehensive and multisectoral.

To sum up the different stages of the multilateral efforts: It started as a WHO activity. By 1990 there was a shift toward more bilateral funding and also other UN agencies establishing AIDS program.   There was more competition for funding.   The multilateral response has on the whole remained on the same level over the last years; about US$ 70 million annually for GPA and about 30 million for the other agencies together.

The shift from a pure health approach to one including multisectoral and developmental approaches did not succeed without complications.   Though WHO was designated lead agency there were competition and duplication, agencies supporting more or less the same type of programs and giving conflicting policy signals to recipient governments.   At the same time the pandemic continued to accelerate at an alarming rate.

In order to increase the efficiency and better coordinate the multinational cooperation, the Word Health Assembly in 1993 initiated a process to establish a joint and cosponsored UN Program on HIV/AIDS.   Six UN system agencies; the Development Program (UNDP), UNICEF, the Population Fund (UNFPA), WHO, UNESCO and the World Bank have now undertaken to set up a joint and cosponsored UN Program on HIV/AIDS, on the basis of co-ownership, collaborative planning and execution, and an equitable sharing of responsibility.   WHO is to be responsible for the administration of the Program. Thus, the Program will be located in Geneva and does not constitute a new separate UN agency.   The establishment of the new Program was endorsed last month by the UN Economic and Social Council.   The Program will start in January 1996.   During the transition period, the ongoing HIV/AIDS activities of each of the six agencies should be maintained.   The transition from the current GPA of WHO and the separate activities of the other agencies to a joint Program will be overseen by a Committee of Cosponsoring Organizations.   The Secretary General, will appoint the director of the Program.

The establishment of a joint and cosponsored UN program is a result of Member States wishing to have more coherent and broad-based technical guidance as well as a more rational UN response in technical cooperation in countries.   The issue of AIDS support is not a choice between a multilateral or a bilateral approach, but instead one of a coordinated UN system response which can reinforce other development assistance in the context of HIV/AIDS.   The Program's priority activities should be at the country level, where the response to the urgent needs and problems posed by HIV/AIDS should be focused.   But how should the country operations be functioning?   First, it should operate within the framework of national plans and priorities.   Representatives of all UN system agencies should form a theme group on HIV/AIDS.   The chairperson of the theme group will be selected from among the agencies.   The UN representative in charge of coordination will iniatiate the process.   The program will provide global leadership and collaborate with Governments, intergovernmental organizations, non-governmental organizations and people living with HIV/AIDS.

The process of establishing the joint and cosponsored UN program on HIV/AIDS has in less than one and a half year, despite all its built-in constraints, proved our willingness to create a stronger multinational partnership.   This new partnership will entail less fragmentation in the governance of international HIV/AIDS activities, and organizational framework for a rational, pragmatic and constructive cooperation between the UN system agencies at global level and in countries.

AIDS represents an extensive work agenda.   It would be wrong to and there will never be enough resources to create new vertical AIDS structures which aim at covering all the sectors where interventions are necessary.   To a large extent AIDS activities have to be mainstreamed in already existing structures and programs.   A priority of the Program is also to coordinate AIDS activities carried out by the cosponsors at country level whether they are specific HIV/AIDS activities or HIV/AIDS activities integrated within cosponsors' existing programs.   At global level there is a pooling of competence and resources within a joint program secretariat.   This approach is at the heart of the program being co-owned by the sponsors.   The alternative is increased fragmenation, stagnation of resources and loss of a critical mass necessary for impact and efficiency.

The revitalizaion of multilateral cooperation which the joint and cosponsored UN program represents should also include new forms of partnership with actors other than states.   For example, the ECOSOC resolution also clearly points out that through consultation with interested nongovernmental organizations, a mechanism will be established to ensure their participation in the Program.

I will conclude my presentation by underlining the opportunities that the new UN approach offers.   Above all, it will offer a broader multilateral framework to unite all efforts, may it be by multinational and bilateral agencies or private organizations.   It will offer partnerships between developed and developing countries, UN agencies and NGOs. It is not meant to be another bureaucratic strait-jacket but should be used as a flexible framework for all actors.   But the success depends on the will of the participants to cooperate.

The new approach also offers improved potentials for fund-raising.   It is estimated that at least US$ 2.5 billion annually is needed for effective preventive activities in developing countries where the magnitude and impact of HIV/AIDS is the greatest—a twenty-fold increase compared to current spending.   These resources can only be raised by intergrating HIV/AIDS prevention in all developmental efforts.   This will be one of the main challenges to the UN Program.

The fight against AIDS is often spearheading evolution of human efforts as exemplified by the unique initiative to join the efforts of six major UN system agencies.   The joint and cosponsored Program on HIV/AIDS will prove that the UN system is capable of creating programs which are truly collaborative, reinforcing and based on partnership with all actors.   The success of the new program at country level will be crucial to the future course of the pandemic.   There is no alternative!

International Cooperation in the Fight against AIDS

The Role of NGOs

Jeffrey O'Malley

International HIV/AIDS Alliance, London, UK

I'd like to dedicate my remarks today to the memory of Christopher Cockrill, my former lover, who died of AIDS this past October. Chris and I met in 1982, when Gay Related Immuno Deficiency was simply a distant cloud on the horizon of young gay men in Montreal. Chris went on to work for a series of AIDS Service Organizations, eventually becoming the AIDS treatment officer of the Canadian AIDS Society, while I decided to pursue my career working with development NGOs. We both met many of you here today for the first time in Montreal in 1989, at a meeting we organized called Opportunities for Solidarity, the first global gathering of ASOs and NGOs working on AIDS.

Opportunities for Solidarity was organized so that people working on AIDS at a community level around the world could discuss what worked and what didn't work in their programs, create strategies together on how to respond to different problems, figure out where to find money and other resources, plan together for how to navigate the Vth International Conference on AIDS that immediately followed, and get to know each other so we didn't feel all alone. The meeting was about solidarity, and about international co-operation among NGOs.

When the meeting was first proposed, and as we went around trying to find money for plane tickets and conference rooms, we encountered a lot of scepticism, especially from what you might call international co-operation professionals in large institutions. It was hard for them to believe that gay men in Doc Martens with ACT-UP New York, Salvation Army doctors at Chikinkata Hospital in Zambia, do-gooder English matrons with old-fashioned charities, and angry Brazilian PWA activists could have much useful to learn from each other. But we did learn, and while the meeting was by no means the first example of international co-operation among NGOs in responding to AIDS, I still believe that it was a watershed that led to a whole new level of co-operation and understanding.

I am mentioning Opportunities for Solidarity here at this Tenth Anniversary Session, because I think that it is worthwhile to reflect for a moment on where we have come from over these past years, in order to assess what we have accomplished, and where we need to go.

Let's step back for a minute and remember why any kind of international cooperation—governmental, nongovernmental, or intersectoral—is seen as important in the fight against AIDS. I think that we are all familiar with the usual arguments, the justifications for expensive conferences and global summits:

- HIV respects no borders, and the pandemic will not be stopped in one country except as part of a global strategy.
- The pandemic is really a series of discrete epidemics proceeding at different paces, and relatively unaffected populations have the opportunity to learn from the years of experience in San Francisco or Kampala.
- No one is safe from AIDS, so we are all in this together.
- The industrialized democracies have a moral obligation to help finance the fight against AIDS in the South, where the epidemic is growing exponentially.

Now what's wrong with this picture?

The rationales just listed for international co-operation are full of subtle and not-so-subtle contradictions.   It's easy in a conference slogan to say 'Together for the Future', or 'One World. One Hope'.   Many of us still believe it, and that's why we're here today.   But in many places, for many reasons, the easy sloganeering is being challenged:

- The Global Program on AIDS is less and less of a global program, and the new U.N. Program won't be one either.   Its a vehicle for assistance from North to South, and it would be a challenge to find many staff people in Geneva who have more than a cursory understanding of the epidemic among gay men in Paris or injection drug users in Scotland. When resources are scarce, it makes sense to concentrate on poor countries where the epidemic is growing quickly, but what are the risks as GPA's concerns seem more and more distant from taxpayers in the North?
- Earlier this week, I asked the Managing Director of the Global Network of People With AIDS whether his network would be interested in providing technical assistance in PWA organizing to the nine countries around the world where my NGO will be working this year, and while I don't yet have a definitive answer, his first response was that it will really have to be a decision that is taken, and a program that is managed, on a region by region basis.   A global effort just didn't seem realistic to him in a network with so much deversity. Once again, it is easy to sympathize with sensitivity to regional differences but what are we losing if the sophisticated PWA movements of Uganda and the USA are cut off from emerging efforts in Ecuador or Thailand?
- As a last example, at least some members of the International Network of Sex-Work Related HIV Projects felt abandoned and betrayed this year when their calls for solidarity in response to Japanese entrance restrictions on professional sex workers seemed to go unheeded, especially by more established networks like ICASO that had established formal consultative relationships with governments and conference organizers.   I've been involved in Conference organising myself, and recognize the conflicting agendas that have to be balanced.   But is NGO solidarity splintering as some of us gain more and more access to decision makers, while others choose to maintain their distance and autonomy?

I am not criticising GPA, GNP$^+$, or ICASO.   Nor do I have anything but understanding for the countless NGO activists who considered coming to Japan for this week, and decided that their time and the public's money would be better spent in service delivery and advocacy at home, or in sharing experiences at less expensive and more relevant regional meetings.   I am raising these examples because our easy answers as to why we cooperate internationally, and what are the roles of NGOs, are being challenged by a differentiating pandemic, a lack of resources, and an increasing understanding of the overwhelming complexity and scale of the challenges we all face.

NGOs *have* had successes in international co-operation that illustrate why we should not give up and go home. Some of the person to person bilateral exchanges at these conferences have led not only to marriage or co-habitation, but to shared insights into AIDS program strategies and tactics which are more than the sum of their parts. The formal institutions of international co-operation, with their emphasis on member states and diplomatic niceties, have shown an increasing ability to adapt to the important role of NGOs, and have benefited from community insights in program design and policy development. Over the last five years, a series of overlapping international networks of NGOs have filled some of the gaps not addressed by bilateral government contacts and the UN system, with increasing exchanges and solidarity through regional ASO networks in places like Southern Africa and South-east Asia, global bodies like the International Community of Women Living with HIV and the International Council of AIDS Service Organizations, and tremendous engagement and support from some of the oldest systems of international NGO co-operation, like the International Federation of Red Cross and Red Crescent Societies. Let me mention a few concrete examples of our achievements together:

• A huge informal network of NGOs developed in response to the American entrance restrictions on people with HIV, leading to the boycott of the San Francisco Conference a few years ago. While it may seem odd to point to this as a success, as the American restrictions not only continue but have now been formalised, international co-operation among NGOs on this issue not only shaped official WHO policy, but helped to move human rights and non-discrimination from the margins of AIDS discourse to the centre of most policy and program guidelines.

• Despite much initial scepticism about international NGO links built around common interests or identities, we have seen the emergence of shared analyses and strategies among many of these informal networks—from prostitutes adopting workers' rights approaches to decrease their vulnerability and increase prevention, to progressive Christians collaborating on inclusive theologies which embrace difference and allow for non-judgmental care

• Most importantly, while many people dismiss the inappropriate transfer of educational materials and prevention techniques from one population or context to another, we have all grown considerably more sophisticated not in inappropriately *replicating* each others program, but in *adpting* innovative and effective approaches to our own contexts. International co-operation among NGOs has spread peer education, home care, direct-action politics, treatment information programs, and indeed safer sex around the world.

So we have had successes through international co-operation, and continue to do so. But I do believe that as NGOs professionalize, decentralize, regionalize, and specialize, we risk growing further away from one crucial element of that dream so many of us shared in Montreal, and that is of solidarity. Along with our successes, we have seen ACT-UP sputter out and collapse in many cities, we have seen ASOs created by queers and whores be taken over by social workers and psychologists, and many of you, like me, have been transformed from activists to bureaucrats.

Much of this simply reflects the maturation of our responses, as well as of ourselves. But if we lose our connection to social movements, if as NGOs we simply become cost-effective sub-contractors of government programs, we lose our raison d'etre. By losing public support and participation, we will also eventually lose what have now become our jobs, and our abilities to prevent infections, care for the ill, and address the causes and consequences of the pandemic.   We have to continually rebuild domestic constituencies in our own countries and communities, not just for AIDS action locally, but for commitment to broader action on AIDS, health and development around the world.

Not all NGOs are or should be part of a grassroots movement.   The organization I work for, the International HIV/AIDS Alliance, is a good example of a group that emerged more from donor organization than from the field, and I am probably more useful in focusing on the UN system and donor policy than in trying to organize protests.   I think all of us in the NGO movement have a responsibility to think strategically about our involvement in international cooperation, and to approach any of these networks, conferences or lobby attempts with clear objectives, and clear understandings of the strengths and limitations of our own organizations.   We also have to be clear that we are finally accountable to beneficiary populations, especially people with HIV or AIDS, regardless of how close or distant we are from the community.

I look to the successes of the environmental movement and the women's movement for inspiration.   For all of the local action on gender and ecology, these movements and the NGOs within them have not allowed cost-effectiveness studies to create atomization and division.   Nor have they forgotten that at the heart of international co-operation is building bridges of understanding and solidarity between ordinary women and men.   That is my main message today: as much as we can and should learn locally, and from people like ourselves, it is through the struggle of building understanding between nuns and drug users, between doctors and economists, and between North and South, that NGO co-operation internationally really can help conquer this pandemic.

International Cooperation in the Fight against AIDS

The Experience of Zambia

Roland Msiska

National AIDS/STD/TB and Leprosy Programme, Ministry of Health, Lusaka, Zambia

Introduction

Deaths from HIV/AIDS have been reduced to a routine, daily event in Zambia. I will not bother you with figures but today social life for an ordinary Zambian focuses on the hospital, graveyard and funeral home. There is not a single person in Zambia who can say that he or she has not lost a relative or close friend to AIDS, or who currently does not have one who is sick or dying from an AIDS related condition.

The response to the epidemic in 1985 was constrained by one, a downturn in the economy caused by a slump in international copper prices, and two, denial on the part of government. These two factors severely reduced government capacity to respond to the exploding epidemic. When finally in 1986 the government recognized AIDS as a major public health problem, we in government did not develop a clearly articulated plan to respond to the epidemic. Rather we concentrated our efforts on mobilizing support from international organizations. As a result, AIDS specific departments were created in government, parallel to the AIDS-specific departments of donor organizations. But by 1990 it was painfully clear to us in government that this approach was not an effective response to the many challenges posed by the epidemic. Let me explain why we reached this conclusion.

Donor

● Most of our major partners—in particular the bilateral donors—insist that we follow the package of interventions that they have defined. But such packages are inflexible and do not take into account the realities of the local situation within which we work. This rigidity stifles local initiative and innovation.

● These plans are biased towards the use of costly external technical assistance with little or no consideration of local capacity building to ensure sustainability of programs.

● As donors are virtually without exception reluctant to cooperate and coordinate with each other, the result is duplication of activities, while, paradoxically, other critical intervention areas are almost entirely ignored.

● Our capacity to respond effectively is hampered by varied and heavily centralized disbursement and accounting procedures.

● Each donor has its own format and mechanisms for project management. As a consequence it is difficult to harmonize the various donor requirements on reporting, reviews and evaluation.   This immeasurably burdens government program officers who are forced to meet the various donor requirements and targets.   Our honest and conservative estimate is that we spend between 50 – 60% of our time accomodating donor requirements such as review missions, consultancies and evaluations.

● Timely implementation of AIDS prevention activities is often delayed by the long lags between donor pledges and actual disbursement of funds.   The gap is typically as long as six months to a year, and in some cases two years! (By this time we in the government cannot remember what we had agreed upon!)

Local Non-Governmental Organizations

Local NGOs in Zambia by their nature have been in the forefront of developing innovative strategies in the fight against AIDS.   For instance it was a Zambian NGO that as early as 1988/89 recognized that care for people with AIDS was a neccesary condition to modifying sexual ritual cleansing.   Moreover, they have been particularly successful in getting prevention and care to the grassroots.   We in government appreciate their very significant contribution in the fight against AIDS/HIV.   Because we share the same goals, I would like to share some the concerns expressed by our Zambian NGO colleagues.

● Is donor and government funding for NGOs guaranteed and certain for the future? How can we ensure sustainable levels of funding?

● How can we ensure that these innovative strategies benefit all Zambians who need them?

● How can we all agree on the best strategic approaches?

● Given that NGOs are increasingly getting interested and involved in operational research, how can we ensure that standards and ethics are maintained?

The Way Forward

These issues are not unique to HIV/AIDS.   We encounter these very same problems in all other health work.

In order to resolve these sector-wide constraints, the Zambian government has since 1990 moved to develop a health reform policy.   Underlying this policy are the following principles—one, to ensure leadership by government; two, accountability toward Zambia's people; three, the building of partnership with the public, NOGs and donors.   The health reform policy is anything but rhetoric.   Thus, the Government, in full collaboration with our major donors and NGO partners, has articulated a Strategic Health Plan which forms the basis for donor and NGO participation in health.   Several donors have already agreed that they will only fund elements of the plan, and will not continue with their damaging insistence on funding independent projects.

(A)   In order to facilitate the government's working with donors and local NGOs in health, a donor and NGO coordinator has been appointed within the Ministry of Health.

(B)   Donors have agreed in principle to standardize the mechanism for reporting, reviews and evaluation of donor supported programs.   This process has been painfully slow but as the Chinese say a journey of a thousand mile starts with one step.

(C)   In order to improve the financial accounting system and consequently accountability at the district level, one major donor has funded a training program for Accounts Assistants.   Coupled with this bi-annual donor meetings are being held to review progress in implementing agreed upon targets.

(D)   Importantly, the government has agreed to protect and guarantee Ministry of Health funding under agreements reached with the World Bank, which is assisting the Government to improve the economy and social sectors.   In addition, the government has further agreed with the World Bank to implement a multi-sectoral plan in the fight against AIDS.

(E)   NGOs are moving to establish an administrative secretariat to assist in coordination of their activities.

Despite all these efforts—which represent progress on one, strategic planning; two, securing funding; three, building sustainability; and four but not least donor and local NGO coordination—we are still concerned about several vexing issues in our effort to build an effective response to HIV/AIDS.

One, what type of policies can facilitate and sustain behavior change?

Two, how can we impress upon donors the need to support the development and implementation of a multisectoral approach to HIV/AIDS.

Finally, how can we impress on reluctant donors that the need of the day is for intergration of AIDS activities with broader efforts to improve health systems.

Index